The
HEALING POWER
of
NEUROFEEDBACK

The Revolutionary LENS Technique
for Restoring
Optimal Brain Function

STEPHEN LARSEN, Ph.D.

FOREWORD BY THOM HARTMANN

With contributions by Carla Adinaro, A.R.I.A. Cert.
Wendy Behary, L.C.S.W. • Lynn Brayton, Psy.D.
Curtis Cripe, Ph.D. • Mary Lee Esty, L.C.S.W., Ph.D.
Thomas E. Fink, Ph.D. • Sarah Franek, M.T.P. • Beth Hanna, R.N.
Kristen Harrington, M.A., L.M.F.T., A.I.B.T. • Sloan Johnson, M.A.
Robin Larsen, Ph.D. • Joan Piper Mader, M.A. Len Ochs, Ph.D.
Karen Schultheis, Ph.D. • Evelyn Soehner, M.A.
Theresa Yonker, M.D.

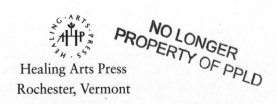

Healing Arts Press
Rochester, Vermont

Healing Arts Press
One Park Street
Rochester, Vermont 05767
www.HealingArtsPress.com

Healing Arts Press is a division of Inner Traditions International

Note to the reader: This book is intended as an informational guide. The remedies, approaches, and techniques described herein are meant to supplement, and not to be a substitute for, professional medical care or treatment. They should not be used to treat a serious ailment without prior consultation with a qualified health care professional.

Library of Congress Cataloging-in-Publication Data
Larsen, Stephen.
    The healing power of neurofeedback : the revolutionary LENS technique for restoring optimal brain function / Stephen Larsen ; with contributions by Carla Adinaro . . . [et al.].
        p. ; cm.
    Includes bibliographical references and index.
    Summary: "An introduction to the innovative therapy that restores optimal functioning of the brain after physical or emotional trauma" —Provided by publisher.
    ISBN 978-1-59477-084-5 (pbk.)
    1. Biofeedback training. 2. Brain damage—Treatment.   I. Title.
    [DNLM: 1. Biofeedback (Psychology)—methods. 2. Brain Injuries —therapy.   WL 103 L334h 2006]
    RC489.B53L37 2006
    615.8'51--dc22

                                                    2005036393

Printed and bound in the United States by Lake Book Manufacturing

10 9 8 7 6 5 4

Text design and layout by Priscilla Baker
This book was typeset in Sabon, with Agenda and Stone Sans used as display typefaces

All illustrations in this book are courtesy of the Stone Mountain Center unless otherwise noted.

Photograph of William James on page iv courtesy of the Swedenborgian House of Studies, Pacifica School of Religion.

This book is dedicated to Dr. Len Ochs:
Inventor, Mentor, Healer, and Friend, and to a
whole emerging generation of biofeedback
clinician/technicians, of which he is an exemplar.

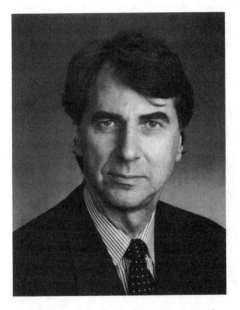

*Len Ochs, clinical psychologist trained
in biofeedback who originally developed
LENS, the Low Energy Neurofeedback
System*

"I am done with great things and big plans, great institutions and big success. I am for those tiny, invisible, loving human forces that work from individual to individual, creeping through the crannies of the world like so many rootlets, or like the capillaries. . . ."

WILLIAM JAMES, A LEADING NINETEENTH-CENTURY
AMERICAN PHILOSOPHER AND PSYCHOLOGIST

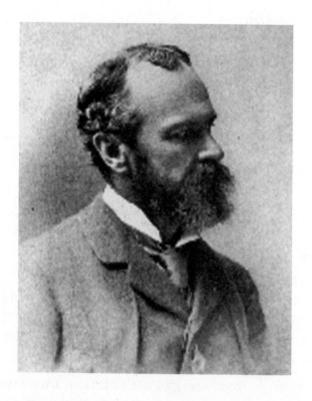

"The greatest thing, then, is to make the nervous system our ally instead of our enemy."

WILLIAM JAMES

CONTENTS

ACKNOWLEDGMENTS

This is a book about a "revolutionary" healing modality: the LENS type of neurofeedback, a gentle, noninvasive approach to healing that is, as of yet, unknown to most professionals and to the public. It is truly the most exciting development I have seen come down the pike in thirty-five years of practice as a biofeedback clinician, but it is far from a monolithic technology. During the second half of the twentieth century, as electronics grew in sophistication and power, so did biofeedback. As new equipment developed, new generations of clinicians sprang up who made better use of it to help people suffering from a myriad of problems. The best of this equipment, such as the hardware and software used in applying the LENS treatments, emerged and continues to emerge from the minds and hearts of skilled biofeedback therapists. The field has thus evolved under our fingers, as it were, as we continue our quest to find newer and better ways of helping people with neurologically based problems, or people who are simply in need of better ways to cope with living in a stressed-out culture.

I wish therefore to acknowledge people from both the clinical and technical domains, who made our journey possible. First Dr. Hans Berger, who died without seeing the flowering from his original discovery of brain waves, and Barbara Brown, who brought this whole new exciting field to the public in the 1970s. Next I would like to acknowledge the great early pioneers and visionaries, many of whom have been both mentors and friends: Elmer and Alyce Green, Steve Fahrion and Patricia Norris, Dale Walters, Matthew Kelly, Barry Sterman, Joel and Judith Lubar, Nancy White, Susan and Siegfried Othmer, Les Fehmi, Joe

Kamiya, Tom Budzynski, Ken Tachiki, Erik Peper, Gary Schwartz, Jean Houston, Liana Mattulich, and Lynda and Randy Kirk.

Many peers and associates enriched my development as a biofeedback clinician in one way or another: Mary Jo Sabo, Jim Giorgi, Adam Crane, Jay Gunkelman, Rob Kall, Sebern and John Fischer, Margaret Ayers, Val Brown, Tom Collura, Joe and Ann-Marie Horvath, Darlene Nelson, Cory Hammond, Jim Robbins, Lynda and Michael Thompson, Tom Brownback and Linda Mason, and Carol Schneider.

I thank my wonderful Stone Mountain staff of "power pixies" and neurofeedback clinicians (I won't tell you who's who) including Carrie Chapman and Alexandra Linardakis, and Beth Stewart; and I also thank Pat Boyer; and Dr. Willie Yee, for his ongoing clinical wisdom in helping us to understand the medical implications of biofeedback treatment, and his wife Elizabeth Lee for advice and counsel on research methods and statistics. I also thank Richard Brown and Patricia Gerbarg for a never-ending flow of interesting cases, and much professional advice and warm friendship.

The Association for Applied Psychophysiology and Biofeedback (AAPB) and the International Society for Neurofeedback and Research (ISNR), as well as FutureHealth's "Winter Brain" conferences, have provided us with a forum for our research and clinical presentations and peer-collaboration in our developing field. The HeartMath Institute, Rollin McCraty, and Carol Thompson, in particular, have helped my training as a licensed HeartMath provider, and helped me to formulate my knowledge of how HeartMath and neurofeedback intersect.

Much of the technical knowledge for the development of the systems used in treatment emerged from Len Ochs's dialogues with Jan Hoover and Bob Grove of J&J Technologies, the manufacturers of some of the best biofeedback equipment in use today.

Many experienced clinicians have joined us for long hours of clinical dialogue and case-conferencing, whether or not they contributed essays or case studies to this book: Mary Lee Esty, Karen Schultheis, Kristen Harrington, Theresa Yonker, Anton Bluman, Carla Adinaro, with her wonderful way with our four-legged relatives, Catherine Wills, Bob DeVinney, J. Lawrence Thomas, David Yourman, and Katherine Leddick, Phyllis Goltra, and Ann Lee. Susan Hicks was enormously helpful with number crunching our clinical outcomes study, as were Jodie

Schultz and Tara Johannesen. I also thank Elsa Baehr, Marvin Berman, Rodney Linquist, Evelyn Soehner, Tom Fink, Curtis Cripe, Sloan Johnson, Lynn Brayton, Robert Boddington, Beth Hanna, David Alexander, Sarah Franek, and Corey Snook.

Mike Quick has been remarkably openhearted about sharing his experience, and helping in many other ways, as have Alan Carey, Joe "Rock," Susan Moran, Walter and Shirley Lechnowski, Joe, Samantha and Nancy Michaels, Gabby Kearns, Craig Linet, Dan McMillan, and Cindy Lambo,

I profoundly apologize to anyone I have failed to acknowledge (due to ADD, or ARCD, age-related-cognitive-decline), who has contributed to this book or the development of the LENS.

Last but not least, I want to acknowledge my wonderful partner and friend, Robin Larsen, who has followed me every step of the way from mythological studies to scientific ones; "through the looking glass" from archetypes to computers and back again. In her management of editorial details, overseeing the art for this book and securing the requisite permissions, she has been nothing less than awesome.

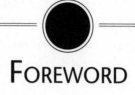

FOREWORD

Thom Hartmann

One of the great sicknesses of our day is the obsession with "normal." Behaviors that for thousands of years were considered merely "odd" or "eccentric" now have labels, and—perhaps more ominously—drugs to treat them and government-sponsored screening programs to look for them. One in ten American adults are taking a psychoactive prescription medication, and the numbers may be even higher among schoolchildren. Parents medicate kids to give them an edge in school, because without a college degree a young person is consigned to a life of flipping burgers or working for Wal-Mart.

In this remarkable book, Stephen Larsen points out that, while there may not be any such thing as "normal," there certainly is a mental and emotional form of "most highly functional," which most of us are born with. However, somewhere along the line—often from physical or psychological trauma—we lose access to some of that function as the result of actual or effective damage to the brain.

The goal of achieving our optimal functional state, Larsen suggests, isn't simply a matter of finding the right drug to balance neurotransmitters—a solution very much in vogue right now, particularly with ADHD (attention deficit hyperactive disorder) and depression—but, rather, can be achieved by restoring flexibility to the brain.

More than thirty years ago, I broke my back in two places in a skydiving accident. For years I was in pain, and my ability to easily move, bend, and stretch was limited. As I got into my fifties, my back pain became nearly intolerable: my back would simply lock up, painful in any position, even when I was trying to sleep.

That was when I remembered the lesson I'd learned doing yoga in my twenties—after my injury had first healed and I was recovering the function in my back. The key wasn't strength; it was flexibility. And to achieve that flexibility, I had to do what seemed counterintuitive: move in ways that it seemed my back was telling me I shouldn't. After about a year of various back exercises involving bending and stretching, I was again able to move into various "normal" positions, as well as to sit restfully without my back hurting.

Although the analogy is imperfect, my experience with my back is similar to that of many people with their brains. Injuries limit flexibility, which impairs function. While the injury itself may always leave a scar of sorts, the brain—being far more plastic and adaptable than my back—can quickly learn to work around this and achieve new flexibility.

But to do this, the brain must be put through a few paces, similar to the bending and stretching exercises I used for my back. Over years of studying consciousness, as well as attention,* and attending dozens of brain and neurofeedback conferences, I have seen a wonderful new world of inner self-management skills opening up.

As a principle, biofeedback is sound, both somatically and ethically. No alien substances are put into the body. Instead, people with central nervous systems of extraordinary capability—who, however, have gotten stuck in certain rigid, dysfunctional patterns—are "broken loose" from their stuckness. In the bargain, they relearn a natural flexibility to deal with the many challenges of life. EEG neurofeedback has proven itself to be a valid way of accomplishing this, and the LENS system of neurofeedback developed by Len Ochs—while controversial—has an *extraordinary* record when it comes to restoring optimal functioning to the brain.

Len Ochs's approach is outstanding, first and foremost because the founder acknowledges that he only found the "philosopher's stone" by "stumbling upon" it (that makes him more genuine in my view). His discovery is unique, even in the fields of biofeedback and neurofeedback, because of the brevity of the treatment, and because of the insignificance of the microstimulus—carried on a wave thousands of times weaker

---

*Please see text and notes to chapter 5 regarding Thom Hartmann's many books on ADD and ADHD.

than that of a cell phone—which makes it incapable of doing any harm to tissues bombarded by far stronger stimuli every day. The fact that the LENS can help very young children, as well as animals, opens mind-boggling new vistas for treatment.

Dr. Stephen Larsen has been practicing the LENS clinically for nine years, as well as biofeedback for thirty years, and psychotherapy even longer. Not only that, but he has written numerous books and introduced or reviewed scores of others. In these pages, it is my hope that you may very well learn some things that will enhance your quality of life, while informing you about this new kind of neurofeedback. Enjoy!

THOM HARTMANN

Thom Hartmann is the award-winning, best-selling author of *ADD Success Stories* and numerous other books on psychiatry and/or learning disabilities currently in print in over a dozen languages on four continents. In addition, he is an internationally known speaker on culture and communications and an innovator in the fields of psychiatry, ecology, and democracy.

PREFACE

Len Ochs, Ph.D.

This is not a rush-to-publish book. The author and his collaborators have waited over ten years to begin to show what the LENS (Low Energy Neurofeedback System) approach can do to restore optimal brain function. I personally believe that we needed to sort things out for ourselves to understand what we are doing well enough to be able to share this information with you. We needed to be able to clearly differentiate the observations made while using the LENS from those regarding the use of other procedures, and to document them in their own right, apart from what goes on with the conventional kinds of brain wave biofeedback in which a light or sound is usually used as a signal to inform the client or patient when he or she is doing a given procedure correctly. The LENS is different in that it pairs the feedback with an invisible stimulation (of radio waves) and spares the person from an experience of success or failure.

Until 1990 all therapeutic stimulation to the brain was of three kinds: it was either a fixed frequency such as a light or sound signal; it could be mathematically varied, as in gradually speeding up or slowing down; or it was a translation of a musical signal. In all three instances, the stimulation was unrelated to whatever was going on in the brain of the person receiving the stimulation. Any resonance of this brain stimulation with a frequency that the brain was already generating was simply a momentary happenstance correlation. Or "resonance" was achieved by making the strength of the stimulation so overpowering that the brain surrendered and adopted that frequency by also generating it.

Then, in 1990, something else happened.

A new idea arose: that of having the frequency of the external stimulus mirror whatever brain-generated frequency was strongest at a given moment, and to change that frequency to match the changes in the brain. This form of resonance was quite different from all preceding forms of resonance, in both concept and effect. Instead of making the brain vibrate *in response* to the stimulation, the stimulation *adopted* the frequencies predominant in the brain.

The idea was neither Eastern-inspired nor Western-inspired. It was just an idea. But it was the first time, as far as I know, that the brain's own rhythm was tied to the stimulation, which then in turn set up a resonant frequency in a living, physical system. With fifteen years of trials and data to support this approach in its current form, the "Low Energy Neurofeedback System," or the LENS technique, has become a revolutionary method of restoring optimal brain function.

Let's examine the claim for its "revolutionary" status. First the technology: Is the Low Energy Neurofeedback System really new? Its first manifestation, in 1990, received a patent in just ninety days, nearly unheard of even then. The patent examiner is rumored to have said that, while there were plenty of biofeedback devices, and many fixed frequency photostimulation devices, there was nothing to join the two together. Over the years many refinements have been made, with the result that the current LENS equipment is now as different from the original 1990 system as *that* was from everything else, insofar as the current equipment uses electromagnetic fields weaker than existing radio waves in the air around us to convey the feedback to the brain.

Second, the domain: The significance of the LENS system is that it treats functional chronic neurological problems—not necessarily structural problems—with one of the least invasive, most rapid, and reliable interventions on the planet today. It leaves nothing in the body, as does medication. No electric current is involved. The LENS helps improve functioning in those with several types of chronic neurological dysfunction such as fibromyalgia, acute and chronic pain, post-traumatic stress disorder, many kinds of mood disorders, some types of seizure and tic disorders, and many dysfunctions that typically accompany Autism and attention-deficit disorders.

Third, the LENS approach opens the communication channels in the central nervous system, thus enabling the nervous system to set its own course and direction. It does not direct functioning in any other way. The approach does not demand hard, conscious, self-regulatory learning on the part of the individual, or active, self-absorbed, micro-management of one's own physiology; it leaves all the work to be done to the brain itself. Individuals who utilize the LENS become more functional and discerning, more flexible in their approaches to life. It allows people to use their consciousness for learning and doing what pleases them. It allows an individual to become more of who he or she truly is.

LENS practitioners have, in a sense, become the midwives of recovery from what are often severe and untreatable neurological conditions. It turns out that the body *wants* to recover from these conditions. For a particular class of physical problems—not easily treated by either modern or "alternative" medicine—very small doses of brain wave biofeedback carried on wisps of electromagnetic fields to the brain allow the rebirth of function.

The Healing Power of Neurofeedback is the first book to tell stories about what happens when this process is applied to the functional neurological problems of humans and animals. As such, it is a harbinger of what kinds of improvements are possible with conditions that may not even be recognized as nervous system problems, and it demonstrates how such improvements give people back their lives.

The authors are taking a courageous risk by allowing others to see what will, to many, seem preposterous: the achievement of significant increases in functioning without medication, shocks, or surgery. This book will be controversial: There will be many who will say that its claims are impossible, if not delusional and mistaken. There will be the usual cries of "placebo." But each of the patients whose stories are told herein has tried numerous other approaches and has had many opportunities for placebo to do its work. The LENS works on people of all ages, from six months and up, and on animals. This eliminates, to my mind, the effect of placebo.

This is not to say that the LENS approach is magic, or that it can by itself make all the changes that are either necessary or desirable. In fact, it both complements the effectiveness of all other approaches and is, in turn, made more effective by them. Time will be the final arbiter of what is true and significant. My experience is that lives have been changed and improved by exposure to the LENS. Consequently, I see that lives will continue to be changed and improved by the brave souls who have written this book.

LEN OCHS, PH.D.

Dr. Ochs is a practicing psychologist and the president of OchsLabs, which is a research and development company exploring the diagnostic and treatment significance of EEG-Driven Stimulation for chronic central nervous system dysfunction.

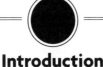

Introduction

FLEXIBLE BRAIN, QUIET MIND

Stephen Larsen, Ph.D.

As the distinguished American psychologist, Jerome Bruner, has said: "Not until we have begun to tell a story about our own experience does it make sense to ourselves, as well as others." This book is the story of my experiences with neurofeedback, an emerging technology of healing, in which EEG (electroencephalograph) processors and computers team up with the brain's own circuits to accomplish remarkable forms of self-regulation. It is also the story of the development and evolution of a particular kind of neurofeedback known as LENS (Low Energy Neurofeedback System), which emerged from the work and research of a dedicated psychologist with an affinity for electronics and an intuitive understanding of the energies of the body: Dr. Len Ochs.

But most of what is presented here are stories relating the actual living experiences of men and women struggling with disorders that affect their nervous systems: parents looking for help with their children afflicted with attention deficit or Obsessive-Compulsive Disorder, people who are depressed or anxious and have run out of medication options, people with a head injury, or the sudden onset of a degenerative disease that has left them cognitively impaired or emotionally unstable. These stories are in the area that the scientifically minded might refer to as "qualitative research," "clinical studies," or "narrative histories." In this book you will also find the stories of therapists who grow as they confront their own challenges in understanding, develop new healing paradigms, and learn how to help people who are very sensitive neurologically.

Although we also cite and rely upon much hard evidence, scientific data, and measurement and use refined, hi-tech equipment that measures the energy of the brain exquisitely, the real heart of what we have to say is about personal hero journeys that transform the self and expand human therapeutic technologies. These stories move the heart as well as inform the mind.

The discipline called "neurofeedback" or "neurotherapy" is itself a subdiscipline of "biofeedback," a term broadly used for techniques of self-regulation.* In biofeedback, a machine is used to generate electronic signals that inform a person about factors such as his or her hand temperature or muscle tension. Starting in the 1950s, it was discovered that, guided by such feedback, a person could learn to raise or lower blood pressure, quiet muscle spasms, or soothe an irritable bowel.

Neurofeedback is simply the application of this same principle to the electrical waves produced by the brain, as recorded on an EEG (electroencephalogram). With subtlety and skill, it is helping thousands of children and adults learn to regulate their own nervous systems—a not insignificant matter, for the CNS (Central Nervous System) determines just how one functions in life!

The field of neurofeedback is not yet well-known enough to have a reputation based on its remarkable efficacy, perhaps because its premises seem closer to the traditional wisdom and spiritual disciplines of the East than to the dominant Western scientific paradigm. But this dominant model is changing, as millions of people instinctively—and wisely—aim themselves toward CAMs (Complementary and Alternative Medical approaches), and as disciplines broadly known as "energy medicine" reemerge into the public theater.

Energy medicine had a fledgling career toward the end of the nineteenth and beginning of the twentieth centuries, but it was displaced by the monolithic and, it should be added, chauvinistic "allopathic" approach that most of us have grown up with. Critics have pointed out that while Western medicine has indisputable benefits, especially in dealing with serious illness and health crises, it has very little to contribute when it comes to staying healthy and avoiding illness.

---

*For the ease of the reader, three glossaries of the medical and scientific terms used in the text have been provided at the end of the book: acronyms; conditions/diseases; and healing modalities.

Neurofeedback is a "people's medicine" that has emerged from the work of dedicated clinicians and their satisfied patients and it is my belief that the work of Len Ochs will come to the forefront of neurofeedback, and that neurofeedback itself will take a significant place in the public awareness among those approaches that are not trying to *displace* Western medicine, but *complement* it (after all, that is what CAM really implies!). So people with conventional medical and scientific educations need not feel threatened by this method. I believe it does more than challenge our current paradigm; it expands it in a healthy direction. In fact the work presented herein is entirely compatible with the scientific method and pragmatic empiricism.

However, I will confess that this book was written by some strange kind of maverick, wearing motley intellectual clothing, always sniffing down the trails of mystery, more committed to journeys than to arriving anywhere. One part of me is a good modern thinker—a psychology professor and a social scientist—as grounded in a post-Newtonian universe as anyone else. The other part of me has always had a fancy for myth and magic, and my published writing includes both scholarly and popular books on shamanism, mythology, and some biographical works, including *A Fire in the Mind: The Life of Joseph Campbell.*

While researching Campbell's biography I found that he also considered himself a maverick. I discovered that we were alike in another way: We both believed invisible things play an all-important part in shaping human behavior. For Campbell it was "the myths," as he called them, "of an immemorial imagination." But my professional focus has always been on consciousness and the energy forms that play within the human brain. Perhaps the two paths of neuroscience and myth may converge in some integrative discipline of the future.

If Campbell gave me mythological and psychological maps of the terrain, it was the Jungian analyst Edward C. Whitmont, M.D., who became my first clinical mentor. A brilliant Austrian Jew, Whitmont fled Vienna escaping the Nazis and came to the United States during the forties. He was the "next generation down" from Jung. Whitmont completed his postdoctoral training at the New York Jung Institute and eventually became its Director of Clinical Training, a position he held for many years. As an M.D., Whitmont had studied homeopathy along with depth psychology, because he believed, along with many European physicians, that some problems were deeper in the genetic and physical constitution than could be addressed by psychotherapy alone.

Based on Whitmont's analysis of a dream, or on a clinical intuition, he would prescribe high potency homeopathic remedies (instead of the psychotropic medications most psychiatrists use) for constitutional problems such as anxiety, depression, insomnia, and so on (see his books on this, including *Psyche and Substance* and *The Alchemy of Healing*, where he describes the remarkable transformations that were achieved utilizing this method). In the hands of a master prescriber such as Whitmont, homeopathy could have laserlike curing abilities. The renowned psychologist and teacher of consciousness studies Dr. Jean Houston personally told me that Whitmont cured her of a lifelong hay-fever allergy with a single dose of a carefully chosen remedy.

I first experienced Whitmont's skill with homeopathy during my early years of personal analysis with him. I had traveled to Mexico and returned with a malaria-like malady that resisted all of the best conventional treatments available in New York, including those of NYU's Medical Center. High potency antibiotics, antimalarials, and antiparasitics had all failed. Regular as clockwork, the 104°F fevers, sweating, and chills returned every three weeks or so. I was so beleaguered that one day during my psychotherapy session with Whitmont I complained about how miserable the last bout had been.

Whitmont clucked in his familiar fashion and scolded me for not mentioning it sooner. Then he began to ask me a bewildering variety of questions on every aspect of my condition, further scolding me for my imprecision in self-observation. (How did I feel in the fresh air, did I crave sour or bitter foods, was I "thirsty" or "thirstless," and so on.) He went into his back room for a few minutes, returned with a single dose of white powder, which he put under my tongue, and predicted the return of the fever—without an actual elevation of temperature—that very night.

I was highly skeptical. The malaise wasn't due back, in its nasty cyclical form, for another two and a half weeks. Nevertheless, that night it returned. I took my temperature. It was 98.6, though I was shivering and sweating in the unpleasant manner to which I had become accustomed. Call it "placebo" if you wish, but he was right in every respect and, after taking its violent departure—called an *aggravation*, in which the symptoms get worse for a little while—the fever never returned.

Whitmont drew clues from personality problems, or from a patient's dreams, to pinpoint and prescribe homeopathic remedies; he used homeopathic character profiles, especially intergenerational familial ones, to help understand psychological problems. He became known as "an analyst's analyst," and a much sought after homeopath who specialized in dramatic cures of obscure and complex illnesses. He wrote groundbreaking analyses of contemporary culture (see *The Symbolic Quest* and *Return of the Goddess*).

His unique genius was to draw insights from different domains of knowledge and come up with a synthesis in which "the whole was greater than the sum of its parts." One of his later books, *The Alchemy of Healing*, combines insights from psychotherapy and homeopathy, as does his clinical text on dream analysis, *Dreams, a Portal to the Source*. Whitmont created, out of the materials at his disposal, a new standard of holistic healing and of symbolic analysis. He was still working with and training a small handful of us when he died in 1998.

Even during the time I was training with Whitmont, I had become involved with biofeedback—in the late 1960s—which probably should put me in some "grandfather" category by now. As a high school student in the fifties, I had tried to devise EEGs out of the electronic radio parts I had all over my room. I became obsessed by the idea that you could learn something useful from brain waves, although at that time there was virtually no cultural or educational support for such a strange idea. My EEG machine never materialized, because, among other problems, I could not figure out how to safely isolate the human subject from the 110-volt electricity in the circuitry. (I was grappling with technical problems that it has taken a whole generation of neurofeedback researchers and clinicians to solve, as well as requiring new breakthroughs in solid-state electronics and computers.)

As an undergraduate, and later graduate, psychology student at Columbia University, I found no brain wave or biofeedback devices, but lots of rats, pigeons, and operant conditioning devices. I had to content myself with devising experiments on human perception, and in graduate school did psycholinguistics research, as well as experiments that measured response times in how well people's brains process specific types of linguistic utterances. Meanwhile, I would sneak off at night into the stacks at Butler Library to study mythology, or catch Joseph Campbell's lectures at the Jung Foundation. I also took up the martial arts and began regular Zen Buddhist meditation.

After graduation, when I began teaching psychology courses at State University of New York (SUNY), Ulster, I soon set up a program in "consciousness studies," and a lab where students could have hands-on experience of this marvelous new thing called "biofeedback." The field was just breaking loose, and there was tremendous excitement in the human potential movement at something that offered to link up the fuzzy edges of consciousness with something measurable and describable in scientific terms. A consciousness revolution was trying to be born.

My students had hands-on experiences with electromyographs (EMGs) where they could be hooked up to a little machine that informed them about how tense or relaxed their muscles were. There were also skin galvanometers (GSRs), still used in the core of polygraphs, which showed a read-out of changes in the skin's conduction of electrical stimuli, a way of measuring stress. My students loved those—they could bring their boyfriends or girlfriends to the lab, hook them up, ask them questions, and try to tell when they were lying! They could

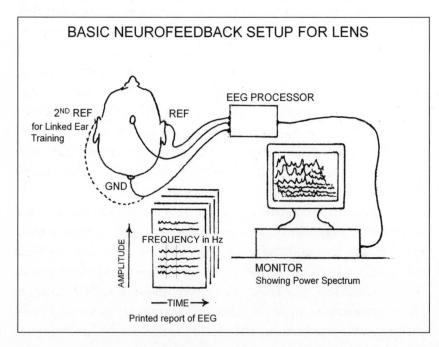

Fig. I.1. Electroencephalography Recording System

also use them on themselves to tell when they were relaxed or tense.

With the EEG biofeedback machines, wires were attached directly to the student's scalp, thus measuring the tiny brain waves somehow making it through all the layers of bone, skin, and hair to the surface; the students could then directly observe an electroencephalograph showing their brain waves moment to moment. Simply by paying attention to themselves—while hooked up to "the little robots," as we called the machines—students lowered blood pressure, decreased anxiety (especially test anxiety), and were performing more smoothly in athletics.

They were introduced to meditation and EEG biofeedback at the same time, and sometimes I would find them sitting cross-legged in meditation in front of the EEG machine, with wires on their heads and a low monotonous tone coming out of the machine (evidence was already accumulating that biofeedback could accelerate the process of meditation). They could try any technique they wanted, from "progressive relaxation" to autohypnosis, or "autogenic training." But it was the biofeedback machine that would give unmistakable evidence about whether they were successful or not.

Ah, the endless fascination of the brain! Many of the students who did the EEG training told me that they "felt smarter," and that their academic scores were going up. Some said that, for the first time, they felt they had a clue as to whether they were actually paying attention in class or daydreaming. I was struck by this finding. Although the high frequency brain waves known as "beta" (12 Hz and above) are characteristic of a strongly engaged mind, the students who used the biofeedback machine and other techniques to induce their brains to spend more time in the restful, nonaroused state characterized by lower frequency brain waves in the range called "alpha" (8–12 Hz) or the even slower "theta" waves (4–8 Hz) still became better students!

Theta is a slowed state associated with hypnagogic imagery and access to unconscious emotions, and alpha—or so we thought in those days—mainly a neutral, "time out" state. How could alpha and theta waves help concentration, which is conventionally associated with beta? I now know that it was the exercising of the brain to move in whatever direction they chose, rather than "training" the brain to produce a specific type of wave, that made the students feel and perform "smarter."

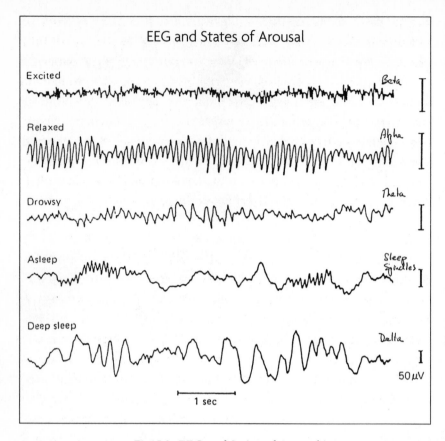

Fig. I.2. *EEG and States of Arousal*

The students recorded their scores on the machines, session by session, and kept a psychological journal of their experiences as they went along. (Incidentally, as the work of James Pennebaker has shown, journal-keeping itself is a kind of "biofeedback" that can be self-revelatory and self-healing.[1]) When I read the first semester's "journal summaries" from the students, I was astounded at the results. First of all, the quality was much higher than the endless psychology research papers I had been accustomed to reading.

Why? Because it was personal and real, not abstract, like so much in academics. I had never really imagined the full potential of Jung's simple idea: "The self-liberating power of the introverted mind." Looking within and using what is found there is also what the Buddhists call "skillful means." As each semester unfolded, I could just feel the students going through psychological growth and maturation. *It was the opposite of what is most deadly about education.* It felt alive! Above all, my students told me they felt a sense of personal empowerment from the experience.

The consciousness program continued to be a popular feature of the campus for twenty-six more years, attracting returning adult students (my favorite population), other faculty who were also fascinated by the subject matter, college staff including administration and even clerks and janitors with anxiety or phobias. People came in with medical problems such as high blood pressure, headaches or panic attacks and got relief, lowering or eliminating their need for medication.

My Apprenticeship with Len Ochs

During the eighties I had begun to realize the tremendous clinical potential of biofeedback, and begun introducing it to my psychotherapy patients whom I saw in clinical settings outside the college lab. With biofeedback, people who had been immobilized in therapy for years or had reached a plateau in their process suddenly started moving again. They were empowered by what Elmer Green called "the voluntary control of internal states."

By 1990, I had sold my partnership in the Green Street Center, a private, humanistically oriented clinic in Kingston, New York, and founded Stone Mountain Center on our rural Hudson Valley property. In 1994 I hired several clinicians and set up a full-service biofeedback and neurofeedback program. Adam Crane, an old friend and one of the pioneers of biofeedback, had told me about Len Ochs; and Chris White, one of my clinicians, also heard him talk in New York City and was enthralled. I invited Len to lecture and teach neurofeedback at Stone Mountain Center.

At that time I had not yet recognized the "maverick mythos" in my personal journey. But the work I had done with Whitmont prepared me for some of the unusual things I would hear from Len, such as: "Less is more"; or how to notice the effects of a remedy or a treatment in a person's psychology; and, perhaps most important, how to notice improvements or regressions in *all dimensions* of a person's functioning, in other words, "holistically."

During the 1990s the field of neurofeedback was exploding and there was no end of exciting things to learn. Before Len came to Stone Mountain Center I had already studied or taken courses with some of the great names in neuroscience and neurofeedback, whom you will meet in the brief history of neurofeedback given in chapter two: Karl Pribram, Maurice (Barry) Sterman, Joel Lubar, Siegfried and Susan Othmer, Elmer Green, and Nancy White. Each was a brilliant scholar or researcher in his or her own way. Each had a vast command of technical knowledge, and lots of experience.

But I was totally unprepared for Len Ochs. Tall and dark-haired, with intense, twinkling eyes, he looked out at the audience, a very serious expression on his face: "No one has done less for the field of biofeedback than I have." (A very few of us, who had heard about his "less is more" approach, got it and laughed—he twinkled a little more.) He looked at us intently, saying, "Everything I have learned has been by accident, by trial and error—and I can't count how many mistakes I have made—and how many mistaken ideas I have entertained. And yet I have this 'cockamamie' procedure that I have stumbled upon—and I don't understand *how* it works—but I do know *that* it works! People really get better. You're smart folks, maybe you'll help me figure it out. So I don't know what I have to teach you—but I can tell you my own experience. Let's have a talk. . . ."

I found myself in some sort of amused shell-shock at such Woody Allen-like honesty in a biofeedback professional. But I also felt myself warming to him. In those days (and into the present) Len joked compulsively—nervously at times—as he taught. In fact, it seemed that the "nervouser" he got, the funnier he got. Soon I found that the man could not teach without making fun of himself, the method itself, and all orthodox and categorical thinking, especially cognitive pomposity or rigidity. Aha! He was one of those trickster-shamans that seem to keep turning up in my life! Underneath it all, though, there was the kind of mirthful genius I had met in some Tibetan and Japanese Zen masters. It is a "presence" of consciousness if you will, nonjudgmental, amused, that cannot hold itself back from making fun of clunky, orthodox thought, in oneself and in others.

I've always thought there were two approaches to overcoming primordial human unconsciousness, with the ultimate goal of becoming more free and creative: The Way of Discipline, or the Way of Laughter. I think they both work, but I noticed as I listened to him that the influence of the second was growing. Len was helping me grow through laughter.

His presentation was discursive, but never dull, because it was so very human. It was unstructured but flowed from topic to topic in a natural way, taking most questions and weaving them into the discourse. Sometimes he would dismiss what he thought was a wrongheaded question with a quip, and sometimes it was a little maddening how he responded to questions by asking the questioner another question, or puckishly saying "I don't know" a few too many times. The more I listened to Len, the more I found I was getting a course in honesty. He really didn't want to talk about what he didn't know. People could get irritable and try to pin him down with questions, whereupon he would deftly change the topic. (I realized sometime later that he was modeling the vaunted neurological flexibility bestowed by his treatment.) To me it looked like the graceful, focused movements of *tai chi chuan*.

My clinician's eye discerned years of training in family systems, Gestalt therapy, and Ericksonian hypnosis. His method reminded me of Jung's dictum, passed on by Whitmont: "Learn every psychological system you can. But when you are in the presence of the actual patient, forget them all—just see what comes in the here and now!"

It really is not an easy thing, to avoid all our "good ideas" and glimpse the splendid and paradoxical nakedness of things as they are. In this regard, the clinician and the scientist are united: theory must take second place to the empirical method. And that method is inextricable from the method that Len Ochs teaches.

When Len was faced with a truly belligerent curmudgeon, or someone with a severe case of "hardening of the categories," he would wave a conceptual cape—like a bullfighter—in front of the guy and let him do himself in. The marvelous thing was that these people often got some kind of insight or awakening. They would actually glimpse the mythmaking tendencies of their own minds. It isn't that he dislikes myths generically, he just doesn't like substituting them for reality. I have done my own analysis on *him*: I think he's allergic to fundamentalists—including, and especially, "scientific fundamentalists." He'd rather know what you have found to be true than muddle around in all the best theories about it.

I particularly resonated with Len when he began to tell clinical stories from his practice. I knew how genuine healing looked and smelled from thirty years of psychotherapy practice, and from watching the work of some of the great masters in the field, including: E. C. Whitmont, Fritz Perls, Charlotte Selver, Alexander Lowen and John Pierrakos, Stanislav Grof, Arnie Mindell, and Ilana Rubenfeld. What Len was describing rang true from my own therapeutic experience, and what I had witnessed when people open themselves to an authentic healing encounter. And the kinds of changes Len Ochs was reporting exceeded some of the best work I had seen, especially as it pertained to the calming and balancing of the central nervous system.

It was only after working with Len for some time that I realized how my own mythology had played into my apprenticeship with him: I hadn't yet seen his motley beneath the casual attire. He was clearly another of those mavericks I seem to seek out: People who are not restricted to a single vision of reality ("Newton's sleep" as Blake put it); people who embrace homeopathy as well as analytical psychology, for instance; people whose fields of expertise include electronics, computer technology, clinical psychology—and subtle energy medicine besides.

There are no more da Vincis. We are in the age of the specialist, in which no *one* person can encompass all of the knowledge of our time. One supposedly must hold one's nose to the metaphoric grindstone of specialization, mastering all that is currently known on the subject by following one narrow corridor of learning. And it is truly amazing what knowledge has been discovered, synthesized, even created by such bloodhounds of knowing.

But I have always been drawn to people who demonstrate what might be called "polyphrenia," or knowing based on "multiple intelligences" (Howard Gardner's important concept). Benoit Mandelbrot, who discovered the mathematics of "Fractals," called such people "nomads by choice" and saw them as "necessary to the intellectual welfare of the settled disciplines,"[2] due to the fact that they cross-pollinate and enrich each one. Under Len's tutelage I found myself becoming a more practical and empirical clinician—as well as a more accomplished paradoxical thinker.

I completed my initial training with Len Ochs in about a year, but have stayed in supervision with him ever since the beginning (a total of ten years). In my experience, he is one of the most discerning and accurate clinicians I have ever met. He notices things about people—energy, mood, posture, reactivity, or sensitivity to stimuli—that other therapists might ignore or gloss over. He has the same almost X-ray perception I had seen when Whitmont worked with patients directly, or with the cases we brought to him for clinical supervision. I got the feeling that it was this level of subtlety that made Len's work seem "difficult" or "esoteric" to some biofeedback professionals.

When he described how his clinical thinking had been shaped by both the good results and the bad—such as when head-injured patients had "overdose" reactions of either tiredness or "wiredness" to the amount of neurofeedback stimulation they had received—I was all ears. Len confessed that he himself had had a head injury at birth. In fact, many traumatic brain injuries (TBIs) come from perinatal damage through chemicals or damage during delivery, since the human head is so inconveniently large. In Len's case, it came when an enthusiastic obstetrician grabbed him by the ankles to turn him upside down for the obligatory "spanking," and dropped him on his two-minute-old head! Because of this event, young Len suffered for years from learning and attention problems, and at times his teachers claimed he was ineducable.

I got it: Len Ochs was a "wounded healer," an extraordinary "cyber-shaman" who had used his own wound—along with his training in (and frustration with) clinical psychology and a compulsive relationship with computers—to design an unprecedented healing method for head injuries, thus healing himself in the process. He was a truly splendid maverick genius. The result of his unique work is an awesome new technology, which practitioners use (in their own idiosyncratic ways) to do tiny, skillful things that make for big positive changes in many patients' quality of life.

Had I Had a Head Injury?

Hearing about Len's experience, and how it led him to work with individuals with head injuries, I began some self-examination. After years of psychotherapy with many different therapists—Jungian, Bioenergetic, Rolfing, even Past-Life Regression—I still suffered from mood instabilities, including spells of anger, cognitive confusion, sleep disturbances, restless leg syndrome, attentional problems, and diminished but still gnawing anxiety. (Lest I sound highly dysfunctional I should say I was carrying on a successful academic career alongside a clinical practice, writing books, and giving lectures. I think all the therapy, yoga, meditation, and so on had really helped!) But the clinician in me knew there was some stone left unturned in my own healing process, and I also knew how common were the blind spots of some of the most discerning therapists.

I wondered: Had *I* had a head injury? Well, in my checkered past there were childhood bike accidents, falls out of trees, a few high fevers, and some skiing bonks. Oh yes, and there was that time that the horizontal bar detached—some other gymnast's ADD (attention deficit disorder) in failing to cinch the safety-clamps no doubt—just as I was starting a giant swing; I slammed to the gym floor, seeing lots of stars. Oh, and there was that time I was rock climbing and fell about one hundred feet, hitting my helmetless head on the way down. (Come to think of it, when I got out of the hospital after a week or so, it was kind of hard to concentrate on my graduate studies at Columbia.)

And there was a more recent incident: my collapse in mile twenty-six of a marathon. (The weather was 95°F and there wasn't enough water available to me to stay adequately hydrated. I fell down within sight of the finish line, my temperature shooting over 106°F, requiring—drat!—another visit to the hospital.) I had sustained all of these injuries, yet, like the majority of people when asked if they had had a head injury, I still wondered: Would you consider *that* a head injury? Hmmm.

I had been troubled by the fact that—after all my work on myself—every time I sat down and tried to do conventional EEG training, whether it was alpha, theta, SMR (sensory-motor rhythm), or beta, I fell asleep within a few minutes. This was actually embarrassing because I taught the stuff—and yet there I was—asleep on the job again! What I now know is that I *did* have a profound layering of head injuries, accumulated over many years. But I can happily say that, thanks to the LENS, the layers are mostly unraveled. I am functioning better in my sixties than I did in my forties. The restless leg and the sleep disturbance are gone. Memory is better, mood is more stable, sleep is better; cognition and multiprocessing are much better. And I get over real or imagined insults (microtraumas?) much faster. Now if I sit down to do conventional neurofeedback training, I don't fall asleep, I just do the training—

easily it seems, and well. For years, when I sat down to meditate, the first half-hour would be spent trying to quiet my yammering disc-jockey mind. Now it "hushes down" more quickly.

But the real shift has been in my anxiety level. My anxiety had always been there—when meeting with influential people, giving speeches before large audiences, or doing anything new or unusual—I would encounter my old friend: anxiety! It was sometimes low-grade, sometimes acute. I couldn't concentrate if something out of place disturbed me. I know that at times I knit-picked with my family, sometimes obsessing over problems. (OCD, Obsessive-Compulsive Disorder, is really an anxiety-system problem, and being a "fussbudget" is probably often more about central nervous system dysfunction and irritability than a feature of a person's character.)

These days my anxiety is a pale shadow of its former self. I sometimes measure it by how "tweaked" I feel before trying a new or exciting trick on the flying trapeze, the weird sport I have taken up in my sixties (following another mentor and friend, Sam Keen). I also look at how free and creative I feel during the trick. I know that my current ease of performance, inner flexibility, and ability to multitask were not fully developed before I started the LENS training on myself. I feel quieter, more centered, and have more freedom and ease of functioning in most activities of life.

Feeling these changes in myself, I am more sensitized to the improvements as well as impairments in my clients, especially the clients with head injuries. I recognize the truth that CNS (head or spinal) injury is a true "chameleon." It can mimic every pathological problem in the DSM IV-r (the current version of the endlessly revised *Diagnostic and Statistical Manual of Mental Disorders*). When I began my internship with Len, the majority of my practice was psychotherapy, a smaller percentage was biofeedback. Today the majority of our clients do the LENS training combined with, in some cases, HeartMath, a technique developed by Doc Lew Childre for emotional self-management, or other feedback modalities, and psychotherapy as well, where indicated. I have noticed that the ones who do the LENS make the most progress. When the nervous system is free from gross distortions, or "static," people are able to confront their own "psychodynamic" problems and issues much more clearly and successfully.

As a psychotherapist, I had often felt defeated by the same modalities that other therapists complain about: nothing we could do seemed to help with endogenous depressions, heritable bipolarity, constitutional (or trauma-induced) severe anxiety problems, panic attacks, ADD/ADHD in children and adults. These are the very categories that have psychotherapists and psychologists turning to the psychiatrists or the neurologists for medicine—or even ECT (electroconvulsive or "shock" therapy) due to the fact that the symptoms seem resistant to the best psychotherapeutic efforts. But we have employed LENS with all these problems and collected overwhelming clinical evidence that, in the hands of skilled professionals, it truly helps.

When queried, my wife Robin didn't seem to think—at least at first—that she had had head injuries. And she generally functions in an awesome way. But in the first "mapping" we did of the brain waves generated by different areas of her brain, I saw a hot spot in her right frontal area, indicating that she had suffered a head injury at some point in the past. "What could *that* be?" we wondered aloud. She couldn't come up with anything.

Then, during the week she approached me with a funny look on her face (a not unfamiliar scenario in our line of work) and told the following story: Thirty years before, riding an unfamiliar horse at a brisk canter down a country road, she had come to an intersection that required a sharp turn. The horse took it too fast and slid out on the gravel. Robin hit her head on the hardpan in the exact spot where we had noticed the "hot spot" on her brain map (riding helmets were not commonly worn in those days). She was taken to the hospital unconscious, and for days she didn't know who she was, where she lived, or what she had been doing before the accident. Her memory returned only very slowly over the course of a year. She had been in college, and it was with great difficulty that she resumed academic activities that had seemed easy to her before. She remembered feeling "a little cloudy" at that time (although she did manage to finish school before going on to graduate school at NYU).

Then we remembered a later injury, probably more diffuse in its effect: During the seventies Robin was on her way to sit in on my evening college class when a guy in an uninsured pickup truck, driving at twilight with his lights off, broadsided her car. She spent a couple of days

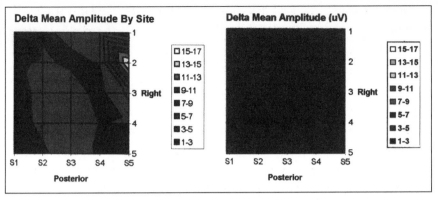

Fig. I.3. Two Map Comparison: Robin Larsen. Left, initial assessment map, 12/29/96. Notice the "hot spot," caused by the concussion, in the right upper corner. Right, 11/21/03, during several years of occasional treatment, the hot spot has disappeared.

in the hospital. "Don't you think that was a head injury?" I asked her.

"Well," she answered, "I was still picking little bits of window glass out of my forehead several months later. Yeah, I guess that qualifies!" Robin's two brain maps are shown side by side in figure I.3. You'll notice that in the later map the "hot spot" is completely gone. Please remember it had been there for thirty years, and the two maps are a couple of years apart.

As Robin did a cognitive self-appraisal, she noted that despite her high level of functioning, she had been having some memory problems, word-retrieval lapses, and feelings of "overwhelm" when confronted with too many possibilities. These issues are now much improved—after about twenty sessions of the LENS.

Thirty years ago, one of my first biofeedback instructors, Dr. Steve Fahrion, then of the Menninger Clinic, said to me: "Train yourself. Don't ask your clients to do anything you haven't explored thoroughly yourself." I have never regretted taking his advice. In the case of the LENS training, it has not only benefited my clinical practice; the LENS has improved my quality of life and that of my loved ones. Members of my office staff and members of our local community, many of whom have received head injuries in auto accidents, or doing extreme sports, have benefited. There is no mistaking improvements so close to home!

In addition to our experience, clinicians and healers from many disciplines have been attracted to Len Ochs's work over the past decade and have profited from it. In this book I present certain of his cases, some of my own, as well as other compelling accounts collected by colleagues. (Please know that, unless another clinical practitioner's name is noted, the stories have been written by me.) We are grateful to our clients for giving us permission to tell their stories and, in some cases, for providing their own words and comments, their own honest self-appraisals on subjective rating scales. In some cases they have asked to have their own names be used, and in others, to change their names to protect their privacy. The stories are as faithful as possible to the real-life clinical events as they unfolded.

You will find their stories grouped in chapters specifically devoted to the treatment of:

- Traumatic Brain Injuries
- Childhood disorders such as Autism and Attention Deficit Disorder (ADD)
- Fibromyalgia and Chronic Fatigue Syndrome
- Anxiety and Depression
- Epilepsy and Tourette's Syndrome
- Chronic Pain and Post-Traumatic Stress Disorder
- Stroke, Alzheimer's Disease, and Parkinson's Disease

There are also later chapters on combining the LENS with other modalities, optimal performance, the physics of low energy treatment, and our work with animals.

In this book you will find the transformational tales of "urban shamans," as we might call our clients who have passed through a challenging ordeal of some kind—head injury, psychological trauma, a congenital illness suddenly showing up—and, in some time-honored way, been positively transformed as well as healed.

Joseph Campbell always encouraged his students, like the Grail knights, to go into the forest "where it was darkest, and there was no beaten way or path." This book is certainly an account of such an adventure, from the *agnosia* of feeling lost, blind, and ignorant about the dark land hidden inside the skull, into *micrognoses,* little awakenings, little clearings in the forest where the light shines through. Myths from around the world agree that the gold, the treasure, or the magic talisman is often found precisely where you lose your way, or where you stumble.

The wish-fulfilling-gem can be glimpsed in the improved clarity and quality of life that our clients report, their renewed energy, their more vibrant perceptions, their freedom from emotional turbulence and anxiety, their improved cognition, and their recovered—or enhanced—creativity. This book is hopeful about humanity, the value of collaborating in one's own healing process, and the fact that we have untapped sources of wisdom, transformation, and rebirth inside ourselves. When the nervous system is quiet and balanced, the mind, or more accurately, the psyche, is a truly awesome instrument. *Transform the brain and you transform the world!*

1

THE LENS IN CLINICAL PRACTICE

Stephen Larsen, Ph.D.

In my personal experience with CNS biofeedback, the shifts in my brain's electrical activity reflected in the graphs were accompanied by equally dramatic physical, emotional, social, psychological, cognitive, and spiritual alterations. I do not believe my experiences have been unique in any way. . . . Every patient who undergoes it may experience a kaleidoscope of reactions to the experience, ranging from joyful excitement to profound bewilderment and even distress.

JOAN PIPER MADER, HEMIPLEGIC VICTIM OF STROKE,
WHO RECOUNTS HER STORY IN CHAPTER 10

> The method of neurofeedback that we introduce in this book has been known by several names, corresponding to its stages of evolution. It was first called EEF (EEG Entrainment Feedback) in 1992. Around 1994, when it was pointed out that it actually is a *dis*entrainment process rather than an entraining one, the name was changed to EDF (EEG Disentrainment Feedback) or EDS (EEG Disentrainment Stimulation). Around 1995–1996 it was also called ILT (Interactive Light Therapy), the name by which it is still known in Australia. Around 1998 the name was changed to FNS (Flexyx Neurotherapy Stimulation) and in 2002, it was changed to the final version (we hope), the LENS (Low Energy Neurofeedback System). You will learn more about what these terms mean in the following chapters (2 and 3) on the history and development of the LENS approach.

Eight Years of Experience at Stone Mountain Center, New York

I retired from a twenty-eight-year teaching career and began an intensive period of training in neurofeedback with Len Ochs. Soon I was shifting the main thrust of the biofeedback center I had founded in 1994 toward the system that was then called Flexyx and is now known as the LENS technique. We began to acquire a professional biofeedback staff, including Jim Giorgi, a school psychologist and neurofeedback specialist who in the past had worked with Mary Jo Sabo at her Biofeedback Consultants in Suffern, New York. (Jim went on to help design and implement the impressive Yonkers School Project using neurofeedback for Attention Deficit with Hyperactivity or ADHD students.) Over the years, we have trained many clinicians at Stone Mountain Center, including our own senior clinicians Carrie Chapman and Alexandra Linardakis, who help to operate our satellite office in New York City and affiliates in Kingston and Red Hook, New York.

During the past nine years we have seen a fairly high volume of patients (between forty and sixty per week) at Stone Mountain. Our patient population has included children struggling with disorders such as Autism and Asperger's Syndrome, in which the child seems "locked away" inside, Cerebral Palsy, and Pervasive Developmental Disorder (PDD), in which a child may face a lifelong struggle to achieve the developmental milestones that come easily and naturally to other children. In addition, we see lots of children with attention disorders such as Attention Deficit Disorder (ADD) and Attention Deficit Disorder with Hyperactivity (ADHD), in which the children dance to a different drummer than their peers and their teachers, as well as those with Reactive Attachment Disorder, and conduct and antisocial disorders, usually the outcomes of child abuse or neglect.

Our clientele also includes a spectrum of adult clients, including Vietnam veterans; those recovering from Workmen's Compensation injuries or industrial accidents; persons dealing with dysfunctional family issues including physical, sexual, and emotional abuse; ambulatory schizophrenics not long out of the hospital; and people with anxiety and substance-abuse problems. We see quite a few traumatic brain injury (TBI) and Post-Traumatic Stress Disorder (PTSD) victims (especially since 9/11), and some with problems like neurological Lyme Disease, Chronic Fatigue Syndrome, and fibromyalgia. During the past two years we have taken on several Parkinson's patients with startlingly good results. Many clients are people who have become habituated to, but disillusioned with, psychotropic drugs prescribed by their doctors, and have been looking, sometimes desperately, for an alternative.

In a one-hour intake interview, I meet with prospective clients and go over the extensive paperwork they have already filled out regarding their backgrounds, or rather, their "story," including their detailed medical and psychological history and a history of traumas and injuries, including birth and vaccination-related crises. They take the CNS Questionnaire, a screening instrument devised by Len Ochs, which elicits information regarding problems pertaining to sleep, mood, energy, cognitive clarity, pain, and sensitivity to stimuli (see chapter 11 for the CNS Questionnaire). The results offer a good indicator of whether or not they can be helped by our treatments: generally, the higher the incidence of positive responses, the more likely the treatments will help. An informative conversation is conducted about the benefits and limitations of neurotherapy, and the prospective patient is invited to question us as completely as we question them about how we work and what to expect.

If they decide to go ahead with treatment, we invite them to work together with us in a collaboration to help them improve their functioning and become more at ease with themselves. They are asked to identify five or more aspects of themselves in which they wish to have improvement such as: sleep onset problem, excessive anxiety, fatigue, cluster headaches, or problems with organization and planning.

Our clients are told that in this treatment—unlike in reward-based "volitional" biofeedback—they will not be asked to "do anything" during the session. However, they are also told that their participation in the form of being self-observant about how they feel after each treatment is an important part of the process that contributes to our being able to do our job well. As the best therapies feel like a partnership and like a peer healing adventure, we feel it is most important, and highly empowering, for our clients to *participate in the healing process.*

Clients can also choose to have psychotherapeutic sessions at the same time as the neurofeedback treatment, because the LENS seems to have a stimulating effect on personally significant material. If the client is already undergoing psychotherapy, we ask them to apprise their therapist of our treatment and to extend our offer to work synergistically with them in any way that might be productive for the client. Each case is presented in conference with Dr. Willie Yee, our supervising psychiatrist, and any issues involving medication and the possible use of nutraceuticals (natural supplements or herbs), diet, and lifestyle are also discussed and noted.

In the first session, we ask our clients for permission to touch them to apply the EEG sensors and usually hook up three: a ground on one ear, a neutral on the other, and an active sensor, which will be applied to different sites, one at a time. The initial session, known as the "offset," is an exploratory procedure in which the active sensor is applied to the site known as "FZ" (located at the center crown of the forehead just behind the hairline). A computer is used to record the activity of the client's brain at this site while he or she sits at rest, eyes closed.

Then four invisible and gentle radio-wave stimulations are given. Each burst is separated by a minute of observation and recording of the changes in the brain waves brought about by the stimulation. The ultimate goal is for the brain to be calmed through the feedback of its own energy. The underlying premise of this treatment method was already known to the ancients and is known in Latin as *similia similibus curantur*, "like cures like." In this paradigm (similar to that of homeopathy), the patient is given back just a little of "what ails" them, imprinted on the radio carrier wave. Then the brain takes the information into account and adjusts its operations, subtly, but almost always a little for the better.

In the next session a topographic brain map will be made of nineteen sites, by moving the active electrode from site to site. The map shows us the "terrain" of the brain and tells us where to begin placing our sensors during treatment. It is part of Len Ochs's genius that he invented the idea of beginning treatment where the brain is healthiest (indicated by the sites where brain wave activity is at the lowest amplitude), and only gradually sneaking up on the problem areas (usually where the amplitudes are highest). (See color insert pages 1 and 4 for examples of LENS maps.)

Using these two procedures—the Offset and the topographic Brain Map—along with what we have learned from the CNS Questionnaire (see chapter 11 for the CNS Questionnaire) and other measures, we then set a unique, tailor-made protocol for each patient. This includes the sequence of sites to be stimulated, the number of seconds of stimulation at each site, and the most effective offset frequency to lower the amplitudes of the brain waves. A typical client will receive a weekly treatment consisting of stimulation of the selected sites, perhaps along with psychotherapy, or other therapies if they have elected to do them.

In the beginning of the treatment there is often a "honeymoon" phase in which the client feels miraculously better. In some cases this turns out to be a permanent change, justifying the "expect miracles!" slogan some neurotherapists have in their offices. In these cases we could say that the vital and self-healing forces were already available in the person and that the treatment merely catalyzed an internal healing process. This occurs most often with people whose main problems are more "functional" than "structural," that is to say, their problems stem more from the brain's own protective (functional) responses to trauma, rather than from "broken neurons" (which would be a structural problem). The "fix" for the first kind of problem is the restoration of dynamical functionality to the system, while the second demands the biological repair of tissue, a task requiring much more time.

Initially there may be a blissful period after each treatment, then a gradual sliding back in symptoms over the week or two until the next treatment. As treatments accumulate, the effect seems to last longer, and the treatments are spread farther apart. The ultimate goal is for the client to be balanced enough to no longer need treatment.

In the spirit of Len Ochs's commitment to the Hippocratic Oath— "Do no harm!"—we have cultivated an attuned sensitivity to the outcomes of our treatment. We have initiated something in relation to a person that wouldn't have happened to them otherwise; it would be careless or inattentive not to track the outcome. We also treat nature, including human nature, as if it were sensitive, intelligent, and responsive, doing the *minimum* to set it on the course of self-healing.

This is the opposite of what happens in allopathic medicine's "heroic" treatments, where extremely drastic measures may be invoked to take care of what is perceived to be a serious problem, but then the patient gets worse or dies from the treatment itself. This is known as *iatrogenic illness,* illness caused by doctors, a hallmark of our time, which doubtlessly contributes to the high rates of malpractice insurance. In the fields of biofeedback and neurofeedback—where the patient or client is enlisted as a *partner* in the process of getting well—malpractice suits are virtually nonexistent.

As clients heal, their fatigue abates, they sleep better, mood swings stabilize, pain diminishes, cognition and clarity improve. Instability patterns stabilize, although not always immediately. Clients who are underaroused (depressed or fatigued) pick up their pace, and those who are overaroused (driven or hypervigilant) slow down. Naturally, the younger and more resilient the client, the quicker their recovery. Recovery is also more rapid if the nervous system is free of disruptive influences such as medication, alcoholism, poor nutrition, or other bad habits. Recovery is also clearly fostered by a healthy family or social environment. The beneficial effects of neurofeedback treatments seem to be amplified in people who maintain a rich organic chemistry of vitamins, minerals, and amino acids in their diet, either through natural sources or supplementation. And those who do self-help techniques, such as Pilates, yoga, Feldenkrais, massage, martial arts, and so on, also seem to progress more quickly.

We have discovered, not surprisingly, that people who had a healthy and vital lifestyle prior to their injuries not only recover more easily but are also more strongly motivated to get well. They will actively participate in the healing process, even to the point of being very assertive about keeping their appointments and driving great distances to get to them.

Those with chronic problems, multiple problems overlaid on each other, or who are replicating old family patterns, make much slower progress. Our findings here agree with Ochs's general approach to prognosis: The longer a person has had the problem—or if their parents or other family members have it or something like it—the longer the treatment is going to take.

Still, people who have been "given up on" by traditional medical science, or who have endured years of oppressive medical regimens, multiple medications, or even electroconvulsive ("shock") treatments, can indeed be helped, as the case studies we share with you in these pages demonstrate.

We begin with two cases from my own practice: that of a seven-year-old child who began treatment with enough DSM IV symptoms to make us think about rewriting the manual, yet now is symptom free; and that of a vibrant young teacher who was shot in the head by a mugger and who, post-treatment, was able to resume her teaching career in addition to telling her own story, eloquently, on NBC television. These two individuals demonstrate how an actual course of treatment typically progresses, introducing many of the themes explored in later chapters of this book.

Jacob: Reconstructing Batman

A seven-year-old boy we shall call Jacob was brought to our center near New Paltz, in the Hudson Valley of New York. He was small, elfin, and with a kind of fixed, pixyish smile. His concerned parents had brought Jacob to us because his behavior had gone haywire. He had started washing his hands very often during the day. Four or five times each night he would come stand by their bed and ask if something was going to fall out of the sky onto their house, or if the germs that had been trying to get him might make him die in his sleep. He wondered if terrorists could have put any poison in the food the family had eaten at the restaurant that night! His parents described how they would patiently answer, "No, everything is okay, dear," and put him back to bed. But he would reappear again with the same questions an hour later.

They told us that Jacob used to be more playful. His favorite game was playing Batman: He would fly off overstuffed easy chairs into Gotham City, or get his dad to impersonate some bad guy whom Jacob would then subdue by wrestling. But his Batman cape was sadly hanging on its peg in the kitchen and he was dwelling in a preoccupied-seeming apathy, occasionally punctured by tantrums or other forms of "acting out."

While intelligence tests showed that Jacob was well above average intelligence, he had become inattentive to what was going on in school and no longer seemed able to keep track of his assignments. And he was impulsive, having recently given his five-year-old sister a spontaneous haircut with sharp scissors! When Jacob's parents rebuked him for his misbehaviors, Jacob seemed "absent," as if no one were home or, if the issue was pressed, he would throw a terrible little tantrum. He complained of bad headaches, which initially frightened his parents toward pediatric neurologists, and MRIs, and CAT scans. But these tests had shown nothing out of the ordinary.

The neurologist, however, had uttered the ominous phrase: "Attention Deficit with Hyperactivity (ADHD)," and suggested that Jacob be given a prescription for Ritalin. He hinted that they should see a pediatric psychiatrist because of their son's OCD (Obsessive-Compulsive Disorder) symptoms and mood swings. They had seen a psychiatrist, who had interviewed them closely, probing for the sources of the significant pathology Jacob was exhibiting.

Had there been sexual or emotional abuse? No. Marital conflict or divorce? No. The parents seemed warm, concerned, involved; their relationship appeared to be a stable one. The psychiatrist suggested medication for Jacob: SSRIs (selective serotonin re-uptake inhibitors) such as Prozac for the OCD, perhaps along with the Ritalin for the ADHD. But the parents did not want to take that route. They had heard bad things about the personality changes that befall some children on psychotropic drugs, and the newspapers had been full of stories about grade-school children trading their Ritalin and Prozac with other children. Although they were distraught, Jacob's parents stood firm in their resolve not to medicate their son.

To make Jacob comfortable during my initial interview with his parents, I invited him to play in the sand tray that I have in my office. I have found that "Sandplay"—following the work of English therapist Margaret Lowenfeld and Swiss psychologist Dora Kalff—is a therapeutically and diagnostically useful technique that children naturally gravitate toward. My office shelves and closet are stocked with hundreds of figures and objects: little people of all kinds, small churches, houses, castles, and many types of animals.

The sandplay technique, the symbolic play the child engages in, is treated like any other projective technique in psychology. Is his world coherent or incoherent? Are there frightening monsters? Are there things buried? The kind of play the child engages in tells us much about his inner world.

Although Jacob was seven, he played like a three- or four-year-old: Objects were randomly chosen; he banged things into each other and crashed cars into buildings, then filled the mouths of little rubber reptiles with sand and dumped it out in a gleeful, but infantile manner. When the clinical intake interview was over, we went into the adjoining office where the neurofeedback equipment is kept. I asked Jacob to sit in a comfortable chair while I gently pasted on the sensors.

Jacob fidgeted while we did the EEG, but we saw more or less what we had expected to see on the colorful screen. Jacob's *delta* waves and

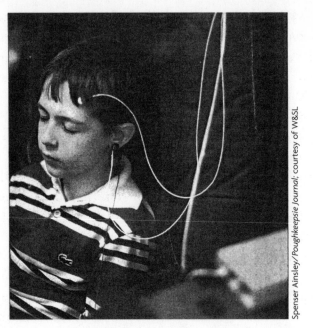

Fig. 1.1. Jacob, age seven, being treated on the current version of the LENS. (Note the lack of glasses, only radio waves are being used for treatment.)

theta waves were higher than 20μv* in amplitude. Jacob was "low-frequency bound" indicating that he probably couldn't have paid attention even if he was trying his very hardest.

Jacob's brain waves told us that, as is true of many ADHD children, he was really more asleep than awake—that is, he was more attuned to inner realities than outer ones—and that life for him was sort of like a big daydream. (That is why the well-meaning doctor would have given Jacob Ritalin: to speed up his metabolism and wake up his brain. And on speed the lad might have been able to function better, but at what cost?)

We noted that Jacob's family was an exception to the stereotyped norms often found with inattentive, hyperactive children. Jacob was not adopted (the rates of ADHD and bipolar disorder seem to be higher among adopted children). Nor was Jacob a male child being raised by a single mother (often a very difficult situation psychologically and emotionally). His parents did not use corporal punishment, nor shame nor guilt-predicated techniques. There was no known mental illness in the

---

*μv = a microvolt is one-millionth of a volt

family, nor bipolar disorders (which seem especially associated with ADD and ADHD), although a couple of grandparents had suffered from alcoholism, which can sometimes signal depression or bipolarity in earlier generations, when such genetically-linked problems were not readily diagnosed.

As the treatments gently began to take, over a period of weeks, Jacob sat more calmly in the chair. We heard from his parents that there were fewer nocturnal awakenings. His mother tracked that as well as other variables from week to week in a little notebook, providing a very helpful adjunct to the therapy. For his sandplay sessions, Jacob started bringing little figures of his own to act out the characters of *101 Dalmatians* (a Disney movie), indicating that a more mature cognition seemed to be emerging.

Soon friends and relatives were commenting on Jacob's improvement, and although Jacob's parents ultimately would be amazed and pleased at their son's overall progress, at this point, Jacob's scientifically oriented father retained some skepticism about it all. This is not an uncommon response among intelligent patients (or their parents) in the beginning of treatment, because the treatment itself is invisible and the explanations are sometimes hard for people to grasp. Also, the therapeutic results often show up little by little, organically rather than dramatically (except in some of the single-session "miracle" cures reported by Ochs and others). But in Jacob's case something untoward happened, which revealed the progress that had been made.

One day, because of computer problems with the machine we usually used for the neurofeedback treatment, we had switched to an older machine that gave stronger signals. I was out of the office, and one of our office clinicians, following the written protocol, gave Jacob his accustomed treatment of four seconds: one second each at four different sites. (No adjustment had been made to temper the stronger signals.) The family had scarcely gotten out the door when Jacob exploded with some ferocity. He literally went "off the wall."

All of his old "bad behavior" came back with a vengeance over the next day, revealing, in stark contrast, how much better Jacob had already gotten in about a month and a half of treatments. After forty-eight hours Jacob's father phoned the center with some urgency. I apologized for the disruption and asked him to bring Jacob in the following day. When they came, both Jacob and his dad regarded the treatment chair uneasily, but I reassured them we would almost surely "do better." I had consulted with Len Ochs in California and followed his advice to reduce the treatment to one second only at one site.

Immediately his parents saw Jacob's good behavior return, as their son's brain balanced and quieted again. After that, most of the treatments we gave Jacob were no longer than one second's duration each week, and he seemed to flourish.

After a few months, Jacob's headaches were a thing of the past. He stopped awakening and awakening others in the night. He reported vivid, cartoonlike dreams (dreaming is a good sign, and cartoons are what he lives for!). Jacob became much more helpful around the house and seemed more thoughtful of everyone's feelings. The reports coming back from school were much better. His grades went up. The Batman cape came down off the wall. He seemed more like himself.

As the spring yielded to summer, even better reports started coming back from his school, and his hand-washing compulsion and associated anxiety about germs seemed to be waning a little (although this was one of the last symptoms to yield). Since Jacob was doing so well, he was given a reward after each neurotherapy session. He was fascinated by horses, so we would walk half a mile together to visit them in the barn at the other end of our rural therapy center. As our walks continued from week to week, Jacob demonstrated more energy, running up the hills and jumping off rocks or out from behind trees to ambush me, wearing his Batman cape. He seemed far more like an average seven-year-old than he had in the beginning, when he was so distractible and frightened of his own shadow.

But the first horse feeding was a disaster. As Jacob gave a hay cake to the horse it gratefully slobbered all over him. We both instantly remembered Jacob's contamination fetish and our eyes met. I broke the impasse with a joke: "Hey," I suddenly said in a strange voice that made him laugh, quoting the movie *Ghostbusters*, "He *slimed* me!"

"Yeah," Jacob replied in the same voice, "he *slimed* me!" I handed him a towel, and the tense moment passed. (This incident demonstrates something that is reported in the LENS treatments again and again: old emotional responses may not completely disappear, but neither does the person remain stuck in them.)

Ironically, Jacob's fears about "the sky falling in" and large-scale disasters had just abated when the attacks on the World Trade Center in New York took place, about eighty miles from his home. We all feared that Jacob would have a full-blown regression. After all, this was what he had been afraid of all along! And indeed there was a wicked little resurgence of symptoms. He became fearful again, and the sleep disturbances resurfaced. But then, to everyone's astonishment, Jacob seemed to be "over it" in a couple of weeks, and his trajectory of improvement continued.

But Jacob still asked his "questions," as the family called them: "Is this restaurant food contaminated?" The focus seemed to be mainly on food and germs. Two psychotherapeutically relevant experiences were contemporaneously raised and explored in therapy. The first had taken place just before Jacob had been born when he had defecated and then aspirated some of the fecal matter trapped in the amniotic fluid. This had almost killed him, according to the obstetrician. (Of course the event was long before Jacob could *consciously* remember anything). As an older child, though, he had had a couple of incidents of projectile vomiting on the whole family in the car, where he had "messed-up everything" and felt terrible about it.

Simple therapeutic reprocessing of these events didn't seem to help much. So with my guidance, the family began a determined behavior-modification program in which Jacob received rewards for each day that he asked no questions having to do with contamination. Progress was slow, but by the end of summer Jacob met the criterion set by therapist and parents: two weeks of *no* contamination questions. (These last details are shared to allow the reader to see how the LENS treatment works interactively with other modalities, particularly psychotherapy.)

Jacob had earned the experience he had been daydreaming about for months: to actually get on a horse and ride it around! At first he was stiff with excitement, but then he relaxed nicely and followed instructions. He didn't even complain when—while giving the horse his own reward, a hay cake—the horse not only slobbered all over him but also pissed copiously, splattering all over the barn floor, and Jacob's feet, highly "organic" events that would previously have had Jacob in quite a state. Jacob's father, with his video camera, and his mother both held their breath, but the moment was defused by talking about what it means to "piss like a horse."

Jacob concluded his sand tray career by working interactively with the therapist to make a large and complex castle from "legos," a project that took real concentration and perseverance. The finished castle was proudly exhibited to his family, who marveled at its intricacy, and all agreed it was something Jacob would have surely been incapable of nine months before. His old, dysfunctional self had been coaxed, by a very gentle method, to give birth to a more highly functioning, more flexible self. Jacob was off and running into the rest of his life.

The local newspaper *The Poughkeepsie Journal* (June 11, 2001) got hold of Jacob's story and reporters came to our center and interviewed everyone, including Jacob's parents. The parents were outspoken about the efficacy of the treatment, and, it seemed, proud of themselves for having resisted the "quick fix" represented by medication. They had been vindicated in their instincts and their holistic values by their outcome.

Our center does an "open house" every other month, where the families of patients and curious members of the community assemble to talk about the mysteries of the brain, and watch a film or see demonstrations. After the newspaper coverage, Jacob and his family were celebrated guests at one of these open houses, and they told their story to the assembled audience. Jacob's father proudly showed his home video of his son's culminating horseback ride. He had not only been converted to seeing the value in the LENS by our success with his son, he became an outspoken advocate of it, later making the following statement:

When my son was 6 years old he came down with a severe case of compulsive obsessive anxiety disorder that bordered on ADD. After a number of psychiatric counseling sessions that went nowhere our pediatrician urged us to consider drugging our little boy so he would not fail first grade. Although we spent sleepless nights shedding tears over the anxious suffering of our child, my wife and I both refused to give in to this quick fix. We painstakingly searched for an alternate means of therapy for our son.

Our prayers were answered when we found Dr. Larsen and the neurotherapy that he used to treat Jacob. After 17 months of treatment, our son was virtually cured of his anxiety disorder, and has not needed any more treatments or drugs of any kind for the past 3 years. Today Jacob is 10 years old and finished 4th grade on the

Honor Roll! These treatments are nothing short of a miracle for those of us who seek drugless and permanent cures.

Postscript: According to Jacob's family, he did very well for three years after concluding the treatment. Then, in May of 2004, they saw a few of his old symptoms return. He was still doing pretty well in school, but at home he seemed a little self-preoccupied, "hyperfocusing" as it is called, or obsessing on computer games, rather than interacting with his family. At times he was excessively timid about trying new things and spent much of the day, even in nice weather, lurking in the house.

Remembering Jacob's former sensitivity, we restricted our treatment to about four seconds of lo-stim (a stimulation whose energy field is several thousand times weaker than that of the customary stimulation) at a couple of sites per treatment. It only took about five or six treatments to bring Jacob around. He became far more social, adventurous, and flexible. His grandparents had been visiting and commented on the changes they observed in him. At one point his father noticed that instead of paddling around the shallow end of the pool in a desultory, anxious way, suddenly Jason was doing "cannonballs" into the deeper end of the pool—and then swimming energetically to its edge. The benefits of the earlier course of treatment were in no way lost; Jacob had grown into the changes in a very real way, and today is a normal twelve-year-old sixth grader.

Learning from Jacob

Part of the success of this treatment can be attributed to Jacob's youth (and more malleable nervous system); to the fact that he was unclouded by drugs during the whole course of treatment; and to his family's cooperation with the therapy. We believe we were able to head-off a potentially pernicious Obsessive-Compulsive Disorder at the pass, and that without the flexibility imparted by the neurofeedback, the behavior modification alone would have been far more difficult, if possible at all.

Jacob's story is symptomatic of our times, when ADD/ADHD and Autism/Asperger's and Obsessive-Compulsive Disorder (OCD) are listed as major epidemiological problems. Both school authorities and such influential organizations as CHADD (Children with ADD, a fine national organization formed to support parents of children with ADD) have heretofore knuckled under to the pharmaceutical paradigm, indicating to parents that medication is really the only option, especially considering the interests of running an orderly school. The climate has, however, begun to change, as more parents assert their civil rights to choose the treatment of their choice, and the efficacy of the neurofeedback and biofeedback approaches is recognized. We support parents' right to choose!

Jacob's case demonstrates that ongoing therapy is not necessary once the nervous system has come into balance (though occasionally, as in his case, a little "tweak" a few years later might be helpful). The ability to conclude the therapeutic process is in sharp contrast to the medication approach; *the neurofeedback alternative frees a person from chemical dependencies.* A flexible brain produces a quiet, productive, well-adapted mind. The brain self-regulates through the prompting of tiny electronic stimuli, rather than being overwhelmed by the massive invasion of ECT (electroconvulsive therapy), or the ingestion of great amounts of chemical bulldozers. This is a vindication of the underlying principle of all biofeedback: the ability of intelligent systems to self-regulate.

Ginny's Story: Learning about Courage*

The capacity of neurofeedback to gently promote self-regulation in the brain is dramatically demonstrated by the case of a pleasant and jovial young woman, whom we shall call "Ginny," who had been attacked and shot point-blank.

In 1995 and 1996 in the Brooklyn neighborhoods of Park Slope and Boerum Hill there had been an unexplained series of push-in robberies, rapes, and murders. The perpetrator particularly liked to shoot people in the head. One of his victims, Sylvia Lugo, was shot in just that way, before he raped her roommate and lover, who had just witnessed the

---

*Originally presented as a paper, "Extreme Trauma: Victims of Shootings Helped by Biofeedback/Neurofeedback," at the the Association for Applied Psychophysiology and Biofeedback national meeting, Colorado Springs, April 2004. The patient herself agreed to appear at the meeting to tell her story of tragedy and recovery, and to meet another young woman, Julie, also the victim of a shooting, whose case had first been presented by Lynda Kirk at the 2002 Association for Applied Psychophysiology and Biofeedback annual meeting in Las Vegas, Nevada. Both women shared their stories with each other, the conference participants, and—through interviews done by NBC TV—with television audiences.

shooting, right next to Sylvia's still-warm body. The two were lesbians, and after this and other horrible crimes, the gay and lesbian community of Brooklyn had gotten up in arms, claiming that these were hate crimes against gays, and that the police were doing nothing because they had disdain for the victims.

But they were wrong. The man who was finally apprehended had no particular rancor against gays. His misanthropy/misogyny was far more widespread. The perpetrator, whom the press identified as a young Hispanic man, Alex Villenueva, would as soon have "offed" a straight person as a gay person if the impulse had struck him. He had, in fact— though coming from a Roman Catholic background—recently killed a much-loved neighborhood priest, and stolen the church's collection box, along with everything else of value he could find.

Late on the night of March 29, 1996, he and a younger companion saw vivacious, cheerful Ginny, a young teacher in training, carefully park her car on a Brooklyn street. She was thrilled to find the parking spot, because that "darned alternate side of the street parking" was in effect, and she had been driving around for quite a while, listening to an inspirational tape on how to have courage. And then there was suddenly a spot in front of her apartment.

"Oh, boy, am I lucky," she remembers saying to herself. As she locked her car, she saw the two young Hispanics with an odd "vibe" coming down the street. Ginny instinctively started to walk the other way but then remembered that she was "courageous," just like the tape had been encouraging her to be. She headed straight for her apartment. The rest of the events are a blur to her, but there were other people on the street, some of whom witnessed what followed. Villenueva walked up to Ginny.[1] Suddenly and viciously, he clobbered Ginny on the temple with his gun. She fell to the ground. But then she jumped up and shouted at her assailant: "What'd you do that for?"

Villenueva, not used to such impertinence, stuck his pistol in Ginny's right eye and pulled the trigger. Now she was good and mad: injury added to insult! She continued yelling loudly and indignantly at her mugger—whose eyes were wide with disbelief that his two lethal attacks not only had failed but had earned him a good scolding. She even used many foul words! Lights came on and windows flew open. People started screaming, and the two young men bolted while onlookers gathered in shock and disbelief. Soon an ambulance arrived on the scene and rushed the still indignant, but by then slightly delirious, Ginny to St. Vincent's Hospital in Manhattan, where she remained conscious long enough to describe the events to the astonished emergency room doctors. Then she lapsed into a coma and was listed in critical condition. Ginny was given a very small chance of coming out of the coma, or even surviving. The situation was almost intolerable to her parents, who some eleven years before had lost Ginny's fifteen-year-old brother to AIDS. (He was hemophiliac and had been given contaminated blood.)

The following is quoted verbatim from the June 5, 1996 report on the injury prepared by the Center for Head Injuries, the JFK-Johnson Rehabilitation Institute, in Edison, New Jersey. It is presented, not to horrify the reader, but to detail the extent of the injury Ginny suffered.

> Prior medical history is unremarkable. . . . Ms. K. suffered a traumatic brain injury secondary to a gunshot wound to the head. The entry of the bullet was through the right superior lid just below the supraorbital margin. The casing of the bullet was lying in the frontal sinus. The anterior and posterior walls of the frontal sinus were shattered. The anterior part of the superior sagittal sinus and falx was lacerated and separated. There was extensive subarachnoid hemorrhage, multiple contusions, lacerations, hematomas and torn bridging veins in the frontal poles bilaterally. The damage was particularly severe on the orbital surface of the bilateral frontal lobes. Both olfactory tracts were totally destroyed and there was subarachnoid hemorrhage in the cistern around the optic chiasm. On 4/4/96 Ms. K. underwent a bifrontal craniotomy with a bilateral partial frontal lobectomy, debridement, excision of bone and bullet fragments and skull base reconstruction. Once stabilized she was transferred to the Brain Trauma Unit at the JFK medical Center which she entered on 5/9/96. CT's of the head completed on 5/11/96 revealed post traumatic and post operative changes involving bilateral frontal lobes with left frontal lobe contusion and bullet fragments in the left frontal lobe.

Amazingly, Ginny came out of her coma in a couple of weeks. Through some miracle not completely understood, her right eye remained intact, the bullet having just grazed past the eyeball on its way to doing the damage described above. Many pieces of the bullet still remain in her brain (so she is not a good candidate for an MRI in which powerful magnets pull on any metal fragments in their field). (See LENS map on page 315.)

By June, two months after the shooting, Ginny had recovered enough to be transferred to the Transitional Living/Cognitive Rehabilitation Program. She spent nine weeks receiving physical, speech, memory, social, and cognitive therapy. But then life at the program began to wear on her, and Ginny asked to be released to the care of her parents.

Ginny had truly passed through the "valley of the shadow of death," but at last she was home. Her parents hovered around her anxiously. Months passed as she convalesced. All she remembers is that this time was very difficult. Her father enthusiastically told her, "They say you'll have a complete recovery now!"

"No, I won't," said the still-pragmatic Ginny, "I will be living with a brain injury. You're never quite the same, and you have to adapt to that reality." (People with very serious head injuries are often astonishingly insightful, as well as candid and accurate about their degree of impairment.)

There is a famous case—read by most Psychology 101 students—of a man named Phineas Gage, a nineteenth-century worker who somehow survived a metal dynamite tamping rod being blown through the front of his skull (he tamped a little too hard). Previously a polite and well-spoken man, he became profane, coarse, and careless of the feelings of others. Even though, like Gage, Ginny was damaged in her frontal lobes, she had regained her conscience and empathic ability. However, she did acquire an irritability that at times became explosive. In the classroom she had previously had a special way with difficult, but very bright students. She had, in fact, demonstrated a high tolerance for these quirky kids. Now she found herself feeling highly sensitive to criticism and hypercritical as a result.

At home she was often argumentative, as her mother attested. Ginny also reported something else frequently experienced by persons with Traumatic Brain Injuries (TBI): sensitivity to light. She saw haloes around lights—particularly halogens—and most light caused her discomfort. This symptom was so extreme that she found it impossible to use yellow highlighters to underline sentences in textbooks. Dilantin began to damage her liver and she was allergic to Tegretol. She said Depakote worked better.

Meanwhile, some very interesting things had been going on in Brooklyn. Ginny's cousin, a police detective, was outraged by what had happened. He put out the word that he *wanted* those guys, and some of the city's best detectives were assigned to the search. These sleuths knew the way their quarry habitually behaved. Eyes and ears waited for the inevitable bragging—and it happened. The young Hispanic men who had been involved in most of the incidents were arrested. Once in custody the young men were, at first, full of denial. But then more and more crimes seemed to be connected to Villenueva.

The police came to Ginny and asked if she would testify, letting her know that her testimony would be the key piece that could put these murderers away, even though—as friends and relatives warned—it is dangerous to testify in a murder trial! Ginny said she didn't remember much, but yes, if it would help to put away a potentially dangerous person, she *would* testify. That was all the detectives needed. They went to Villenueva's companion and told him that Ginny remembered the whole incident, and would testify. They also said that if he would tell the truth about the guy who pulled the trigger, he would get a lighter sentence. He spilled, and the Park Slope murderer was brought down by a woman who wouldn't die.

By the year 2000, four years had passed since the incident, but many of Ginny's symptoms were not going away. Strangely, the migraine headaches, which had afflicted Ginny *before* the incident, had disappeared for a while. In 2000, however, they returned as painful tension headaches, which were almost continuous. As her doctors upped her doses of medication, including pain medications, antidepressants, and anticonvulsants, Ginny suffered insomnia at night and sleepiness during the day, leaving her feeling "drugged" and dysfunctional while at work.

Furthermore, she was still seriously depressed, medication or not. Her self-esteem had plummeted after the accident. Following her outbursts, especially if they were at the children she was teaching, she would become, as she said, very "upset at myself" for having "lost it" in this horrible way, saying that the children "didn't deserve it!"

SELF-ESTEEM IN THE TRAUMATICALLY BRAIN-INJURED

A problem with self-esteem frequently arises with TBI, along with other major CNS irregularities. It is not only that in PTSD psychology, victims frequently blame themselves—they often do—but a person's own self-image is formed in a kind of virtual "feedback loop" of how they find themselves behaving. If they behave badly—explosive, oppositional, moody—their self-image suffers. It is therefore especially important to help young people with learning disabilities, explosiveness, oppositionality, or impulsiveness, who feel terrible about themselves because of their disorder, to realize that these disturbances are less in their control than they believe them to be.

Neurofeedback treatment helps to restore their sense of control, because they participate in "fixing" themselves, even if they have no idea how it works. When their extreme emotional reactions have stabilized (with the neurofeedback), then their positive self-image is likely to be restored. Psychotherapy and counseling can be used to help children or adults through this process. If they are already in psychotherapy, neurofeedback can breathe energy into the process.

Ginny tried to return to graduate school but felt mentally cloudy all the time. She could not bring herself to complete one particularly important group of reports, on which her grade depended. The task felt insuperable to her. She was ready to give up on everything. But somehow she found her way to Dr. Richard Brown on the teaching staff of Columbia-Presbyterian Medical School. One of the top psychopharmacologists in the country, Dr. Brown manages cases given up on by most other doctors.

In addition to the Depakote, Dr. Brown suggested small amounts of a stimulant. He then used small amounts of a stimulant, Adderall, combined with Rosavin (Siberian Rodea Roseola), and Idebenone, a Japanese equivalent of CoQ10 (nutraceuticals) to improve her energy and clarity by stimulating her dopamine and cholinergic pathways. This regimen began to help Ginny almost immediately. She finished her paper, and the course, in pretty good style. Still, all medications seemed to exacerbate Ginny's growing gastrointestinal problems, so he referred her to us.

As we initially mapped Ginny's brain, we expected to see high, spiky waves as a result of the trauma she had undergone, but the medication was masking the underlying post-traumatic instability. Naturally, her highest amplitudes were in the frontal lobe area where the bullet had entered, fragments still resided, and the partial frontal lobectomy had been done. As we moved the sensor from site to site to make our topographic map (using the lo-stim setting at which no deliberate stimulation is sent but the energy of the reading itself has a mild effect), Ginny "felt things," notably an annoying twitch on her right side, and other twinges and localized aches. However, these disappeared within a few minutes of the reading, just as responses in sensitive patients do after an actual brief stimulation.

For her protocol, we limited ourselves to treating no more than three sites per session, one second each, on the lowest intensity. Together with Ginny, we chose to track five clinical dimensions or symptom areas where she felt the most stress. These were: sleep disturbance and headache, both of which she ranked a "10" (the worst); mood instability, a "7"; ADD/distractibility, a "6"; and energy level or fatigue, a "5." Later, after she began to improve, Ginny came to the sudden insight that she had initially been far "worse off" than she had thought, and that very high or "bad" ranks would have been appropriate for all of the areas. (This is very common among brain-injured people, especially regarding the cognitive dimensions; as they begin to get better, they become clear enough to realize just how bereft they have been.)

Client ID: Ginny					
Prominent Symptoms		Begin Date	2	3	4
	Session dates:	10/9/2001	10/18/2001	10/26/2001	10/31/2001
1	Sleep Dis	10.0	8.0	7.0	6.0
2	Headaches	10.0	6.0	5.0	0.0
3	Mood	7.0	7.0	3.0	4.0
4	ADD	6.0	6.0	8.0	8.0
5	Energy Level	5.0	5.0	4.0	4.0
6					
7					
8					
9		7.6	6.4	5.4	4.4

Fig. 1.2. Ginny's subjective symptom rating chart showing her progress (generally declining scores) over her first four sessions. (See color insert page 3 for Excel graph based on subjective symptom rating scale [SSRS].)

Over a couple of months of regular neurofeedback, Ginny began to revert to some version of her preshooting self. She reported that she was sleeping better, often getting through the night without awakening. Her mood stabilized, and she reported that she was more able to handle the ups and downs of the classroom environment. On week four, her headaches, which had shown a slow decrease over the preceding period, suddenly dropped to "0": she had no headaches at all! Ginny was ecstatic.

When patients are not forthcoming about their own responses to treatment, or when the patient is a child or a teenager, it is very helpful to have a family member weigh in with a "second opinion." When we asked Ginny's mother to share with us her assessment of how Ginny was doing, she was very forthcoming—after all, it was she who lived with her daughter and drove her the seventy-five miles each way every week to her LENS appointments! She said that Ginny was definitely becoming "easier to live with," exhibiting fewer instances of "picking fights," fewer explosions (which may actually have been subclinical seizures).

During the Christmas and New Year's season Ginny missed three weeks of treatments and regressed a little, but once she resumed regular sessions she got back on course fairly quickly, a pattern we have often observed: If treatment is stopped when healing is incomplete, there is a tendency to regress, but seemingly never to the worst levels of previous dysfunction. When treatment is resumed, progress is readily made. As time went on, Ginny's general vitality began to improve; she appeared more energetic and buoyant. Her droll sense of humor started to re-emerge, fostering her return to the more jolly, less testy creature she once had been.

It was around this time that we suggested Ginny begin HeartMath training, one of the best-documented biofeedback modalities, to boost her emotional self-management and cognitive clarity still further. She showed a very ready aptitude for this method, which is based on learning to control one's own heart-rate variability. (More is explained about HeartMath, and how Ginny mastered it, in chapter 12. See figure 12.1a and 12.1b)

Dr. Rollin McCraty, one of the main research scientists at the HeartMath Institute, has said that HeartMath training is the ideal precursor to neurofeedback, because it has a calming and stabilizing effect on the nervous system, thus enabling the patient's subsequent EEG training. In this case, the inverse was true. The LENS training helped Ginny become calm and stable enough neurologically to derive a lot of benefit from the HeartMath training.

Within a few weeks, Ginny was hitting ninety percent entrainment (a beautiful smooth sine wave that shows that the sympathetic and parasympathetic branches of the autonomic nervous system are entrained). She reported feelings of calmness and well-being following the sessions. In between sessions she described herself as having better emotional balance in the hectic school environment in which she worked.

Learning from Ginny

Being shot by another human being is an intimate kind of trauma; in addition to the obvious damage, it is usually an intentional act, in which a deadly weapon is pointed at the victim and discharged. Such an act naturally gives rise to questions such as: "What did I do to deserve this? How can human beings *do* this to each other? Why aren't there more protective laws?" In such instances psychological, emotional, and physical traumas seem to be intertwined inextricably. Biofeedback and neurofeedback are gentle, noninvasive treatments of choice for victims of these three kinds of violence, as they allow the person to participate in the healing process, and to pace their rate of treatment and recovery.

With brain damage of the severity that Ginny suffered, it is natural to wonder why she responded so significantly and so rapidly. One factor was her age: she was only thirty-two years old at the start of treatment, so she was both young and resilient, which—along with her previous high level of functioning—helps to explain her remarkable improvement. She also had a concerned and skilled neurosurgeon, who took a personal interest in her. She went to some of the best head-injury centers and rehabilitation programs in the country. She had a supportive family and home environment. She went to a wise physician who titrated her medications down, and listened carefully to how she was responding. In addition, she had an innately wonderful, generous, and jolly spirit, and a real love for her work.

People have said to her, "Don't you want to start carrying a gun?" "Don't you just hate that guy rotting away in jail?" "Aren't you angry?"

"No," Ginny responds. "I don't want a gun and I don't want to make myself angry and stay angry. What's the point in hating people? In fact, you know, I think that's the way you could guarantee you'll never get over it, never really recover. There's so much to do in life, and I want to do lots of good things. I think you have to heal from within!"

Ginny's story is an inspiring modern hero journey wherein she experienced a sudden, unexpected departure from the familiar world, a journey to the dark underworld, and a successful return. Her case not only proves that the gentle biofeedback principle can work, even in extreme cases; it is also a demonstration of the remarkable ability of the human body and nervous system to heal itself. Above all, it is about the resilience of the human spirit, and a testimony to Ginny's courageous self!

In the pages to come, we will share many more stories with you about the dramatic changes brought about in our patients' lives by the gentle practice of neurofeedback. But first let's take a brief look in the next two chapters at the history of its development and in chapter 3 the "wizard" responsible for its formulation as LENS: Dr. Len Ochs.

2

A Brief History of EEG Neurofeedback

Stephen Larsen, Ph.D.

The ultimate biofeedback may well be brain wave biofeedback. Certainly, the brain electrical activity of human beings is the greatest potential resource for understanding the dynamics of all human behavior. . . . Human beings can learn control over a wide variety of extraordinarily complex brain functions. With brain as the substrate of the mind, the potential of biofeedback techniques for regulation and modification of mind and consciousness looms enormous.

BARBARA BROWN, AUTHOR OF *STRESS AND THE ART OF BIOFEEDBACK*

The Roots and Dendrites of "Brain Waves"

The earliest mention I have been able to find regarding the existence of "brain waves" is in the remarkably advanced eighteenth-century writings of Emanuel Swedenborg. Swedenborg was a Swedish nobleman who spent the first half of his life on scientific research and publications related to the sciences of his time: chemistry, mineralogy, geology, astronomy. As he got older, Swedenborg became more interested in physiology, including brain physiology, and psychology. By the age of fifty-five, Swedenborg had a series of visionary experiences that opened inner senses, which he felt were "spiritual" in nature. But Swedenborg's later spiritual perceptions also seem to include insights cultivated in his earlier scientific studies. In effect he hoped to learn about the body from the spirit and the spirit from the body.

Whatever the source—anatomical studies or direct visionary experience—Swedenborg was the first person to postulate the existence of neurons (he called them *cerebellula*, "little brains," which make the microscopic decisions that add up to the overall functioning of the whole brain). He was also the first to recognize the importance of the cerebral cortex in cognition (in his time the "grey matter" of the cerebral cortex was described merely as a gland that nourished the real brain, the "white matter" or nerve cells under the cortex).

Swedenborg averred that the frontal lobes of the cerebral cortex were the seat of the highest mental activity and cognition. He noticed that the left and right hemispheres had different cognitions that were related to thinking (the left) and feeling (the right). Perhaps most amazingly,

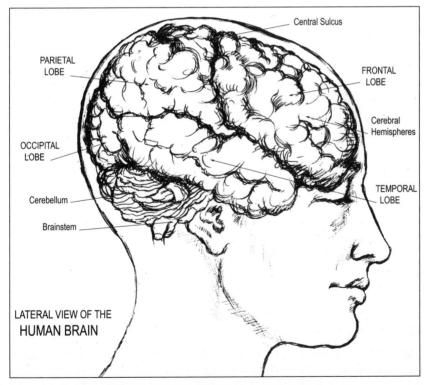

Fig. 2.1. The right hemisphere of the cerebral cortex (the outer layer of the cerebrum, which handles many higher intellectual functions). Each hemisphere is made up of four lobes, which coordinate areas of functioning.

given the state of anatomical knowledge at the time, Swedenborg said that he noticed, from firsthand experience, that the brain propagated its impulses by wave forms or "tremulations," and that the rhythms of the brain were synchronized with those of the heart and those of respiration, relationships that have been validated by modern research.[1]

Luigi Galvani has generally been recognized as the first scientist to announce the specifically *electrical* nature of the nervous system, based on his measurements of the electroconductivity of the leg nerves of frogs in 1791. During the nineteenth century would-be researchers exploring skin conductivity, or the presence of nerves, used "galvanometers" named after Galvani. By the 1870s and '80s Dr. Richard Caton was using a "reflecting galvanometer" to demonstrate the presence of electricity in the exposed brains of cats and monkeys, which he stimulated. He also used an oxy-hydrogen lamp to project the resulting images of an activated animal brain on theater walls for the public. Caton probably did the first scientifically documented piece of electroencephalography.[2]

Most histories of biofeedback fail to mention an early twentieth century explorer who studied the nervous system and paved the way for modern biofeedback: Carl Jung. Often described as "Freud's runaway psychoanalyst who became a mystic," Jung actually gave the first scientific, physiologically based evidence of the existence of Freud's "unconscious." Using a stopwatch and skin galvanometer or GSR, Jung measured subjects' responses to emotionally loaded stimulus words in his "word-association experiments." Words with a high emotional charge affected the autonomic nervous system (not available to conscious control, hence "unconscious"), demonstrated by changes in the person's skin conductivity, as well as by delayed cognitive responses.[3] This is the principle at the heart of the modern *polygraph* or "lie-detector." The involuntary nervous system "betrays" what the conscious mind, the cortex, refuses to reveal.

The regular measurement and recording of brain waves, as well as their naming, did not occur until 1924 and is credited to German physician Hans Berger. Berger called the first rhythm that he was able to record with his primitive string galvanometer "alpha," after the first letter in the Greek alphabet. This range of brain wave frequencies (8–12 Hz), now so familiar to EEG specialists, dominates many people's mental activity, particularly when they are cognitively "idling" or have their eyes closed. He called the next range to be discovered (12 Hz and greater) "beta."

Two other ranges were later identified: "delta" (0–4 Hz), associated with trauma, deep sleep, or coma; and "theta" (4–8 Hz), usually signaling profound reverie, emotional recall, or hypnotic trance.[4]

(Although typically theta is considered a state of underarousal, when in high amplitude, it is also associated with seizure activity.)

In the beginning, doctors used the EEG measurement of brain waves only for the most basic kinds of clinical purposes: to establish brain death (by their absence) or epilepsy (during which the waves went "tidal," with huge spikes). Berger died in 1941, disappointed that the medical world had been so slow to make use of his astonishing discovery. (His unfulfilled hope began to come true only in the decade after his death and is still unfolding, as we learn increasingly more interesting neurofeedback technologies based on brain waves.)

Surfing the Waves

During World War II, pioneer W. Grey Walter was exploring devices for measuring brain waves in all frequency ranges (1943).[5] These were the first precursors of modern electroencephalograph machines, with filters (known as band pass filters) that could separate out the different brain wave ranges from the raw EEG. Then, in 1949, Gibbs and Knott studied the growth and development of EEG through the life cycle and showed that the brain waves of children, functional adults, and the elderly differed profoundly.[6]

By the 1960s researchers had begun to focus on something that now most neurofeedback practitioners—and probably most intelligent laypersons—take for granted: namely the fact that *brain waves* can be shown to *correlate with states of consciousness*. Most conventional neuroscientists of that time—and some still to this day—were skeptical of anything involving "consciousness," regarding it as a mere "epiphenomenon" of brain physiology.

The continuing reluctance of some neuroscientists to grasp the obvious fact of the correlation between consciousness and brain waves is a remarkable sign of how entrenched "parallelism"—the post-Enlightenment approach that says subjective consciousness must always be held apart from its physical or neurological correlates—still is. For materialistic science, the EEG patterns that Berger worked so hard to elucidate were relegated to being seen as a function of brain oxygen and carbon dioxide levels, glucose metabolism, or blood flow (with all of which they may be correlated), without any causal or explanatory mechanism being established. [7]

Then in the late 1960s Basmajian's remarkable premonitory work with muscle cells showed that people could learn to control units as small as a neuron, without knowing how they did it.[8] "Such learning," wrote Barbara Brown in her comprehensive 1977 book *Stress and the Art of Biofeedback,* "is truly amazing, since it has been amply demonstrated that the learning involves selective (but unconscious) manipulation of motoneurons (cells) in the spinal cord."[9] Suddenly, the word "will" was back in psychology for the first time since William James, having seemingly been banished by behaviorism since the early twentieth century. Biofeedback was exciting to many people because it moved the opposites of "consciousness" and "behavior" one step closer, by showing that "covert" as well as "overt" "behavior" could be measured, and thus were equally "real."

It would be hard to overstress the importance of Karl Pribram's groundbreaking work in helping to eliminate the literalistic neurology that lingered until the 1960s. This old-time fallacy implied that there *must* be some sort of *isomorphic* relationship between brain and behavior, that specific neurons could be found to account for each feature of psychology and behavior.

Pribram's article in *Scientific American* of 1969 shattered that model with the concept of the "holographic brain," his own development of his mentor Karl Lashley's observation that when sections of the brain are damaged, the person may lose precision or quickness of memory, but does not lose specific memories. Storage of memory was not restricted to definite locales but distributed *holographically* throughout the brain. (The analogy to the hologram is based on the fact that each piece of a hologram contains information about the whole picture.)[10] This work encouraged neurofeedback researchers to study brain waves, that is, the patterns of energy that sweep through the brain, rather than the specifics of neuroanatomy.

Joe Kamiya's pioneering studies, stretching as far back as the 1960s, had already shown that experimental subjects could subjectively identify brain wave states. Could they then, perhaps, bring them up at will or learn to prolong them, thus altering the way their nervous systems functioned? Barbara Brown replicated some of Kamiya's findings and came up with elegant new research designs that showed that subjects could learn to tell what brain wave "state" (alpha, theta, or beta) they were in when a light of a certain color was presented at the same time their EEG was being monitored remotely.[11] Subjects also were able to "control" the states at statistically significant levels. The science of "the voluntary control of internal states" (in the words of pioneer biofeedback researcher Elmer Green) was born.

Kasamatsu and Hirai recorded noticeable EEG differences between beginning versus experienced Zen Buddhist meditators, as well as differences in "habituation" (ignoring a repeated stimulus) between Zen and Yoga meditators. In one of their studies, "blinded" EEG specialists were simply handed the charts and asked to rate the waveforms of meditators on symmetry and amplitude. Their ratings were then compared to the meditation master's evaluation of the student's depth of meditation, from least to most advanced. The two ratings were found to be highly correlated.[12]

It was not long before the clinical implications of some of these findings were explored and found useful. Different practitioners began to select one or another frequency as desirable, and to be encouraged through reward-based training. Some encouraged alpha, others beta or theta, and still others a combination such as alpha and theta or beta and theta. In all cases the mechanism to achieve this was similar: different colored lights were used to inform the patient about the type of brain waves they were producing.

The early "alpha-enthusiasm" began when it was found that an abundance of brain waves at this particular rhythm (usually thought of as 8–12 Hz), more generally found in the occipital and parietal regions, was equated with a subjective state of well-being. Alpha could thus be used to help people with anxiety, which often manifested in the beta range of 15 Hz and up. An abundance of alpha also showed up in the EEGs of people lightly intoxicated on alcohol (one to two drinks) or experiencing the "highs" of marijuana and the opiates. However, a heavier dose of alcohol or opiates produced theta (4–8 Hz) or—if well beyond the legal limits of intoxication—delta (close to passing out or completely unconscious).[13]

TYPES OF BRAIN WAVES

Common interpretation is offered first, uncommon or paradoxical aspects in parentheses, because all interpretations of brain waves need to include location, specific frequency and amplitude, coherence (whether there are a lot of the same type of wave in one area), synchrony, and even the shape of the waves themselves. Being locked into any one wave state in a large area of the brain probably represents an anomaly, whereas a mixture of all of them in moderate to low amplitudes, and in a flexible, constantly altering relationship, is found in "healthy normalcy. (See color insert page 3.)

0–4 Hz Delta: Sleep, coma, sign of injury or trauma, depression (but also very deep types of meditation, Cosmic Unity or "Oceanic" transpersonal experiences, some kinds of ESP).

4–8 Hz Theta: EEG slowing, ADD, ADHD, psychosis, seizure activity when in high amplitudes (but also creative reverie, trance, "gateway to the unconscious," spiritual or religious experience, important kinds of memory storage).

8–12 Hz Alpha: Mental idling and well-being (but also mental rumination, obsession, anxiety, and pain). There is also a strange nonalpha that registers in this range called "mu."

12–15 Hz SMR (sensory-motor rhythm): "High-functioning Alpha," alert stillness, an antiseizure, antihyperactive frequency (per Sterman and Lubar), (but also restless rumination, aspects of insomnia, anxiety).

15–22 Hz Mid-Beta: Active sensory focus, mental activity, problem-solving, alertness (but also insomnia, rumination, high-anxiety, panic, phobia).

22–28 Hz Hi-Beta: Hypervigilance, high-anxiety, anger, rage, prodromal seizure activity (but also some high levels of creativity, genius, multitasking, problem solving). Muscle artifacts often show up here.

28–70 Hz and up Gamma: An area whose exploration is a "work in progress." Associated with the "binding rhythm" that integrates all cortical activity (but also exceptional mental states, genius, "enlightenment").

Then along came Elmer and Alyce Green's intriguing work at the Menninger Foundation during the 1960s on alpha, theta, and altered states of consciousness. The Greens found that when they taught subjects how to stay in theta, the perpetuation of theta brain waves would often precipitate the recovery of memories from childhood, or deep spiritual or creative experiences. Some of the experiences recovered were profound enough to be life altering, and Elmer Green went on to devise the ambitious term, "programming the unconscious."[14]

The Green's work was later carried on by their daughters, Patricia and Judy. One of their daughters, Patricia Norris, and her partner, Steven Fahrion, did research in theta training, finding that training in this range not only facilitates the recovery of buried childhood memories and creative and spiritual experiences but also improves the functioning of the immune system and may aid such paranormal abilities as clairvoyance and telepathy.[15]

Thomas Budzynski, a graduate psychology student during the 1960s, had studied the "Systematic Desensitization" technique of Dr. Joseph Wolpe, a technique used to "de-condition" (or "extinguish" in the parlance of behavior modification) anxiety and phobia problems. The technique was somewhat effective and was very popular in that era. It was used as an alternative to the "psychodynamic" approaches of Freud and his colleagues, which looked for buried traumas and sexual conflicts primarily through dreams and "free associations" on the couch. In this new method, no analysis was needed; a new behavior was simply substituted or "conditioned" in exchange for the dysfunctional old one.

However, Budzynski felt that the technique had a weakness, and that was its failure to enable a person to "transfer" the learned relaxation response from a clinical to a real life situation. He reasoned that if he could find a way to encourage the person's alpha brain waves, known to be relaxing, along with the desensitization process, the effect would transfer better. With a friend, John Picchiottino, an aerospace engineer, he developed an "alpha" training machine to use as a clinical tool.

Budzynski's first case was an ambitious undertaking: A man with an inordinate *thanatophobia*, a fear of death. (You might say "We all have that!" but in this case it kept Ken, the patient, out of his own basement and from being able to drive home after dark.) In the very first session in which alpha training was combined with "desensitization," Ken was able to remember an incident when he and his younger brother (who also had *thanatophobia*) were required to kiss the corpse of a dead grandmother. More sessions were done, and Ken was freed of his phobia. [16]

This interesting cure was a mixture of biofeedback and psychotherapy, a topic we return to in an intriguing chapter (Chapter 13) that explores emerging possibilities.[17] Despite all of this groundbreaking exploratory work, however, Budzynski found that his psychology department at the University of Colorado Medical School "was not impressed. Instead . . . they suggested that we stop trying to relax people by feeding-back brain waves, and simply feed-back muscle tension instead."[18] Budzynski, in fact, spent the next several years doing that and developed impressive EMG desensitization procedures as a result.

Eventually, though, Budzynski returned to his first love: neurofeedback guided by EEG. The Greens had shown that theta training "made the unconscious available" and had asserted it could be programmed; Budzynski wondered if theta training could be used to counteract the interference of the conscious mind, or "ego" as it is sometimes called, with the positive suggestions or "new program" that a therapist was hoping to insert in a patient's unconscious mind. Often, when they were asked to repeat a positive affirmation to themselves, many people also heard a critical inner voice that would deny its validity.

Budzynski learned of the research being done by Foulkes and Vogel "out on the windy plains of Wyoming." They were studying the cognition of individuals as they fell asleep, and it had become "apparent to these investigators that in the context of the Freudian model the individual's defense mechanisms that guard the gate of consciousness were decreased as he passed into sleep."[19] Budzynski related that "One day it occurred to me that we could use the finding that a drowsy state characterized by theta EEG would be one of uncritical acceptance and if the affirmation was presented then, the little negative voice wouldn't get in the way."[20]

Despite beliefs that became popular in the 1960s, people do not learn while they are asleep, but while they are in the "twilight" or "hypnagogic" state that leads to sleep. That is the time for minidreams, little visions, auditory hallucinations, and spiritual insights. Budzynski felt that this state not only would facilitate recovery of childhood memories "too awful to remember" in ordinary states but also would offer a "window" through which to embed positive therapeutic suggestions.

Thus, by the mid-1970s two major uses had been discovered for neurofeedback's special access to the part of brain functioning that was roughly equivalent to Freud's "unconscious." One was simply to gain *access* to the mysterious zone that generated dreams and fantasies, creativity and inspiration; the other was to program and embed suggestions to remediate "bad programs" in the unconscious, whether they were self-defeating neuroses from childhood or simply self-limiting beliefs. Neurofeedback offered a way to gain access to some of the same zones sought by psychoanalysis and hypnosis, in a way more precise than either, because of its utilization of the brain's own signaling system (its own frequencies).

The Garden of Forking Paths: Two Tracks in the Development of Neurofeedback

But another approach was developing in neurofeedback, the result of examining a different set of problems and ways of remediating them. Instead of focusing on production of brain waves in the lower ranges and the "encounter with the unconscious," this other method worked with the brain waves in the higher ranges that characterize mental alertness and problem solving.

This part of the story also began in the sixties, when the United States space program was in overdrive to compete with the Soviets. High-powered rocket fuels containing *monomethylhydrazine* were giving workers and astronauts seizures and hallucinations. (NASA had grown quite concerned when astronauts reported seeing natives on South Sea islands waving at them as they drifted soundlessly overhead!) Antiseizure medications were tried, but these made the astronauts woozy; and being "drugged," quite simply, is no way to pilot a spacecraft.

Dr. Maurice "Barry" Sterman—a UCLA neuropsychologist who had done impeccable research on brain rhythms in cats and rhesus monkeys—was approached by the chemical firm who made monomethylhydrazine to see if he could offer some insight into the problem. By a fortunate coincidence, some of the cats that Sterman had used in his brain wave research he had operantly conditioned to produce the SMR rhythm. The SMR rhythm is a frequency of 12–15 Hz, located between alpha (8–12 Hz) and mid-beta (15–22 Hz) as per the preceeding chart on page 50 of this chapter. These conditioned cats proved to be seizure-resistant and slept well when exposed to the seizure-inducing toxin, whereas cats who hadn't been trained were vomiting and having *grand mal* seizures. Nor were they sleeping well. This chain of coincidences was to lead to one of the most important early breakthroughs in neurofeedback in that it was discovered that brain wave frequencies of between 12–15 Hz could be used to counteract and neutralize seizure activity.

I will never forget my first glimpse of Sterman's research in a BBC film made in the 1970s called *Mind over Matter*. It explores the fledgling but promising field, as the BBC presented it, of *biofeedback*. All the "greats" who were then involved in developing the field are represented in the film: Thom Budzynski and his EMG work with anxiety disorders and "twilight learning"; Joe Kamiya speaking on the remarkable ability of many subjects to "recognize" what brain wave they were manufacturing; Herbert Benson speaking on stress and blood pressure; and Professor Les Fehmi making a brilliant statement on the consciousness-enhancing potentials of biofeedback. (See color insert page 7 for pictures of pioneers.)

The conclusion of this significant film on biofeedback history involves an interview with Dr. Sterman, in which he introduces a seven-year-old boy named "Kevin," along with Kevin's mother, who explains that for many years Kevin had been in the very worst category of seizure-proneness. (Sometimes he was having as many as seven or eight seizures an hour!) Kevin, cute as a button, is invited by Dr. Sterman to play an "airplane game" in which the flight of an airplane is simulated by moving lights on a console (in what now seems a relatively primitive, precomputer-screen EEG display), activated by brain waves at the SMR frequency. As the procedure goes on, Kevin is able to make the airplane "fly" and a bell rings for a reward to show a certain level of achievement, in a very simple operant paradigm.

Kevin grows visibly more quiet over the course of the session, not surprisingly, since SMR rhythm is associated with muscular and kinetic "quietness." He exhibits a kind of rapt attention, much like one of Sterman's cats crouching at a mouse hole, motionless, ready to pounce.

Sterman shows a wonderful warmth and rapport with the boy, but there is clearly more than the placebo effect going on. Later the boy's mother is interviewed. The stress of years of coping with her son's illness is evident on her face, but she is thrilled with what Sterman has accomplished so far. And she is clearly convinced the treatment has "worked," and is continuing to work.

One truly astonishing thing about Sterman's robust findings is the failure of the medical and neurological community to take advantage of them.

To this day, doctors called upon to treat children and adults with seizure disorders just write "a scrip" or go to their sample drawer of antiseizure medications: Tegretol, Depacote, Keppra, and many others. (At least many of these anticonvulsants are cleaner and have less side effects than Dilantin or the even worse Phenobarbitol and other barbiturates that used to be prescribed.)

Most theorists have regarded cortical recruitment; that is, the activation of neurons by other neurons, as the "cause" of seizures, which led to recommendations for surgery, including temporal lobectomies, or "split brains," in serious cases. Sadly, despite the significant negative side effects of medication and operations, the far gentler, subtler, neurofeedback option is almost never suggested, except by doctors educated in complementary and alternative medicine.

Dr. Joel Lubar, who worked with Sterman early in his neurofeedback career, did further studies on seizure disorders, as well as adapting

---

SPLIT BRAIN REPERCUSSIONS

The so-called "split brain" operation was developed approximately fifty years ago, when psychosurgery was more popular. It was a crude way of halting the spread—from one hemisphere of the cortex to the other—of the massive recruitment of neurons that takes place in a seizure. It was effected by severing the corpus callosum, the bundle of nerve fibers that connects the two hemispheres. The operation was basically supported by neuropsychologists, who claimed that the patients who had undergone the procedure experienced very little alteration in cognitive abilities, except for the inability to solve certain puzzles involving spatial relations. In reality, though, think of what it would be like to be unable to think while you felt and imagined, or unable to feel and imagine while you thought. Much affectively-toned cognition is accessible only when the two hemispheres operate reciprocally, in a "stereo" mode that brings out the depth of field in our cognitive/emotional worlds.

the use of the SMR protocol for ADHD children. He felt there were analogies between the theta waves that were typically predominant in children with ADHD and the massive theta waves visible in readings of children suffering from seizure disorders.[21] In his work, Lubar proceeded to focus on the relationship between beta and theta brain waves in children with ADD and ADHD. He discovered that at one particular site, CZ (the "vertex" or crown of the head), a particular ratio of beta to theta was a clear indicator of ADD and ADHD.[22]

He reasoned that if neurofeedback could help the ADHD or ADD children to increase their beta waves and lower their theta, then they could improve their mental focus and powers of concentration to make global improvements in learning and development.[23] Lubar went on to refine and develop this training into a complete protocol for ADD and ADHD, with very robust and replicable results. (Recently Lubar worked with the application of this protocol in the public school system in Yonkers, New York, along with Mary Jo Sabo, Jim Giorgi, and Linda Vergara.)

Another student who worked with Sterman was Margaret Ayers who, in 1976, would go on to found the first clinic specializing in EEG biofeedback in this country. Ayers would develop her own protocols, with specialized EEG processors she had designed, with a very small delay between the brain event and the feedback stimulus. She developed a reputation as a "miracle worker" for patients with TBI or "closed head injury." She was also one of the first people to initially treat sites all over the brain, as well as perform neurofeedback on animals (see chapter 14).

Based on an early study of some 250 patients who had a variety of diagnoses, (and using her specialized equipment and protocols), the following results that her patients displayed were reported—clearly benefiting their lives:

1. An increase in energy and a decrease in depression and temper outbursts in the first six sessions.
2. A decrease in light/sound hypersensitivity and an increase in attention span in the next six-session period.
3. A decrease in dizziness and vascular headaches in the third six-session period.

4. An increased libido, less reversal of letters and words in the final six-session period.

There were EEG changes as well:

1. Phasic spikes decreased in first six sessions.
2. All spikes gone but theta-slowing still present in the second six-session period.
3. A reduction in theta in the third six-session period.
4. Most theta eliminated in the final six-session period. [24]

Budzynski says, in a 1994 article summarizing the state of the art in brain wave research, "Margaret Ayers's work over the last 20 years or so has certainly documented in clinical fashion the successes of neurofeedback in the area of brain injury."[25]

Siegfried and Susan Othmer worked with Ayers (see Jim Robbin's discussion of this developmental relationship in *A Symphony in the Brain*), then branched off and started their own company called EEG Spectrum. Grappling with seizure and learning disorders in their own children, the Othmers drew from the work of Ayers, as well as that of Sterman and Lubar, but developed their own protocols. Whereas Sterman and Lubar had tended to favor neurofeedback that trained their patients to produce more SMR waves (12–15 Hz), which had the effect of lifting epileptic and ADHD patients out of their underaroused "theta doldrums," the Othmers found that beta training at the C3 site in the central part of the left hemisphere had a powerful positive effect on mental energy and concentration. They routinely used beta protocols in which the desired training range was 15–18 Hz. However they also made the ingenious discovery that if the beta training "wired" the subject too much, they should switch to SMR training at the C4 site (the equivalent site on the central right hemisphere), which had a tendency to calm the brain.

The Othmers went on to shine in the domain from which they had begun. As they had helped their own children, they were able to help thousands more as the company they founded offered comprehensive training opportunities for hundreds of clinicians in EEG procedures. Siegfried Othmer cites just one case that is exemplary of the kind of results they were getting:

A boy of 15 came to us for problems of attention and reading. He had exhibited early hyperactivity, for which he had taken Ritalin for two years. He also had a lot of other support, including psychotherapy and educational therapy. At session six, he reported that he was able to pay attention better in school. At session twenty, he reported his best grades ever. At session 22 he said he was more organized; he established a budget for himself; he dismissed his tutor, and organized his own homework schedule. He completed the training at 32 sessions. His Wechsler IQ score improved from 90 to 127. He improved four grade levels in reading. He went from borderline to superior according to the Benton Visual Retention Test. He went on to a highly academic residential high school, which would not have even considered his application prior to his treatments (given his unremarkable academic behavior pre-treatment). The clinical psychologist who did the testing on this boy reported that he had never seen a more dramatic improvement in test scores in twenty years of working with learning disabled children. (He encountered many more surprises as he tested additional children who underwent the training.)[26]

Beta training worked not only for ADD children. Adults interested in improving their mental abilities were able to try it too. In a very droll article published in the 1994 *Megabrain Report*, entitled "The Church of Brain Wave Training! Wherein the Author Is Converted and Sees the True Path Forward," Dr. Julian Isaacs (an innovative biofeedback provider and professor of parapsychology at John F. Kennedy University) describes the benefits of a regimen of beta training upon himself as subject.[27] Isaacs also claims that the training helped ameliorate the aftereffects of early trauma, which was shown by high amplitude theta waves in his EEG chart, and an emotional volatility he calls being "Limbo-man": driven by the limbic, or as he puts it, "reptilian brain."

The net result of the beta training, as he described it, was to turn him into "Thalamo-man (the thalamus being associated with sending messages to the "higher brain" or cortex), more in touch with his rational, logical side, and "associated with all the cognitive and cultural goodies we associate with being human." Isaacs also added a caveat, however, echoing the mixed results obtained with the kids who were overtrained at beta. He suddenly took on a personality that he described as: "Mr. Beta-head . . . decidedly weird, somewhat like a robot, with a very unpleasant, 'hard,' forced compulsive quality of attention that I could not shift out of."[28]

This interesting firsthand phenomenological account is very valuable, an example of the importance of Steve Fahrion's advice that a therapist should not ask a client to do anything that the therapist hasn't done himself.

Healing from the Depths

During the seventies and eighties, the work on neurofeedback and accessing the unconscious begun by the Greens at the Menninger Foundation went on. One of the people inspired by their findings was a dedicated researcher named Eugene Peniston. Peniston, who worked both at Fort Collins, Virginia, and at the Sam Rayburn Memorial Veteran's Center in Bonham, Texas, used traditional biofeedback mixed with neurofeedback to treat very difficult populations of patients. He wrote in 1994, "My associate Paul Kulkosky and I have found that combining alpha and theta brain waves with temperature and visualization training, contributed to sustained prevention of relapse in alcoholics and PTSD (Post-Traumatic Stress Disorder)."[29] (Temperature training involves learning to warm the extremities, and is a frequently used early biofeedback procedure. The visualizations were probably based on Autogenic training, involving images of warmth and relaxation.)

Peniston described the impact of the new treatment he called "BWT" (brain wave training) on patient populations that had been recidivist and very resistant to traditional psychotherapeutic treatment. He wrote:

The original experimental study of chronic alcoholics compared thirty subjects in three groups: (a) alcoholic—BWT, (b) alcoholic—traditional therapy, and (c) non-alcoholic controls. Subjects were matched on age and were evaluated for alcoholic history, number of prior hospitalizations, IQ's, and socio-economic status. Before and after treatment, subjects were administered the Beck Depression Inventory (1961) (BDI); the Millon Clinical Multiaxial Inventory (MCMI) (Millon, 1983; Craig et al, 1985); and the [Cattell]

16 Personality Factor Scale (16PF); and were tested for EEG characteristics, and serum beta-endorphin levels. The beta-endorphins are stress related hormones and are elevated during the experience of physical or emotional stress. Successful treatment would stabilize beta-endorphin levels, so that stress related increases would be less likely to occur. . . .

80 percent of those receiving the EEG training were able to quit drinking following a 30-day program . . . after checking in with these same patients three years later, 10% had relapsed but that was it. Such success had never before been achieved. . . . All replications have resulted in similar success: 70 percent to 80 percent of treated patients are able to give up their addictions, with a minimal relapse rate.[30]

Peniston was able to apply the same protocol with the highly damaged and recidivist population of Vietnam veterans, who were affected not only by the traumas of the war but also by returning to an adversarial social environment that did not value their considerable sacrifices. Peniston wrote:

Alpha-theta brain wave neurofeedback was next employed for Vietnam theater veterans with combat-related PTSD. The 15 experimental patients receiving BWT showed significant decreases on the Minnesota Multiphasic Personality Inventory (MMPI) clinical scales within "normal limits." These patients also showed a reduction in recurrent anxiety-provoking nightmares/flashbacks, and a significant reduction in their psychotropic (i.e., anti-depressant and anti-anxiety) medications. In contrast, the traditional control group of (14) patients, which received treatment modalities such as rap groups, group therapy, psychodynamic therapy, psychotropic meds and individual psychotherapy showed only a significant decrease on the MMPI scale labeled Schizophrenia, and did not show a reduction in recurring anxiety-provoking nightmares/flashbacks; nor did they show a reduction in their psychotropic medications. . . .

After thirty months, twelve of the fifteen combat veterans who completed alpha-theta training were maintaining normal functioning and sustaining long-term prevention of PTSD relapse, whereas all 14 traditional therapy control patients had relapsed.

The application of alpha-theta brain wave training to addiction, depression, post-traumatic stress disorder, and other emotional dysfunction is proving to be one of the most efficacious treatment modalities for these disorders. Such neurofeedback therapy has produced both significant-related symptom diminution in combat-related PTSD and/ or PTSD symptomatology, and even significant pre- and post-test psychometric changes on standardized instruments. It has also permitted recall of significant experiences not previously accessible by traditional behavioral and/or psychotherapy. Without such specific brain wave training, many combat veterans have been unable to specifically identify crucial antecedent events. When able to identify and abreact to those experiences, much relief is obtained. Follow-up studies also indicate a markedly reduced recidivism rate, implying at least moderately long-term prevention, and reduced dependence in the use of psychotropic medication. It is noteworthy that concurrent medication appears to be no barrier to the success of treatment and that BWT may eliminate the need for medication.[31]

By the investigators' estimation, this neurofeedback that trained patients to produce both more theta and more alpha waves was the *most successful* therapeutic intervention ever tried with this refractory population. The increased production of theta waves was believed to facilitate recall of traumatic memories, and the increase in alpha waves soothed the anxiety associated with the recall. Although later criticism questioned Peniston and Kulkosky's methodology and the replicability of their remarkable early results, their work was highly influential on other researchers in the field.

In Arizona and New Mexico, Matthew Kelley was seeing comparable results in his work with alcoholic and addicted Native Americans. Perhaps not surprisingly, the alpha-theta training took the Hopis and the Navajos back to their shamanic cultural roots. They had visions of ancestral helping spirits and "power animals" that appeared as allies to help in their healing.[32] Kelley's results also were robust with this population of original people whose reality system had been devalued and trampled upon by an alien race. After treatment, the Native Americans showed signs of cultural adaptation that had previously been lacking, along with a stronger connection to their own cultural roots.

Texas psychologist Nancy White has also done work focusing on alpha and theta. Specifically, her investigations have hovered around that delicate point on the brain wave spectrum called "the crossover," where alpha shades into theta. (Interestingly, this often is seen as being at 7.8 Hz, which is the same frequency as the oscillation of Earth's magnetic field, known as the "Schumann rhythm.") White worked on a daily clinical outpatient basis with a difficult population of multiply diagnosed patients. She was also trained in transpersonal psychology and believed, as did Jung, Grof, Wilber, and others, that an encounter with the sacred can be healing. She writes:

> With alpha-theta training, we are working with an interactive system of mind/brain, body, psyche, spirit. As we discharge negative emotions and rigidly held beliefs from our past woundings, neurochemistry seems to be altered, our brain waves are normalized, our ability to move from state to state is enhanced and our psyche alters. Trauma is released and the more desirous programs are dropped into the deep unconscious.[33]

Some early researchers continued to emphasize the value of neurofeedback training for alpha more than theta. Among them was James Hardt, who had been a subject in Joe Kamiya's Chicago lab in 1968. In one of their early sessions, the experimenters had hooked Hardt into the equipment, set to reward alpha, and had virtually forgotten about him (staff ADD is not unknown, even in biofeedback labs!). Three and a half hours later, the whole staff had come running back in alarm, only to find that Hardt, sitting in the dark, soundproof room, had taken an extensive interior journey.

At first, Hardt had noticed that "thinking" and "trying" were both counterproductive, and that the only thing that seemed to work was "letting go." When he had really gotten into letting go, he noticed that he was "floating up near the ceiling." His "out-of-body" experience was accompanied by a variety of mystical insights and reflections. "For two days afterwards," he wrote, "I walked around feeling light and buoyant and not at all sure I was touching the ground."[34]

Over the years, Hardt came to feel that he could use isolation and long periods of alpha training to induce similar experiences in others.

He began, and continues to this day, something he calls the "Biocybernaut Program." Hardt felt that biofeedback could accelerate the processes normally involved in meditation and went on to demonstrate that the theta state eventually achieved by long-term Zen meditators could be replicated in the laboratory in a week of immersion training in brain waves.[35]

Another early explorer who stayed loyal to the alpha model was Les Fehmi. Fehmi had originally trained at the Brain Research Institute at UCLA with the formidable team of Joel Adkins and Donald Lindsley, studying how the brain responds to specific stimuli in monkeys. As he contemplated this research, Fehmi says, he realized that "information processing required simultaneity of activation" of millions of neurons, or "synchrony."

When Fehmi first joined the faculty at the SUNY campus at Stony Brook, in the late sixties, he determined to research this synchrony. He decided to do so in the context of alpha because he knew of Kamiya's work, which said that people could discern brain wave states, and because he knew that alpha was a highly synchronous wave.

In trying to self-train in alpha, Fehmi experienced the same early frustration Hardt had. Similarly, he noticed that *when he stopped trying*, the incidence of alpha waves suddenly shot up. Fehmi then began training in earnest. After a while, he was moved to write about his experiences:

> These increases in brain synchrony were accompanied by many releases, and positive changes in personal experience and perception and behavior. . . . I felt more open, lighter, freer, had more energy, and felt more spontaneous. I felt less urgency and gripping. I experienced more verbal fluidity and seemed to grasp things more easily, as if I had greater perspective, which allowed me to experience a more grand, whole and subtle image. As the letting go unfolded, I felt more intimate, intuitive and emotionally expressive. My interpersonal style changed and became lighter so that people of various ages seemed more inclined to gravitate to and be playful with me. My relationship with my children became softer and more personal. At times I literally felt as if I were walking, gliding effortlessly. All of this was unexpected and occurred without damaging . . . my ability to teach the hard-nosed physiological

psychology courses and "neurophysiological techniques" laboratory courses that my position at the University required. Even chronic rheumatoid arthritis, which had peaked in graduate school was disappearing.[36]

Fehmi came to feel that there were two kinds of attention—narrow and broadly focused—and that both were indispensable to a complete way of functioning consciously. He developed a useful technique to evoke the latter, which he called "Open Focus." He regarded both the exercise, which could be practiced anytime, and his specialized alpha training as prerequisites for ease and flexibility of function. Fehmi tried to train people to do the most difficult things they did in life with a sense of ease, that is, to "do it in alpha."[37]

As the results of alpha wave training became known, the "alpha-craze" of the seventies and eighties was generated. These were real, not theoretical, results. People could *feel* the difference and even began to think that alpha was the gateway to bliss and transcendence. Since bliss and transcendence do not lend themselves readily to scientific evaluation or quantification, a lot of scientists dismissed the entire movement— including all the hardworking, ethical neurofeedback researchers—as new-age and fraudulent.

Some of the claims about brain wave biofeedback were so extremely positive that by 1992, in *Biofeedback* magazine, Dr. Peter Rosenfeld raised an important question regarding brain wave biofeedback training effects: "Why *should* alpha-theta brain wave biofeedback have a positive effect on alcoholism and other forms of substance abuse?"[38] Robert Fried questioned the whole enterprise of a "frequency-based" training, because the "rhythm-generators" were primarily subcortical and largely influenced by the amount of carbon dioxide in the brain. And W. B. Plotkin questioned placebo effects, social reinforcement, and the simple presence of "eyes closed," as neglected factors in developing an experiential phenomenology of the alpha state.[39]

Perhaps even more to the point is the question regarding why protocols for training in *each* kind of brain wave have *all* been beneficial. Positive clinical results have been obtained by training every range from theta to beta, including the vaunted alpha and SMR ranges, all of which have their adherents. The only analogies that come to mind involve blind men and elephants, or spiritual sayings like, "there are many paths to the one truth." What is going on here?

In a thoughtful article written in 1994, psychophysiologist Jonathan Cowan calls attention to a principle underlying training in all brain wave types:

> The EEG is but one of a number of multiple converging indicators of state-context as Dr. Joe Kamiya is fond of pointing out. The multiple rhythms of the EEG are often overlaid on one another at the same time; the amplitudes, frequencies, and phase relationships of these rhythms presumably have some connections to the underlying brain state-context. . . .

It is probably more accurate to state that EEG rhythms roughly reflect one or several dimensions of the focusing and deployment of the student's attention, ranging from the relatively narrow focus associated with some predominantly beta rhythms to the more open or even diffuse attention, divided among multiple objects, characteristic of alpha dominance, as Fehmi has brought to the field's attention.

By training the student to produce more or less of these brain rhythms, we are actually doing something far more complex: teaching her/him to perceive and control a number of different transitions among his/her own unique state-contexts, which differ among themselves in the amounts of each of these rhythms that they produce.

One possible reason for the success of this therapy is that we are training the student better to control many of his transitions between his/her unique state-contexts, by teaching him/her how to control the way he/she focuses and deploys his/her attention.[40]

Cowan himself later developed a "broad-band suppression" technique of inhibiting high amplitudes all across the spectrum, with the observation that this protocol tended to produce global improvements in functioning. In part, he says, the inspiration for his protocol came from Dr. Len Ochs, who in turn, found his method through the unusual, serendipitous play of events described in the following chapter.

THE DEVELOPMENT OF THE
LENS APPROACH

Stephen Larsen, Ph.D., and Kristen Harrington, M.A., M.F.T., A.I.B.T.

We don't want to substitute our "good idea" of what the brain ought to be doing for allowing it to regulate itself, with close monitoring of the effects of the stimulation, the actual change we introduce, to see if the patient is changing within the bounds of comfort.

LEN OCHS, PH.D.

What we have stumbled upon is a bunch of anomalous findings and observations, and they do not fit within the current medical-scientific frame of reference. So I get a lot of skeptical doctors who say, "These results are impossible, so you're really not believable!" But guess what? This is the leading edge of science. This is where science comes from, from the realization of the anomalous.

LEN OCHS, PH.D.

The Discovery of EEG-Driven Stimulation

The furor probably started with a bunch of smart, sassy rats.

Mark Rosenzweig and his colleagues at the University of California, Berkeley, were exploring the relationship between learning and chemistry. Since the 1920s it had been noted that some rats were better at running mazes than others. The Rosenzweig team was exploring the role played by concentrations of a certain brain enzyme, acetylcholinesterase (AChE); they found, as they had suspected, that the smarter rats did indeed have more of it in their brains. Then they decided to approach the problem the other way around to see if the amount of the enzyme was affected by performance.

They placed rats in three environments. The first was the equivalent of a rodent "slum," with opaque walls, dim lights, reduced sound. This was called the *impoverished* environment. Then there was your ordinary middle-class laboratory cage, called the *standard* environment. The third group got all the toys of privileged existence: the company of other rats, "a large, well-lit multilevel cage filled with swings, slides, ladders, bridges . . . frequently changing stimuli, and a variety of challenges." This was called the *enriched* environment.

The hypothesis that the amount of AChE in the rats' brains would be affected by their experiences was confirmed when the rats were sacrificed: the rats who had been in the enriched environment had the highest amount of the enzyme, while those in the impoverished environment had the least. But an unexpected discovery rocked the neuroscientific establishment: the brains of the stimulated rats were larger and heavier. This flew in the face of neurobiological fundamentalism, which said that once a brain developed all of its neurons (at about two years of age in human beings) the job was basically done, that *neurons don't grow or increase in number through life!*

Some scientists did, in fact, claim the results were impossible: "Skepticism or frank disbelief were the initial reactions to our reports that significant changes in the brain were caused by relatively simple and benign exposure of animals to different environmental experience."[1]

However, the Berkeley group teamed up with the neuroanatomist Marian Diamond, who had obtained samples of Einstein's brain, analyzed them and found that the number of glial cells *per neuron* was higher than in ordinary brain tissue.[2] Glia, from the Latin for "glue," usually outnumber neurons by about ten to one. Traditionally regarded as mere "scaffolding," or kind of dumb "helper cells" for the all-intelligent neurons, glial cells are now regarded to have far more complex and fascinating roles in brain maintenance and function.[3] Thus the great physicist did not have a *larger number of neurons*, but the ones he had were very well fed and cared for. The brains of the rats in the enriched environment consistently showed a number of factors that indicated higher functional capacity.

Increased thickness in the cerebral cortex.

Greater weight of the cortex compared to the rest of the brain.

A fifteen percent increase in the actual size of individual neurons in the cortex.

An increased number of dendritic spines per unit length of dendrite.

An increase in the number of synapses (where neurons come together to talk).

A fifteen percent increase in the number of *glial cells* that support and surround the neurons.[4]

For the entire neurofeedback community, the outcome of Rosenzweig and Diamond's work was very exciting. Above all, it showed that the brain was responsive to *stimulation* and was able to make use of it to *change itself.* As Tom Budzynski wrote, "Dr. Diamond's research indicates that novel stimulation produces increased dendritic growth with a resulting increase in the brain's functioning. This probably does occur, but there are also higher order organizing processes taking place, i.e., new, more efficient reprogramming is taking advantage of the new 'circuitry' of increased dendritic growth."[5]

The discovery that the brain was able to change itself in response to stimulation was one of the ingredients in the mix that led Dr. Len Ochs to a remarkable breakthrough. Ochs had been a precocious "electronics buff," during his high school and college days. He felt an intuitive rapport with computers and became attracted to neurofeedback when it was still in an embryonic stage. During his early career, in the 1970s, Ochs rubbed elbows with many of the pioneering researchers and clinicians: Barry Sterman, the Othmers, Ken Tachiki, and Joe Kamiya. His earliest interest was in the alpha/theta type of protocol that Peniston had used in treating alcohol addiction. At one point he also trained in alpha/theta protocols with the Greens, and Patricia Norris and Steve Fahrion in Topeka, Kansas.

Ochs also knew Dr. Harold Russell of Galveston, Texas, who—along with his collaborator Dr. Carter (inspired by Rosenzweig and Diamond's work)—had found that audio-visual stimulation (AVS) helped the brains of learning disabled (LD) students. The protocol was fairly simple, based on the assumption that the brain would have a tendency to follow any rhythmically pulsing stimulus. A flashing light was presented at two frequencies: 10 Hz to entrain alpha, and 18 Hz to entrain beta. That the cortex was entrained by the lights, showing increases in alpha or beta according to the stimulation, was confirmed by EEG readings. Russell and Carter also used EEG biofeedback, or neurofeedback in which the subject tries to increase or decrease the abundance of certain rhythms.

The AVS was less expensive (and could be done at home), whereas the EEG was more expensive and had to be administered by a clinician in the lab. The benefits of both, though, were unmistakable. The AVS alone, over forty to eighty sessions, produced increases in IQ scores of five to seven points, while the EEG work produced fifteen to twenty point gains over thirty to seventy-five sessions. Russell and Carter's clinical explorations also included successful cases of using the two stimulation technologies to help stroke patients.[6]

At one point Harold Russell consulted with Len Ochs about helping to design an AVS machine that children could take home. However, Ochs replied that he definitely had a prejudice against the light and sound *entrainment* machines that seemed to *drive* the brain waves. He had observed that there seemed to be an attraction or pull to the stimulation frequency and felt that this was coercing the brain to change frequencies, through a process closer to physics than psychology. As Ochs wrote in 1994, in a *Megabrain Report* article, "New Light on Lights, Sounds and the Brain":

My negative bias and disposition toward these devices showed clearly, even in the face of Marian Diamond's and W. Grey Walter's pioneering work on stimulation. (But) I have, on occasion, heard second-hand stories of these devices producing effects that seem nothing less than miraculous.[7]

It was on the trail of "the miraculous" that Ochs found himself in response to Russell's request. He had been thinking that the fixed frequencies *would not* be good for children. Besides, there were issues of arbitrariness in how the stimulation frequencies were chosen. He wondered *how one frequency or set of frequencies could be good for everybody!*

Then followed one of those creative or visionary breakthroughs that checker the developmental history of science. As Ochs told the author, "In about sixty seconds of very clear intuition, I proposed to Russell that the AVS should *follow* the brain waves, and described how it could be done."

Then all Ochs had to do was to move his insight from his brain's right hemisphere to its left hemisphere (or, as American cognitive psychologist Jerome Bruner would have said, "from the left hand of creative imagination to the right hand of engineering"). (Jerome Bruner: *Essays for the Left Hand*.) Ochs had to "make it happen" in the real world. He wrote:

> I had the EEG processor made by the biofeedback company J&J, the I-330 EEG, and the Synergizer light/sound device from Synetic systems. EEG software was designed to link these two devices allowing the person's EEG to change the frequency of the lights and sounds, and the stimulation, in turn, to change the EEG.[8]

Thus the first EEG Entrainment Feedback (EEF) device was born, using light-emitting diodes (LEDs) inside a pair of welder's glasses, and sound through earphones. Ochs soon realized that the light was far more effective than the sound; the visual pathways are three times as extensive in the brain so the visual stimulation was reaching more areas of the cortex. He dropped the sound component and switched to the ordinary dark glasses with built-in LEDs that became his early trademark.

"I found it much more visually beautiful than the traditional sound and light stimulation," Ochs wrote in *Megabrain Report* in 1994. "It seemed more alive and responsive to my brain waves than was the fixed-frequency or pre-programmed slowly ramping stimulation I had tried."[9] (At that time many people were using light and sound machines with their "ramped progressions" up and down the brain wave frequencies for aesthetic appreciation and to generate "altered states," as well as for therapeutic stimulation.) But Ochs did not yet guess the astonishing potential of what he had created:

> The clinical effects of this system were entirely unpredictable to me. This link had not been attempted before to my knowledge. There was certainly nothing in the literature, which described the

EEG-stimulation link, what the effects of it might be, what problems might be encountered, and how it might be used. [10]

In retrospect Ochs feels that a series of unbelievable accidents and coincidences led him to the discoveries he then began to make, one after the other.

During his professional development he had felt the same quandary many biofeedback theorists have encountered: Should he specialize in the alpha/theta approach, as used by the Greens and Peniston (for traumatic integration and encounter with the unconscious) or, like Lubar and the Othmers, head for the "high ground" of the SMR and beta protocols (to stimulate the brain for "underarousal problems" like depression or ADD)? All the approaches seemed effective in their own way and all had their enthusiastic adherents. Each approach had what its practitioners regard as an "ideal" training range, such as Michael Tansey's legendary 14 Hz that, according to him, facilitates recall of traumatic memories without the "abreaction" or "catharsis" that sometimes happens with the lower frequency (theta) types of recall.[11]

But the discoveries that Ochs made spanned the paradox: neither this nor that, but somehow both! The treatment he had designed included all the brain wave ranges, because it "fed back" to the brain whatever frequency it was producing. That led him to wonder whether it might be capable of addressing a whole spectrum of CNS-related problems. In 1994, he pursued this:

> Interested, but not especially aware of any unusual ability of the system, I introduced it to some patients who had a great deal of psychotherapy, biofeedback and even EEG brain wave biofeedback, but who needed results that were clearer, faster, and more meaningful than brought about by these procedures.
>
> One man had displayed 20 years of rages, many of which lasted two weeks at a time. The family threatened divorce because of the unacceptability of his explosiveness. He was unable to work because of his temper. Another patient was a woman who worked for a major retail chain as an upper-level manager and had been exposed to increasing work pressure over the past few years, capped by threats of bodily harm to her and her family by ex-employees. She

had been unable to go to work and was extremely depressed and anxious. Both of these individuals were very highly motivated and very bright. Both wanted to work again; and both felt the shame of being out of work. The man highly valued his family and wanted to continue in it. What follows are lessons I learned using EEF to work with these two individuals and others.

LESSON ONE: People can be hypersensitive to their own brain waves.

Within two minutes of feeding back EEG-driven sound and light the woman began to complain of back, neck and head pain. I had set the system to lower her EEG by flashing the lights a little slower than her dominant frequency . . . I wondered if increasing her EEG by flashing the lights slightly faster than her dominant frequency would keep her from pain. Contrary to the wisdom of conventional biofeedback, it did.

LESSON TWO: Those with psychological and physical trauma are much more frequently hypersensitive than "normals" are to stimulation. . . . One woman was so sensitive that she found the lights too bright even when they were shielded with poster material and placed on her lap.

LESSON THREE: The people with the worst symptoms are the most hypersensitive to light stimulation. . . . It is astonishing to link sound and light sensitivity to symptom intensity . . . we are not used to documenting central nervous system status with peripheral problems, or brain irritability with consciousness, motivation, mood, and energy problems. It is much more typical to think of psychological reasons for these problems.[12]

In response to his patients' hypersensitive reactions, Ochs developed a "desensitization" protocol similar to the ones used in behavior therapy for the treatment of phobias. He would increase the intensity of the lights and the duration of the session until the person could not tolerate them any more, then back off, then stimulate still more, until the patients' sensitivity seemed less acute. Those he could "desensitize" seemed to improve. But he noted that if he wished the patients to continue improving after they were desensitized, he had to lower the light stimulation markedly.

LESSON FOUR: The people who desensitize get better.

LESSON FIVE: After desensitization the lower the intensity of the stimulation, the more reliable the improvement.

LESSON SIX: There is more than one kind of hypersensitivity. Although the woman (who had been so sensitive to the lights gradually became used to them and) appeared comfortable with brighter lights, she did not resume making progress until their brightness was lowered significantly. . . . After her hypersensitivity to the lights was lost, there was a need to develop other objective ways to alert the clinician that she continued to be hypersensitive, in other ways.

LESSON SEVEN: There appears to be such a thing as optimization of one's EEG. As a patient becomes progressively more functional— that is, mood, energy, motivation, memory, attention, sequencing, prioritizing become more present and reliable—there are predictable changes that appear in the patient's EEG patterns. As the patient learns to "cruise the frequencies". . . lets go and permits (the dominant brain wave frequency) to be pulled however it goes, the activity observed in each of the bands becomes minimized, equalized, and reduced in variability.

LESSON EIGHT: We appear to have subcortical as well as cortical intelligence, fortunately. . . . Those who were brightest consciously before their trauma often do the best, as if their intelligence is a quality that permeates the brain subcortically, as well as cortically.

LESSON NINE: High functioning people who are truly injured and handicapped will do almost anything to get better if there is a reasonable chance that they will show relatively rapid significant improvement.

LESSON TEN: Research, Research, Research . . . all to make sure we are not fooling ourselves and each other . . . The makers of claims need to recognize the desperation of those afflicted with head injuries, strokes, spinal cord problems, depression, obsessions, rages, enormous fatigue, and emotional and environmental hypersensitivity. Only research can define a product's limitations and capabilities.

LESSON ELEVEN: Move to other sites to monitor the EEG. One site most probably won't be enough. An individual's EEG may be optimized at one site and problems still remain. . . . The therapist may need to proceed systematically around the head following the standard 10–20 electrode placement system, which conventionally designates the 19 sites used in most EEG's. (See page one of the color insert for an illustration of the standard 10–20-electrode placement system.)

LESSON TWELVE: Trauma, both psychological and physical, may be a lot more treatable than formerly thought.

LESSON THIRTEEN: Dead may not be so dead. . . . While there is undoubtedly structural and tissue damage in head injury, including stroke and spinal cord injury, the inevitable linking of that damage with the subsequent loss of function may be premature and largely based on the treatment resistance of the subsequent problems using conventional methods.

LESSON FOURTEEN: We ain't seen nothin' yet . . . as long as people are alive, creation has a chance of being a continuous process. Just as this EDF process couldn't have been anticipated and just as the beneficial consequences of this process couldn't have been concretely forecast (disregarding the slogans about the brain being only 10% used and therefore capable of anything), openness to surprise has helped many who were condemned to a hopeless life.[13]

Ochs noted that the procedure clearly had relevance to psychotherapy. It brought up symptoms, intensifying them, including memories related to trauma, such as with the explosive man mentioned above, a Vietnam veteran: "Over a span of two weeks of daily EEG-driven LS (stimulation) sessions, tears would show over the man's cheeks; he felt thermal hallucinations ("It's hot as Nam—whoops—it's gone!") He experienced auditory hallucinations ("I hear the choppers").[14]

After the course of treatment, the man's rages (explosive personality disorder) abated, and he displayed a higher frustration tolerance. His marriage and family life improved. This man had already received forty conventional EEG biofeedback treatments without much improvement, before the two-week intensive EEF, which brought about the far more dramatic relief.

As mentioned among his lessons learned, Ochs noted the sensitivity of TBI and PTSD patients to the treatment in which pulsing lights followed their own brain waves; the flashing lights made them uncomfortable just as he applied the stimulation. In his 1994 paper he noted that nonverbal signs of overstimulation included, "tightening of the chest, restriction of chest motility, lifting or rounding of the shoulders, flexion of the neck, or tightening of the jaw. There were verbal expressions as well, ranging from 'too bright' to 'too much flicker' to 'too much red,' to cries and grunts of discomfort."

It was as if these highly irritable or sensitive individuals were being given a dose of themselves—their own brain waves in a slightly different form—and it was intolerable! The red lights that were initially used (because they were available) seemed particularly irritating to the more sensitive clients. He requested that new glasses be built with gentler green lights, as well as offering him the ability to turn the intensity and bandwidth of the lights up or down.

During this period, two dominant insights were to emerge that would characterize Ochs's thinking throughout. The first was the importance of the clinical criterion regarding the "comfort" of the patient. As he told the author: "That idea of comfort, combined with the clinical experience of working with the most sensitive categories of patients, is what shaped the protocols."[15]

The second pertained to the impact of varying the brain wave feedback by introducing plus or minus offsets in the response: "If the patient looked uncomfortable or sounded uncomfortable, I reversed the polarity of the leading frequency, i.e., alternating between slightly faster and slightly slower than the dominant brain wave frequency."[16] Ochs says that again and again, he was having attacks of incredulity. "An inveterate curmudgeon," he says, "I couldn't really believe that what was happening was happening. I began to wonder if it was a life-punishment, now to have to investigate and develop this incredible healing technique I was certain never should have worked."[17]

Jonathan Cowan suggested to Ochs that he was really doing something like "disentrainment" rather than "entrainment." The flashing light or light and sound devices "entrain," due to the tendency of the brain to follow any rhythmically pulsing stimulus (the reason epileptics should avoid discos with flashing lights). When stimulation is determined by the brain waves (at 0 offset), the process might actually amplify brain waves, creating an instability condition, and maybe even initiating seizures. Using an offset, however, decreased the amplitudes, because the brain waves "tried" to follow something that was close to, but actually different from itself, and hence lost power, or amplitude. Ochs reasoned that whereas the entrainment process could be dangerous for people with seizure disorders, the disentrainment model might break up incipient seizure activity, as well as areas locked up in the wrong kind of synchrony or "coherence." (See color insert page 2 for offset protocol.)

Around this time, Ochs read James Gleick's *Chaos: The Making of a New Science,* which had a major effect on him. Gleick pointed out that entrainment, or "mode-locking," tends to decrease freedom and bind intelligent systems. In neurofeedback, then, mode-locking would amplify the patient's pathology—"A locking-in to a single mode can be enslavement, preventing a system from adapting to change"[18]—whereas disentrainment (applied chaos theory) would break down the locked-up or stuck patterns, opening up functioning, and making new alternatives of behavior available.

Ochs began to experiment primarily with "offset" protocols, and later even eliminated the "0" setting from the equipment, because of the danger of "entrainment" adversely affecting epileptics, or people with tics.

On the machines he designed, offsets could be varied anywhere from minus 5 Hz to plus 20 Hz. Large negative offsets were not used, because the disentrainment of 4 Hz delta at a minus 4 Hz offset results in a 0 frequency. (If the person's dominant brain wave frequency were pulsing at 10 Hz and a +1 offset was used, the signal would feed back to them at

11 Hz; if a +5 offset was used, it would feed back at 15 Hz, +20 at 30 Hz, and so on.) Ochs noticed that whether plus or minus offsets were used, the procedure tended to *lower the existing amplitude,* because the brain would try to follow the new offset, and jump out of its existing pattern. (He assumed that the existing pattern was less than desirable, since the person was suffering from symptoms of CNS dysregulation.) The protocol seemed, in fact, to be the method "par-excellence" for "bumping people out of their parking places," and breaking up dysfunction quickly.

The name was changed to EDF (EEG Disentrainment Feedback). A new machine, called the I-400, was built by J&J Engineering, a West Coast biofeedback company, to work with the new Pentium computers. It featured a pair of the traditional red glasses for the more robust, and a pair of green glasses for the more sensitive patients.

While working with patients referred by neuropsychiatrist Herbert Gross of Los Angeles, a specialist in head injuries, Ochs noticed that he had to lower and lower the intensity of the light he used, and that, finally, "no intensity allowed for the comfort of these highly sensitive patients." Ochs had seen sensitive patients' responses right at the moment of treatment, with grunts, cries, or body language. Now he began to question them more probingly, and observe the consequences of a treatment over the twenty-four hours following it, and then over the course of the week until the next one.

The two most obvious signs that the patients had received an "overdose" of stimulation were that they were "tired" (exhausted or sleepy) on the one hand, or "wired" (hyperactive children became more "hyper") on the other. A definite "irritability" could come along with either condition: small things seemed overwhelming; noises and lights caused adverse reactions. He also noticed that patients experiencing "overdose" never seemed to develop new problems, just a re-presentation, and maybe momentary intensification, of old symptoms.

A third sign of "overdose" was that, over time, the symptoms being treated showed no therapeutically positive movement. In some way, the overstimulation was "locking-up" the recovery process instead of facilitating it. Ochs came to realize: "Sometimes the strongest stimuli evoke the strongest defenses we have, but make it gentle enough and it 'sneaks right under' the defense system's radar."[19] He began to try out lower and lower doses that were less taxing for the patient, but still effective.

At first he tried different offsets, such as +5, +10, +15, or even +20, and found that certain ones seemed to work better for certain patients. In general it was thought that the larger, hence "further away," offsets were less stimulating, but there was no uniform rule or principle.

In response to a suggestion by an early practitioner, Dieter Dauber of California, Ochs began placing opaque barriers, such as manila-folder cardboard or folded plastic or electrical tape between the LEDs and the patients' eyes. Soon he was using six layers of plastic, then fifteen, then thirty over the green LEDs for the most sensitive patients. Naturally, these strange maneuvers drastically reduced light stimulation, but then the question came up as to whether the patients were receiving any stimulation at all. Still—to the astonishment of Ochs and the early practitioners who were using his protocols—the treatments still seemed to produce a substantial therapeutic effect.

The watchword of EDF practitioners became "Less is more." In each case the desideratum was the clinical comfort of the patient: the patient should be free of discomfort during the session, and hopefully during the twenty-four hours following the treatment. If the treatment stayed within these bounds, the positive effects tended to accumulate.

The most reliable and methodical way Ochs found to diminish the "dose" was to shorten the time of stimulation. Soon treatment lengths were reduced from minutes to mere seconds of treatment per site. Each client was evaluated as the treatment progressed, using CNS Questionnaires (see Chapter 11), clinical interviews, and observations of behavior. Ochs continued to find great individual variability between patients, making diagnostic acumen crucial for the treatment process: the setting of the protocol and of the levels of feedback stimulation.

Ochs confirmed with dozens of cases that patients whose treatment did not overtax their resources showed not only the greatest rate of improvement, but more lasting results. To fine tune the treatment to each patient, he developed a computer scoring method to measure the activity and reactivity of each site, using *amplitude* (the height or power of the waves) to measure activity and *standard deviation* (sudden rises and falls of amplitude) to measure reactivity.

Ochs created maps of the cortex using twenty-one sites of the professional standard, as it is called: The International 10–20 system. He found that by sampling the twenty-one sites he could feed data into an Excel chart arranged according to the location of the sites on the cortex, and thus produce a topographic brain map. The mapping procedure he created was analogous to the standard neurological QEEG (or "Quantitative EEG") in which nineteen or twenty-one or more sites are measured simultaneously with a cap connected with lots of wires to a simultaneous processor such as the *Lexicor.*

But, instead of measuring all sites simultaneously, he measured one site at a time, usually adding a little stimulation to see how the brain responded at that site. Initially he used a 120-second (two-minute) sampling at each site but then decided this was cumbersome and unnecessary. Later, a twenty-four second protocol was developed, which allowed the maps to be done more quickly yet still seemed an adequate guide for the development of treatment protocols. (The most recent protocol is a four-second sampling, with or without stimulation, depending upon the person's sensitivity.) It is important to note that Len Ochs himself does not see his maps as "diagnostic," in the way a QEEG might be, but as a guide to treatment. (See color insert page 1 and 4.)

In searching for a rationale about how to approach the various sites in treatment, he converted the topographic map into a series of bar graphs representing the brain wave frequencies for each site. When he organized them by increasing amplitude, he realized that this "site sort" revealed important information about the condition of the brain:

Looking at the low-amplitude sites, I was seeing an area where the cortex is functioning well, exerting a greater inhibition over the sub-cortical rhythmical potentials (that produce the brain waves). And where the amplitude was highest, I was looking at areas where the cortex was functioning the least well. I thought about Barry Sterman's discussion of cortical inhibition being the key to all higher levels of functioning. I saw that we could begin to work with the low amplitude sites, and gradually build up the strengths of the brain as treatment progressed.[20]

That led Ochs to use the site sort as a guide for a treatment: a few sites at a time were stimulated in a graded sequence, first those sites whose brain waves showed the least amplitudes and smallest SDs (standard deviations), and then proceeding to those with the highest amplitudes and highest SDs. The number of sites stimulated per treatment ranged from as few as one or two to as many as six, depending on the sensitivity of the patient.

Eventually Ochs found that sites that had looked like "tigers" on the original map, with high amplitude and spiky, high standard deviations, looked like milder and tamer "kitty-cats" by the time their turn for treatment came in the sequence, that is, after he had painstakingly proceeded through the site sort.

Traditional EEG biofeedback—in which people put themselves in alpha, beta, or theta for a certain period—had already proven itself helpful with head injuries in the work of Ayers, Othmer, and others. From the beginning, this kind of EEG driven stimulation seemed to produce effects that were unmistakable.

With the treatments pioneered by Len Ochs, skillful clinicians, administering exactly the right stimulation or pulse of "feedback," to a receptive client, were able to attain immediate effects. Without the lengthy training protocols used in conventional EEG biofeedback, people were recovering many kinds of functioning that they had lost in the aftermath of injury. Mood, energy, flexibility, and cognitive clarity were frequently seen to improve. Some of the most surprising improvements noted were in the domain of "metacognition": the ability to observe and critique one's own behavior. People got clearer about "outer reality," but also clearer about evaluating their own responses to events in it. Sometimes this touched on a domain we have come to see as vitally important: the ability to "learn from experience," one of the dimensions measured on the CNS Questionnaire (see chapter 11) administered to each client at the intake, and periodically through treatment.

The disentrainment type of neurofeedback seemed to help people become more pragmatic as well as more flexible. They tended to make fewer "mountains out of molehills," big deals out of small frustrations. Even a few sessions were able to help people with the tasks of conventional neurofeedback: putting themselves in an alpha, beta, or theta state for a certain period. It also helped meditators, who claimed there was less "noise" in their brains; they had more ability to still their minds and enter deeper states of consciousness.

Ochs's protocol came to differ from almost all other biofeedback treatments because it included mandatory visits to all sites on the map, two, three, or even four times, where tiny stimulations were given until the amplitudes at "tiger" sites lowered, and the whole brain wave complexion changed enough to warrant a new map. Ochs believed that this procedure offered a far more thorough stimulation of the cerebral cortex than traditional biofeedback, which relied upon five, as he says, "canonically approved" sites (C3, C4, O1, O2, and CZ).*

Ochs kept upgrading his equipment designs and in 1998 introduced the C-2, also built by J&J. It offered a far more effective and precise registry of brain waves, and a two-channel capability, allowing more areas of the brain to be accessed in a single treatment, and the interaction between specific areas of the brain to be monitored. Out of concern for ultrasensitive patients, he introduced new glasses whose emissions were in microlumens, barely registerable by the eye, and that included a switch so there could be a mode of treatment without light. Still, the effects of stimulation by the new C-2 machines seemed more powerful than the old I-400 system. This was because of the precision of the new machines (and other factors yet to be discovered).

After some time he designed yet another generation of glasses, with the lights still weaker, even though the technicians at the manufacturing plant accused him of being crazy for wanting to have the stimulation so low it couldn't possibly have any effect. However, he still observed that some sensitive people were getting overdosed, based on the criteria mentioned above ("tired," "wired," or showing no progress). He moved the glasses out inches and then feet from the patient's face, as far as the wires would reach in an office, and there still seemed to be some effect for the most sensitive!

Finally a research grant† enabled Ochs to take the equipment to the Lawrence Livermore National Laboratory for a series of tests aimed at discovering what stimulus was really reaching the patient. There they discovered that the I-400 machine had no measurable emissions, other than the light of the LEDs in the glasses, but that the C-2 machine had

---

*This has begun gradually to change, as conventional biofeedback clinicians find training at other sites to be equally effective, or more effective for certain kinds of problems, a problem discussed at a recent *Futurehealth* conference (2001).

†The investigation was made possible by a generous donation obtained by Dr. Mary Lee Esty from Rush-Presbyterian-St.Luke's Medical Center, described later in the book.

radio frequency emissions—very weak, but still measurable—emerging from the EEG processor. J&J had used a crystal clock inside the C-2 as a timing mechanism.

The radio frequency emissions were coming from it, then traveling down the wires to the glasses and the leads to the patient's head, which were acting as radio antennae. These emissions had not been controlled for in building the equipment because they had been deemed too small to have any effect whatsoever, being in the "nanowatt" per square centimeter range, thousands of times weaker than those of cell phones or walkie-talkies. Nonetheless, the clinical reports about clients who received treatments *without glasses,* who were exposed only to the radio frequency emissions received by the lead wires, indicated that something significant and beneficial was indeed happening to their nervous systems.

Once the penetrating power of the radio frequency emissions was discovered, standard radio frequency emissions (RFI) filtering devices were added to all leads coming into and out of the C-2 EEG. This seemed to make a few seconds of treatment tolerable even to the ultrasensitive. Glasses with LEDs were generally not used any more, except for the extremely robust patient, and then still with mandatory RFI filters on the leads to the glasses.

To further minimize the chance of overdose, a new EEG processor called the "mini C-2" was developed in partnership with J&J engineering in 2002. Its processing unit emits radio frequencies sufficiently weak (several thousand times weaker than the C-2) that the RFI filters could be dispensed with. In this form of treatment, the patient has no conscious registry of the feedback; it does its work "subconsciously," or subliminally. That, however, does not diminish its effectiveness. The biofeedback delivered subliminally seems to do its work on those preverbal, affective, and arousal dimensions that we are never normally aware of, but nonetheless represent adjustments and accommodations of the organism to information that is made available to it, and may also represent subcortical learning.

Under the guiding principle of "Less is more!" Ochs has refined the equipment until it is so minimalist and so gentle as to be in danger of total devaluation by contemporary science, because of the difficulty in imagining how stimuli as small as it uses could do anything at all. Lest at this point the reader thinks that the results obtained must surely be due to a "placebo" effect, or perhaps even "entrainment of the belief system of the therapist on the patient," or even unconscious misperception or manipulation of the data by clinicians, let me recount an event that happened, which affected the main office in Walnut Creek, California, our own center, and a number of the treatment facilities around the country.

From time to time, Len Ochs would develop new versions or "upgrades" of his software programming for conducting clinical sessions, and send them out to practitioners. On one of these upgrades the programmer (who was unaware that he had developed a brain aneurysm) inadvertently made a significant mistake. The result was that instead of tracking a patient's dominant frequency at a given site, and providing stimulation at the prearranged offset, the equipment stimulated everyone only at a fixed frequency between the delta and theta ranges (4 Hz).

This generated an inadvertent double-blind study, in which neither the subjects nor the experimenter knew what was going on. Within days, however, Ochs started receiving reports from practitioners that were very different than the varied, but usually positive, ones he was used to getting. People were regressing, complaining of headaches, depression, pain returning, sleep disturbances, and many other things, all negative.

Our own office at Stone Mountain Center was one of the afflicted ones, where patient after patient was giving negative reports that went directly against the grain of what we had been receiving and were used to expecting. Finally, while one patient was hooked up, I pulled the black tape off the LEDs and observed the ominous flashing of the single signal of 4 Hz, instead of the varied, pulsing dance of an alive signal we had been used to! It was a scary moment.

We called the home office and learned that others had been experiencing the same thing. The source of the error was discovered. In short order, a corrected version of the software was prepared, the patients were apologized to with considerable chagrin, and the usual course of treatment continued. Once again the patients reported a steady rate of improvement.

Although purposeful double-blind ABA studies—in which a variable intended to make a subject better (A) is applied, followed by its opposite (B), and then by a reapplication of the first (A)—are frowned on by ethics committees because of the possibility that the B factor might do lasting harm to the subject, this inadvertent "study" demonstrated that the treatment results cannot reasonably be ascribed to a placebo effect.

Another factor makes it doubtful that placebo could explain all of the results obtained with Ochs's method: They are long-lasting (unlike with a placebo effect). And the improvement sometimes follows a unique and idiosyncratic course of recovery that the patient him or herself wouldn't or couldn't have predicted. The steady progress of the spectrum of improvement is only elicited by the clinician's thoughtful questioning and unbiased recording of "worse" along with "better."

Ochs the Clinician

Ochs is notable as an innovator in many respects, but especially in his astuteness as a clinician: tracking the subtle changes of many symptoms of his patients resulting from his therapeutic interventions, but always with an eye to the overall health and functionality of the patient. He has been able to identify several constellations of symptoms that—when present in one form or another and usually in combinations—point to a pervasive underlying CNS dysregulation. These include:

1. Mood disturbance: emotional lability, depression or anxiety, irritability
2. Energy depletion: also sometimes described as chronic fatigue or fibromyalgia
3. Chronic Pain: localized or generalized, including headaches and muscle spasms
4. Sleep Disturbance: from sleep onset to nocturnal awakenings, to daytime sleepiness
5. Cloudy Sensorium: the world seems inaccessible or far away, the person is unresponsive to cues
6. Memory Problems: forgetfulness, short and long-term disturbance
7. Cognitive Problems: regarding clarity, focus, planning, sequencing, and/or organizing
8. Problems initiating behavior and pursuing to completion

Ochs developed the CNS Questionnaire mentioned above (and reproduced in chapter 11) to include specific questions that touch on all of the above. These symptoms not only show the existence of an underlying CNS dysregulation but can also be used by the clinician as ongoing measures that will indicate the degree of the healing process. Ochs observed that if there were an exacerbation of symptoms during treatment, it would be along the lines of familiar symptomatology; it would probably be something recognizable to the patient from his or her history.

The neurotherapy seemed to evoke, and then resolve, knots or impasses in the nervous system, and thus in the psyche. If there were an aggravation (along the lines of what happens in homeopathy, where the patient gets "a little worse" before getting better) within twenty-four hours the clients usually reported the opposite: an upswing of energy, relief from pain, and so on.[21]

Nonetheless, Ochs held to his criterion: The neurotherapist should try to cause the least discomfort possible at every stage of the treatment process. "The medical establishment," he wrote, "and to a certain extent the psychological establishment, have taken a 'bully-exercise, gain-through pain' approach to rehabilitation, which I, too, almost began to apply to FNS (LENS) work, until I saw that the opposite was the only approach that worked. It has turned out the more sensitivity is favored, and the treatment made as gentle as possible in ways I couldn't even begin to imagine, the neuronal strength of the patients has been supported, and recovery follows far more often than not."[22]

The Wizard Is In

Ochs went on to develop and perfect his technique and, on a pleasant fall day in 2003 I accompany him to his office in Santa Rosa, California, to observe him in clinical practice. We drive over the freeways, still in autumnal bloom, to a sedate professional treatment office in Santa Rosa; a complex that houses physicians, psychologists, and social workers, as well as CAM (Complementary and Alternative Medical approach) practitioners. Len's office is plain enough, but in addition to the LENS setup, there is a photonic stimulator, and a large and impressive-looking Bales Thermal Imaging Camera. (He and his partner, Cathy, a nurse, use it to help women find a noninvasive way to search for signs of breast cancer.)

Dr. Ochs asks each client, in turn, his or her permission for a colleague (me) to sit in on the session: a construction worker with terrible anxiety problems, a retired seaman with a head injury, someone with bad cognitive symptoms as a result of mercury poisoning, and others. Len gives full attention to each client, asking many questions about the previous week: How they are sleeping? How is mood, energy, clarity? There is an almost palpable warmth in the sessions, and it is clear that each of these clients feels cared about and cared for by their therapist. And, I can tell by their conversation, they also care about him. (In clinical lingo, the *transference* is solid. The therapeutic environment seems safe, and supportive.)

The construction worker, a handsome, muscular man of about forty, has been about 50 percent better since starting treatment, and he really can't believe it, because, well, frankly, he thinks what Len is doing is pretty weird stuff—but he shrugs his shoulders and they both laugh. Just a couple of neurofeedback sessions have made this patient able to attend family functions without embarassing panic attacks. His sexual "performance anxiety" is also much better, he says smiling and almost winking. He's gotten back on his mountain bike again after a long layoff; he felt so bad, not physically, but mentally and emotionally, before.

"Good," Len says. "We'll go on with a few more sessions. But I was struck by something you said; could we go into that a little more?" The man talks, rambling on a little, as Len perfunctorily changes the sensor sites and attends to his computer screen.

It seemed that this man's serious anxiety problems had begun at a very specific time. Up until aproximately that time there had been no death in his family. But then it began: grandparents, uncles, and very unexpectedly, one of his younger cousins. Tears well up, as the man begins to talk more. Len mostly says "mm-hm" but shakes his head and smiles sympathetically. When the neurofeedback treatment is over, and the sensors are off, Len looks at the man. "Have you done any bereavement counseling?" he asks.

"No," the man replies.

Len is all attention and empathy. "Your world crashed down about you, and yet here you are, alive and functioning—amazing! I think you and your wife should do some bereavement sessions—maybe even work with someone skilled in Hospice work."

The man nods, looking relieved. I have just seen an example of psychotherapy woven deftly into what seemed a simple neurotherapy session.

The older man with the head injury—and the onset of Alzheimer's-like problems—is in his seventies and is accompanied by his wife. He hasn't been the same since falling down the hatchway of an oceangoing vessel; his soft head encountered lots of hard steel. Now he is clearly forgetful and distracted—and irritable. He glowers at his wife if she dares to contradict him. She is assertive enough in the session, though, sensing that the doctor wants to hear a second opinion on this somewhat refractory patient.

"He's been much better since the last treatment," this man's wife reports. "He's less forgetful, less moody. In fact," she adds, brightly, "he is less hard to be around." She looks at him, and they both sneak a look at us. The patient sits without much change in his expression but a slightly contemptuous amusement about all this "fuss" being made over him. (Here we have an instance of that familiar male attitude where "Nuthin's wrong.")

The wife has been asking her husband not to drive, because he's definitely not as "sharp" as he used to be. He's distractible, and she's scared to death he'll cause an accident. He argues back in a surly way, saying in fact, that "Nuthin's wrong."

Len looks at the man directly and says: "I don't think you should drive!"

The man looks startled, and then even grumpier: "You're on her side," he says accusingly.

"No," says Dr. Ochs, "I'm on my own side. I drive on these roads, and I really want to feel safe, thank you."

When the session ends, it does so with a trenchant jest: "Honestly, would you feel safe if the likes of you were on the road?"

The man snickers. Nothing more is said, but I later learn the therapeutic ploy was effective. The man is letting his wife, or other friends, drive. (And, come to think of it, he never would have been that flexible or compliant before the LENS treatments . . . hmm. . . .)

Len's third patient has been mercury-poisoned and, to her horror, she thinks by a family member—which only makes the problem worse, because she is trying to digest the implications of that! Since the poisoning, her immune system has run amok. Her memory, procedural and short-term, is shot. She has fibromyalgia-like symptoms and her life is awash in unaccomplished tasks. She procrastinates. She doesn't sleep well and feels tired in the morning.

Len gives her the very lightest of treatments. She says she knows she feels better after them and has noticed that she's taking a little more initiative these days, and sleeping a little better. A creative artist, she then shyly takes out a drawing based on a dream she had. It is of a key.

Len defers to me, telling this patient that I had been trained in symbolism by Joseph Campbell. The woman, highly literate, becomes animated. We have an amazing discussion about keys and locks, and what a dream like hers might open up for her. Len sits back with interest and amusement. She acknowledges that the LENS neurofeedback has been a "key" for many things locked away inside of her, and that she now is opening up to them. It is an hour-long and energy-filled session. The client leaves, grinning from ear to ear. She got her neurofeedback treatment and a little *Jungspeak* too! Her creative mind got exercised.

She carefully writes a check before leaving. I see the amount: $15. My eyes meet Len's, because we both know that his current hourly fee is well over $200. He shrugs, "I know, I know! She has no insurance, and she couldn't get this treatment any other way."

I smile at my maverick friend and love him for his inconsistencies. (Almost all the biofeedback practitioners I know chide each other for "giving away treatments" and insist that we must be professional, and be rewarded appropriately for our work, Len among them!)

Wizard though he be—and I have met his ilk before—the thing that will really tell the tale about this esoteric form of therapy is: "Is it replicable? Can other people work the magic of a gifted innovator like Len Ochs?"

The few dozen qualified and certified LENS clinicians (maybe 200 worldwide) all reply with a resounding, "Yes!" and I am very happy to say that I am one of them.

The Proof Is in the Clinical Results

The success of the method that Len Ochs had "stumbled upon" was proven recently in an overwhelmingly confirming way when, together with my colleague Kristen Harrington, I presented the results of 100 patients evaluated in the clinical setting of our Stone Mountain Center and its satellite offices to a peer group of clinicians and researchers at the annual meeting of the International Society for Neurofeedback and Research, (ISNR) held in Denver, Colorado, in September 2005. Though the presentation was scheduled at an unpopular time (8 A.M. Saturday Morning, the third day of the conference) the room was full of attendees and presenters—probably 80–100—and was very well received. It eventuated in our being asked to include it in a future issue of the *Journal of Neurotherapy* (the professional journal of the ISNR) dedicated entirely to the LENS, and a future volume on the LENS to be published by the Haworth Press (a press that specializes in neurology and brain research) sometime in 2006. A condensed version of the study is included below, edited to be understood by the general reader. In the words of our independent statistician, Susan Hicks: "These results (of the study) are a statistician's dream. Most symptom areas achieve significance below the .0001 level, which means that there is overwhelming evidence that the results are showing a true difference. The lowering of the EEG amplitudes at both CZ and HAS are both highly significant."

The Low Energy Neurofeedback System (LENS): A Study of 100 Patient Clincial Outcomes, with a Comparison to Changes in the EEG

An Abstract presented by Stephen Larsen, Ph.D., B.C.I.A.-eeg, A.I.B.T. and Kristen Harrington, M.A., L.M.F.T., A.I.B.T. (with Jodie Schultz, M.A., Tara Johanneson, B.A., and Alexandra Linardakis, B.A., A.I.B.T.)* at the ISNR (International Society for Neurofeedback and Research) Annual Meeting, Denver, Colorado, September 2005.

Abstract

One hundred patients treated with the LENS neurofeedback were evaluated for clinical improvement based on five areas of a "subjective symptom rating scale" administered at each treatment session. The five areas corresponded to the patient's self-identified most "problematical" symptoms.

---

*AIBT refers to the American Institute of Biofeedback Technologies, a professional certifying body founded by Dr. Mary Jo Sabo in New York during the 1990s. This association independently certifies most LENS practitioners. The BCIA is the Biofeedback Certification Institute of America and is associated with the professional membership body, the AAPB (Association for Applied Psychophysiology and Biofeedback). The BCIA was recently recognized as a valid certifying body for the licensure of Mental Health Practitioners in New York State. LMFT stands for "Licensed Marriage and Family Therapist."

Subject records were also examined for changes in EEG amplitude at the highest amplitude site (HAS) and the Vertex (top of the head or CZ). The Change in Subjective Symptom Averages (subjective measure) was found to be Statistically Significant at the .0001 level, as were the changes in EEG amplitude (objective measure). The changes in clinical improvement were found to be statistically correlated with the changes in amplitude. Conclusion: The LENS treatment exerts a beneficial effect on patient well-being across five preselected areas that reflect "quality of life." The LENS treatment also lowers cortical amplitudes at key sites, which is correlated with the clinical improvement and enhanced functionality.

Introduction to the Study

Over a period of five to seven years, Stone Mountain Center has collected recorded data on approximately three hundred patients who came to our clinic for neurofeedback treatment. Out of these, one hundred were selected by blinded volunteers, and on the basis of whether they met the criteria of: over ten clinical sessions, with clinical data recorded at each session; beginning and ending measurements of CZ (Vertex at center of head site) and the highest amplitude site on a LENS topographic map. Research assistants were educated in HIPAA regulations, and signed an agreement to keep any personal or clinical information regarding patients confidential.

Though most patients carried DSM IV diagnoses, our position is that these are more relevant to the purposes of the clinician or the third party reimburser. Our choice was to study five problem areas *most distressing for the patient*—in effect, *their concerns,* not our diagnostic or labeling concerns. Each one filled out the CNS Questionnaire, designed by Dr. Len Ochs (see chapter 11 of this book to reference this Questionnaire). From their responses to the CNS questionnaire, five problem areas were chosen. Patients were asked: "Which symptoms give you the greatest problems in your life, which interfere most with your freedom or creativity, which would you most like to be helped with?" They were consulted on this scale for each symptom at the beginning and end of treatment, and at each treatment session. They rated their symptoms on a "Subjective Symptom Rating Scale" (0 being no discomfort, 10 being the highest discomfort). The change in symptom severity was measured by subtracting the value of each session score from the value of the first session score. Changes in all five symptoms were also averaged together to get one final overall change score.

Setting

All sessions were done at Stone Mountain Center in New Paltz, New York, or one of three satellite or affiliate offices, in Kingston (Kristen Harrington's work), New York City, or Long Island. Maps and treatments were administered by Dr. Stephen Larsen, Kristen Harrington, or senior clinicians Alexandra Linardakis, B.A., A.I.B.T., or Carrie Chapman, B.A., A.I.B.T.

Population

The population was almost exactly evenly divided between males and females (49–51 percent) and spanned ages 6–80. Presenting problems are listed in the box below:

DSM IV-R RELATED DIAGNOSTIC CATEGORIES
REPRESENTED IN STUDY

ADD, ADHD, attentional problems of all sorts, Learning Disabilities

Affective Disorders, including Monopolar and Bipolar Depression, Dysthymia

Autistic Spectrum Disorders, including Asperger's Syndrome

Anorexia and Bulimia

Dissociation

Epilepsy and Seizure Disorder

Explosive Personality Disorder, Oppositional-Defiance Disorder

Fibromyalgia, Chronic Fatigue, Lyme Disease, Epstein-Barr Syndrome

High Blood Pressure

Headaches (Cluster, Tension, and Migraine)

Irritable Bowel Syndrome, Ulcerative Collitis

Obsessive Compulsive Disorder

Pain, acute or chronic, or both, Muscle Spasms, Dystonia

Paranoia and Schizophrenia

Post-Traumatic Stress Disorder (PTSD)

Tourette's Syndrome and Tic Disorders

Traumatic Brain and Spinal Injury (TBI)

Method

Each of the patients received ten or more sessions of the LENS (Low Energy Neurofeedback System). The goal of the treatment was a positive clinical outcome. Data was collected in this interest, and only secondarily was thought of as potentially valuable for a study. More details about the nature of the treatment are given below. Additional information can be found at www.ochslabs.com.

Some patients received other modalities, such as HeartMath, Interactive Metronome, or Psychotherapy. Some did not. Some were on psychotropic medications, some were not; no attempt was made to control for these extra variables. There was a general tendency of patients to reduce medications during treatment, either at their own initiative or with therapeutic encouragement. All were actively involved in their lives, with the chaos and unpredictability of those variables impossible to account for. Many felt that previous treatments of more conventionally available sorts had failed to address their problems and were referred to our center by psychiatrists who had placed them in the category of "difficult to treat" or "treatment failures." (Thus, in effect, the patients served as their own "control group.") There was no attempt, however, to differentiate "Difficult" patients from "Easy" patients for this study. Many of each category were included.

The only variable the 100 patients had in common was that they were mapped at the beginning—less often at the end of treatment—and received the LENS treatment more than ten times. Each treatment session was preceded by the Subjective Symptoms checklist and miniclinical interview to ascertain treatment progress.

Equipment

All LENS work was done on equipment from J&J Engineering, a West Coast biofeedback equipment manufacturer: the C-2 I-330, the mini-C-2, the GP+, the C-2+, both 6 and 12 input were used, along with Ochslabs proprietary software interfaced with two generations of operating systems: USE2 and USE3. (These are believed to have been essentially the same mechanism of operation in the LENS treatment.) It is important to note that this equipment allows for the extremely fine gradations of treatment, both in intensity and duration. *There was no attempt to standardize treatment for experimental purposes.* Intensity and duration of treatments were determined by patient's response to previous treatments, by their clinical comfort, and by therapist judgment as to the optimal treatment for the particular patient's progress.

Medium of Treatment and Description

Earlier generations of Len Ochs's neurofeedback equipment had relied on flashing lights. After a detailed examination of the equipment by Lawrence Livermore National Laboratory in the late 1990s, it was determined that radio frequencies in the 15–100 mHz band with an intensity of 10–18 watts/sq cm. were the only measurable emissions. From this time on, lights and LEDs were abandoned by most clinicians, and only the radio frequencies emitted by the crystal clock in the EEG processor were used for treatment. Treatment intensities and durations, as mentioned, were moderated to the sensitivity of the patient, but most consisted of a minimum of one second to a maximum of about 21 seconds, rarely higher, of exposure. The active stimulus is based on the dynamic *dominant frequency* of the EEG, with an added *Offset* (an antiseizure precaution) of +5, +10, +15, or +20 Hz.

Patients are seated comfortably in a chair close to the treatment console. A single ground is attached—usually to the neck or shoulder, and a reference to an ear. A single active electrode is placed at a site on the International 10–20 system, as determined by a topographic brain map, always moving from the lowest amplitudes toward the highest as treatment progresses. As many as seven sites may be treated in one treatment session for the robust patient. Sessions are usually weekly but may be as close together as 24 hours, or as far apart as several weeks.

Hypotheses to Be Confirmed Were:

I. The the LENS treatment improves quality of life for patients across a spectrum of symptom or distress areas.

II. That improvement (a drop in scores) is greater in the earliest sessions but continues throughout the treatment.

III. That there is a relationship between change in subjective response scores and change in amplitude of the highest amplitude site (HAS) or "worst" site.

IV. That there is a relationship between change in subjective scores and change in the amplitude at CZ (an arbitrarily chosen site, sometimes used in neurofeedback treatments, that correlates more poorly with improvement than the HAS).

Data Manipulation and Analysis

Data was then sent to an independent Statistician (Susan Hicks) for analysis. Results were then sent back to principal investigators (Stephen Larsen and Kristen Harrington) for analysis and presentation. The design of our study is single group, pretest/post-test. We are using t-test statistics to measure the relationship between different measures of outcome for each client: drop in severity of symptoms from first to last session, drop in frequency of symptoms from the CNS Questionnaire pretest to post-test, and drop in amplitude of CZ and each patient's highest amplitude site.

Results

Scatter plots were obtained for different symptom areas, as illustrated below in Figures 3.1a and 3.1b.

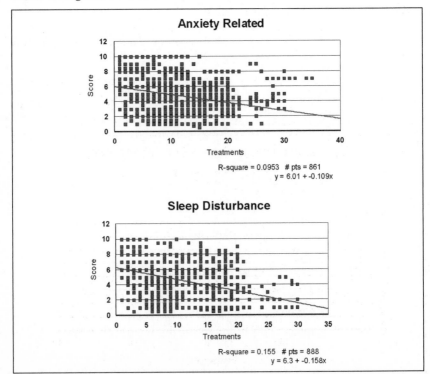

Fig. 3.1. Scatter plots for a) anxiety and b) sleep disturbance.

A statistically significant score was obtained for overall subjective response to treatment, as demonstrated by the decline in symptom severity as seen on the chart below.

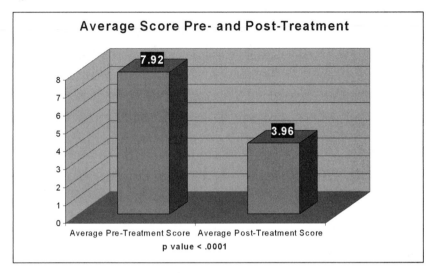

Fig. 3.2. Average Score Pre- and Post-Treatment

We were also able to calculate the drops in the amplitudes at CZ and the HAS or Highest Amplitude Site.

Average Subjective Response Scores in all categories dropped over treatments, with the greatest drop (steepest curve) found in the first five sessions. After that it begins to asymptote (grow shallower).

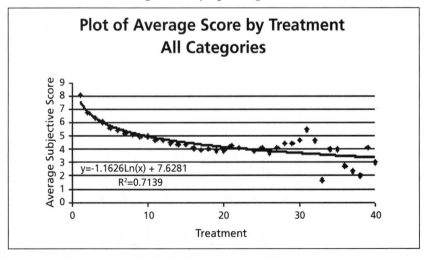

Fig. 3.3. Plot of Average Score by Treatment, All Categories

Finally, a positive and significant correlation was obtained between subjective response scores and changes in EEG amplitudes at CZ and HAS.

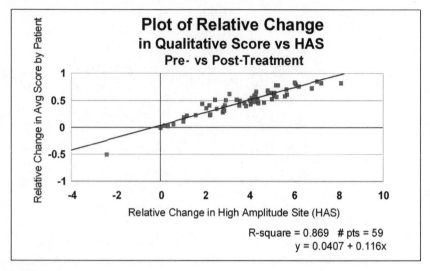

Fig. 3.4. Plot of Relative Change in Qualitative Score vs. HAS Pre- vs. Post-Treatment

Interpretation of Results

In the words of our Statistician Susan Hicks: "These (study) results are a statistician's dream. Most symptom areas achieve significance below the .0001 level, which means that there is overwhelming evidence that the results are showing a true difference. The lowering of the EEG amplitudes at both CZ and HAS are both highly significant."

Summary

The results of this $n100$ clinical outcomes study of broadly based CNS disturbances, including both "neurological" and "psychological" problems, shows overwhelming evidence that the LENS treatment is efficacious in reducing the grip of symptoms on patients, and improving their quality of life across five symptom areas of their most troublesome problems.

When it is further considered that this is an extremely gentle, non-invasive procedure, with no side effects, and in which people's overall quality of life is enhanced; this is a truly groundbreaking finding.

TRAUMATIC BRAIN INJURY (TBI) AND SPINAL INJURY AND THE LENS

Stephen Larsen, Ph.D., Mary Lee Esty, L.C.S.W., Ph.D., and Len Ochs, Ph.D.

While we know enormously more about the brain than we used to, even with PET and SPEC scans and MRI's, what we know is a drop in the bucket compared to what there is to be known. I think that people can have dysfunctions in any and every domain, with a head injury.

LEN OCHS, PH.D.

If what he [Len Ochs] is saying is true, everything we think we know about head injury is wrong.

CATHERINE WILLS, M.S.W., R.N.

You know, for years, I've been looking into Complementary and Alternative methods: Acupuncture, herbal medicine and the like—this is the only truly new thing I've seen.

DR. JOHN SPENCER, OFFICE OF ALTERNATIVE AND COMPLEMENTARY MEDICINE (A DIVISION OF THE NATIONAL INSTITUTES OF HEALTH) TALKING TO DR. MARY LEE ESTY

It should be clear by now that neurofeedback is a clinically driven enterprise. That is to say, the problems in human suffering that we are trying to solve actually invite and direct the type of inquiry and the solutions that are implemented. We think of PTSD and the Peniston alpha-theta work, epilepsy and Sterman's protocols, or ADHD and Lubar's "inhibit theta and reward SMR" protocols. Recently, at the 2003 Annual Meeting of the International Society for Neurofeedback and Research (ISNR), Margaret Ayers was honored for the importance of her work with traumatic brain injury patients.

Ayers had come into national prominence after the well-known comedian Rodney Dangerfield suffered a bad stroke and, at his wife Joan's request, Ayers was invited to try neurofeedback on him. Dangerfield had been in a coma for thirty days at that point. After several treatments he was able to awaken and consciously communicate his love to his wife before he died. Joan Dangerfield was quoted as saying that Ayers's work was "truly astounding" and that she was "forever grateful for giving me those moments."

To other clinicians, and certainly to the broader medical community, Ayers's reports may have seemed grandiose because she was claiming a 95 percent success rate of improvement with TBI victims, while also claiming these improvements to be relatively permanent. But for the specialized community of professional LENS practitioners, her results are not only believable, but familiar.

Some of these results will be presented in just a few pages but, one brief example is worth mentioning here: Ayers worked with the (helmetless) victim of a motorcycle accident who had been in a coma for seventy-seven days and who, after a course of neurofeedback treatments with her, almost completely recovered!

Ayers attributes her success to her special equipment, which has digital real-time signal processing. This signal processing works with the raw EEG (instead of the FFT or Fast Fourier Transform that most neurofeedback systems use to set training protocols to break the raw EEG into the familiar "ranges" of alpha, theta, beta, etc.). While our equipment is a bit different from Ayers's, the underlying principle and effect are quite similar.

The whole approach to traumatic brain injury that will be opened to the reader in this chapter may be unfamiliar—seeming unrealistic or even audacious. If so, it is because the dominant paradigm sees the brain as an admittedly complex electrical wiring setup with chemical overtones (those annoying but powerful neurotransmitters, and calcium and sodium channels.) If you've had a brain injury, it's like you dropped your portable radio, or cell phone. It may have to be opened and resoldered, or have parts replaced, or massive numbers of chemical ions may be needed to effect or change certain neurotransmitter channels.

But a living brain is different than a mechanical object. We know, for example that after an injury, some of those mobile little *glial* helper cells crowd like repairmen to the pertinent site to fix things, and that dendritic regrowth to compensate for injuries, even in the adult brain, is now accepted as a given by neuroscientists. But there are more far-reaching implications to the successes of the neurofeedback cases and studies you will be reading about herein.

These implications tell us much about the *entire functioning of the brain*, but in different terms than the old mechanistic paradigm. As Pribram pointed out, people don't get a chunk knocked out of their cortex and forget half the members of the family (as if each entity in our experiential world had a specific locus in the brain). But that injury may nonetheless "dim the lights" in a overall experiential sense, as the individual who has suffered the injury finds his or her perception "cloudier," their cognition working more poorly, their memory misfiring, and so on.

We will open this discussion with a look into the "grey room" that some TBI patients complain of inhabiting after incurring an injury. As they attempt to fight their way back to some semblance of normalcy, theirs is a painful process. Oftentimes their claims for insurance compensation are denied because "nothing showed up" on their MRI or CAT scan. But they themselves know, with exquisite poignancy, how diminished their functioning truly is. Their "mild traumatic brain injury" has left them with a bleak and diminished life.

Our work, and neurofeedback in general, vindicates their claims (because what our investigations reveal are impairments of *function*, not damage to *structure*). We work on their functioning, their energy, and how they *live*. Neurofeedback healing for TBIs also validates the new paradigm hovering between the thresholds of physics and physiology: This model is entirely congruent with Pribram's "holographic brain" theory, in which our consciousness is seen more as intersecting multi-dimensional wave-fronts or energy patterns. Subtle interventions, such as Ayers's short and sweet "real-time" feedback, or the absurdly tiny LENS stimulations, perturb this energy field with a small dose of its own energy and set it on a self-rectifying pattern.

As Dr. Jonathan Walker, a neurologist who has replicated most of Ayers's clinical findings, says of TBI, "Most of the time neurofeedback improves symptoms, or completely eliminates the problem. . . . There's no effective drug treatment, no effective treatment at all, except (EEG) biofeedback."[1]

TBI: The Gift That Keeps on Giving

According to The Centers for Disease Control, 260,000 people a year are hospitalized with a traumatic brain injury, and the annual costs of combined forms of care are $37 billion in direct and indirect costs. Multiple injuries are not uncommon, because after the first TBI, the risk of a second injury is three times greater than for normals, and after a second injury, the risk of a third is eight times greater.[2] After that, the rate becomes exponential. Like it or not, our wounds (the Greek *trauma* means "wound"), particularly to the brain and spinal cord, seem to multiply, repeating themselves again and again.[3]

There is remarkable agreement in the "subjective sequellae" of TBI and spinal injury. We hear of acute chronic pain, muscle spasms, mood swings, explosive disorder. Sleep is often disturbed. The perceptual world seems removed or muffled. Then there are cognitive impairments that people know they have, but have lost the ability to explain. They know things are "not right" but feel helpless to improve them. (It is amazing how subtle some people can be in their self-appraisals, even in the midst of impairment, showing that, even with all their impairments, some proprioceptive—self-discriminatory—systems are intact.) They may blunder about, forgetting appointments, getting lost, making bad business or personal choices, self-medicating in bad ways—and then be truly horrified at the ensuing chaos they have caused.

Doctors may quibble over diagnosis from a list of literal terms and descriptions that, while seemingly complex, are actually quite crude as, in the meantime, the sufferer is limping along, living in a chaotic world that "just doesn't feel right." While managed care, lawyers, and the courts stand in the role of arbiters of *what is real or not,* the individual in question lives in quiet desperation in a world only he or she knows—the subjective one, which now seems grotesquely distorted and almost impossible to communicate about.

Despite the mantle of authority worn by these tribunals, here we must invoke civil rights; the rights of the psyche, of the soul, to its own ultimate "diagnosis," or sense of what is truly right or not right in its own domain. Ultimately, no one else can intimately know one's own state, and the closest approximation we can even imagine is the discerning but empathic human witness: the clinician or therapist.

Early EEG researchers soon found that the locus of injury tended to be characterized by low frequency high-amplitude brain waves. The presence of slow waves indicates a failure of the cerebral cortex to inhibit powerful subcortical rhythmic impulses and explains the symptoms of depression, cloudiness, exhaustion, etc. Thus the basic assumption bears out: if the cortex, the "higher brain," was healthy, it would be able properly to manage the subcortical impulses—the amplitudes would drop, and the frequencies would go up. This gives rise to the idea of helping to solve the problem by speeding up the brain waves, whether by stimulant medication or by biofeedback. Neuroscience has learned an enormous amount about the brain through systematic comparisons of the impact of brain damage on changes in personality, as in the famous nineteenth-century case of Phineas Gage, (whose character and behavior, as we have mentioned earlier, seemed radically altered after a steel tamping rod was blown through his frontal lobes). Later, observations were made of people who had undergone frontal lobotomies: individuals who formerly had been models of social appropriateness had become oblivious to the most ordinary social proprieties.[4] Here we are making a case for a treatment that effects both gross, and exceedingly fine, levels of processing, and involves all of the subtleties of cognitive, affective, and even spiritual dimensions that make us truly human.

Why, in this domain of TBI above all, should "less be more?" As Ochs explains it, the "too-strong" stimulus (of whatever kind) provokes the *global defenses* that the already highly sensitized nervous system has marshaled to protect itself. This should not be so hard to understand from a medical point of view, because most of the "symptoms" that we become aware of, from fevers to allergies and other "auto-immune" disorders, are not the direct experience of a pathogen, but the body's defensive reaction to (a real or perceived) one. Some research and clinical evidence suggests that TBIs (as well as emotional traumas) can compromise the immune, digestive, and hormonal systems. As we take up later in this book, Ochs believes that the field of neurofeedback—and bio-feedback in general—needs to acknowledge and include this "sensitivity-reactivity" dimension.

LESS IS MORE: LEN OCHS ON SENSITIVITY AND REACTIVITY

As we refine our language in neurofeedback, it is really reactivity that we wish to decrease, as when a tiny insult provokes an outrageous and inter-minable response in someone, or the presence of a small amount of irritant that has no seeming effect on others causes severe allergic paroxysms in this particular individual. Sensitivity, then, in the special sense we are seek-ing to develop here, would be a positive attribute: the ability to notice, and respond appropriately to, slight differences in sensory input, subtleties, and nuances. TBI patients usually start out reactive, which by definition, and even though it seems contradictory, means "insensitive." It is always a positive sign when they become more sensitive and discerning in the latter, positive sense, and much less reactive.

Aside from Len Ochs himself, no clinician has contributed to the development of this method more than Dr. Mary Lee Esty, who prac-tices in Washington, D.C. And her specialties, as they came to evolve organically in her practice, were TBI and fibromyalgia. (Fibromyalgia is a condition of neurological depletion, exhaustion, and acute chronic pain, which is often an outcome of TBI; it is discussed later in this book.) We also present excerpts from the experimental study published in 2001 ("Flexyx Neurotherapy System in the Treatment of Traumatic Brain Injury: An Initial Evaluation")—the first of its kind that we know about—which documents the effectiveness of neurofeedback in cases of head injury. It was written in a collaboration between Esty, Schoenberger and Ochs, among others.

In the following section, Dr. Esty tells us about TBI in the same inci-sive way she has presented to many professional audiences.

Traumatic Brain Injury and Its Treatment with FNS

(The Flexyx Neurotherapy System is a forerunner of the LENS. The name changed from Flexyx to LENS in 2002.)

> *Many professional papers and presentations were condensed into the following writings. The most important of these are cited.*
> MARY LEE ESTY, L.C.S.W., PH.D.

Most people are surprised to learn that a relatively low level of force is enough to cause minimal brain dysfunction and that every mild insult that succeeds the first one has a cumulative effect on a brain's response to life's demands. Slightly slower processing and reactions times are the first effects of a mild injury, even without a loss of consciousness.

An intact skull injury is considered a "closed head injury." While sounding tame enough, closed head injuries can be quite serious, with whiplash and "contra-coup" syndrome, etc. Concussions are in levels, and clearly not all concussions are the same. The "dings" that occur in sports, the confusion following the blow to the head that made us see

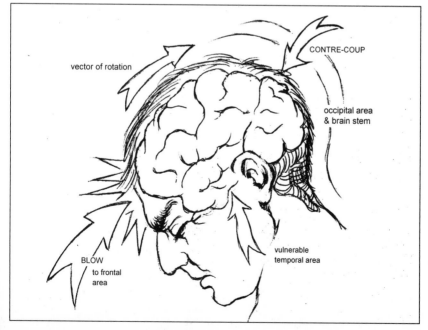

Fig. 4.1. TBI: Concussion and the Brain

stars, the "mild" rear-ending that made your glasses fall off, all have varying degrees of consequence on the physical structure of the brain and its function. The effect of these incidents becomes cumulative until that seemingly inconsequential event that becomes the tipping point as it is followed by symptoms that interfere with memory, sleep, mood, pain, and the ability to get along with people. (See the accompanying box for a clinical definition of brain injury and a discussion of concussions).

BRAIN INJURY

A Clinical Definition of Brain Injury: An insult to the brain, not of degenerative or congenital nature, caused by an external physical force that may produce a diminished or altered state of consciousness, which results in an impairment of cognitive abilities or physical functioning. It can also result in the disturbance of behavioral or emotional functioning.*

Definition of the Three Grades of Concussion:

Grade I: Concussion resulting in a short period of confusion—up to 15 minutes.

Grade II: Concussion resulting in amnesia related to the confusion without loss of consciousness—lasting more than 15 minutes.

Grade III: Loss of consciousness with post-traumatic amnesia lasting 1–24 hours, with a Glasgow Coma Scale (GCS) of 9–12 during the first 24 hours, and intracranial lesions or focal neurological deficits.[5]

---

*(Brain Injury Association, www.biausa.org)

How Common Is Brain Injury? (Or, "Surely It Hasn't Happened to Me!")

Each year 1.5 million people in the United States experience a traumatic brain injury. Fifty thousand die, and eighty thousand begin living with long-term disabilities. The remainder struggle with a puzzling array of cognitive problems, fatigue, mood problems, and difficulties in relating to others.

An eye-opening comparison with other illnesses shows the lack of public perception about the extent of TBI. In 1999, there were 176,300 cases of breast cancer, and 43,700 deaths from it. Incidence of breast cancer, multiple sclerosis, HIV/AIDS, and spinal cord injuries cases combined totaled 241,381. This number is a small fraction of the incidence of TBI; yet very little research money goes to finding treatments for TBI. There is no celebrity or poster person championing the cause of this problem, and most of us don't recognize the importance of traumas that we've had.

Most people are unaware that they have had a brain injury. For example, in a retrospective study of Canadian Football League players in 1997, 44.8 percent of them experienced concussion symptoms, but only 18.8 percent realized that they had had a concussion.[6] The following interactions demonstrate the point.

I. Mary Lee Esty Questions a Prospective Patient

Q: "Have you ever had an injury to your brain?"

A: "I fell off the roof of a two-story building when I was ten. I was unconscious for a while but was only in the hospital a few days. I guess I was okay after that; I don't really remember, but I don't think that was a brain injury. I mean, was it?"

II. Mary Lee Esty Questions a Patient with Post-Traumatic Fibromalgia

Q: "Have you ever had an injury to your brain?"

A: "I had football concussions in high school that paralyzed me—but only temporarily. Oh, I did have nine teeth knocked out with a baseball bat. Would you consider *that* a head injury? There was also a basketball incident that split my forehead open. I don't think it broke the skull, but I was unconscious for 40 minutes. When they read the MRI they said I had an inflammation of the brain stem."

Here the respondent sounds dubious. "Do you think those would be head injuries?"

You get the idea.

Clinicians working with many kinds of problems are finding that the prevalence of TBI is shockingly common. It appears that TBI is a common factor in causing major depression, and learning problems.[7]

How Does the Brain Get Hurt?

There are more TBIs than ever, due to motor vehicle accidents and falls during sport-related activities—snowmobiles, skiing, sky diving, etc. Despite the use of helmets, TBIs from bike accidents and comparable sports are on the rise, probably because people, thinking they are protected, take more risks. If helmets are worn properly, they may protect against fracture, but they give no protection whatsoever against whiplash action. (Our fragile jellylike brain is not well suited to moving rapidly through space when sudden changes of speed and direction are introduced.) Dr. Muriel Lezak describes what happens inside the skull when there is a trauma while the body is in motion:

> The key to the trauma pattern is rapid deceleration. What happens is that a driver or passenger riding in a car suddenly is hit or hits something and the car stops very rapidly. There may or may not be an impact of the head against anything. What is important is that the head that's been going along . . . at 30, 40 or more miles per hour, suddenly comes to an instant halt. The skull is stopped against a windshield or seat headrest, or the car body. Unfortunately, the contents of the skull don't stop moving because they too have been carried along at the rate of 30 or 40 miles an hour.
>
> When the skull stops, the brain—which in its natural state is kind of a gelatinous mass that floats on a slender stalk in a liquid bath—has all of the momentum of its forward motion added to the sudden impact momentum. This sends shock waves through the brain, and sets up a rotary motion of the brain within the skull. It has been demonstrated that the brain ends up being bounced around onto the bony cage of the skull as it's being forced back and forth with great rapidity. The force of the spin shears and snaps nerve fibers and tiny blood vessels. Knocking about within the skull cage bruises the vulnerable areas of the brain.
>
> Diffuse damage to these areas causes attention deficits, *slow thought processing*, and diminished bilateral integration. Slow processing in head trauma patients can be understood when likening the brain to a most enormous, elaborate computer. This computer has billions of connections and programs that run its various parts

and intermesh with each other. Then mild diffuse damage is created by someone coming along with a little hammer who knocks off a few connections here and a few connections there. When you turn on the machine . . . most of [the programs] would be slowed down, and as they become more complex, processing speed would become slower and slower. Destruction of any single connection would create something like a short circuit that would have to be bypassed and compensatory programs would have to be developed: all of this increases processing time. . . . These patients frequently cannot do two things at once; they are easily distracted from what they do, and their every action involves slowed processing.[8]

A simple whiplash results in astounding activity inside the skull. There are 2.55 million reported automobile rear-endings each year in the United States. Two-thirds of them occur at speeds of less than thirty miles per hour. Most people think of whiplash as being a possible cause of neck or back pain, but what about the inside of our heavy heads? The G-forces generated by an accident occur in four phases:

1. In the first 100 milliseconds the car moves forward from under the passenger, the torso rises causing compression, torsion, and shearing at the cellular level in the brain.
2. At 200 milliseconds the head starts back, causing shearing and compression on a macro level.
3. Between 200 and 300 microseconds after impact, the body starts forward even faster than it went backward, with the head always lagging behind.
4. The head moves forward as the seat goes back. In a collision of 20 mph, at 100 milliseconds there are 18 Gs generated in the skull; at 250 milliseconds there are 2.3 Gs; at 350 milliseconds the force is down to 1.7 Gs and, finally at 400 milliseconds, the G force is at 0.8. In less than the blink of an eye a cataclysmic event has occurred in the skull.[9]

Fibers in the brain become swollen and varicose, leaving the neurons alive but dysfunctional. If the fibers rupture, more permanent damage occurs. In mild TBI the most common damage is called Grade One Diffuse Axonal Injury, and does not result in loss of consciousness. But the physical damage it refers to is also accompanied by neurochemical changes brought about by the damage done to the physical structure of neural cells. These changes result in "paralyzed, dysfunctional brain cells that create increased vulnerability to further injury." There is a neurochemical and metabolic cascade that begins within the first hour of insult and continues for up to 10 days post-injury.

These metabolic changes create cells that are not necessarily irreversibly destroyed but are alive, although existing in a vulnerable state characterized by an increase in the demand for glucose (fuel) and a reduction in cerebral blood flow (CBF), or fuel delivery. Consequently, the neurovascular system is rendered unable to respond to demands for the energy required to return to normal neurochemical and ionic environments. Following a release of glutamate, a neurotransmitter, potassium reaches up to seven times the normal amount, creating an inability for the cell to produce an action potential, making the sodium/potassium pump dysfunctional. The result is increased metabolic stress to damaged neural tissue containing low levels of cerebral blood flow.*

Dialogue between Mary Lee Esty and Stephen Larsen at AAPB (The Association for Applied Psychophysiology and Biofeedback), Las Vegas, March 23, 2002

Stephen: Mary Lee, I want to hear the fascinating story of how you got interested in this treatment for TBI that you do so well.

Mary Lee: I got into the field of biofeedback in 1988 because I had had breast cancer many years before, and my practice included working with cancer patients, and looking for anything that would help them. That led me to read a book on the subject by Patricia Norris and to have my first experience of biofeedback and brain wave training at the Menninger Foundation (in Topeka, Kansas, where much early biofeedback was developed).

I practiced with myself first, and then I started using regular autonomic biofeedback with cancer patients, and occasionally alpha-theta work with other patients. But I really wanted a system that would have

---

*Many professional papers and presentations were condensed to provide the version for this chapter.—Editor's note.

all the autonomic measures on the same screen with the EEG, so I waited until J&J had their I-410. But I got one of the first ones, and they really hadn't finished the software yet, so I couldn't do exactly what I wanted. I mentioned my situation to someone, and they said, "Why don't you visit Len Ochs (in Walnut Creek, California)?" I was going to California quite a bit in those days, so I called him and was able to spend two days watching him treat people.

I was absolutely floored with what I saw, because in my experience people don't just get well that dramatically. It turned out Ochs was using the J&J I-400. My new computer was compatible with his software for the I-400 (the old system with the glasses and LEDs). So I took what I needed back with me and started treating myself—and kept it up for quite a while.

Now, I should give you a little personal history here. I had had a head injury when I was five. I was knocked unconscious for some time—I don't really know how long—but I very clearly remembered the events that led up to it. For months after the injury I would faint in school; a one-room country schoolhouse with seven students. When I fainted, the teacher would wrap me up in a blanket and put me over the heating register; then when I woke up I would go back to my desk. And that was just the way it worked. I remember my mother taking me to the doctor. I was tall for my age, and the doctor said, "It is just because she is growing fast." (But that was around 1943, and what could they have done anyway?)

I had always loved school but eventually decided that I wasn't really very smart, because I couldn't remember much of anything that I read. And often I found I couldn't put what I wanted to say into words. All the way through college I marveled at the people who could just say what they wanted to say—the words would just roll out. And they could read things and remember them! I couldn't do that. But I was a musician, and I could memorize music—play recitals from memory without any problem—but not the other stuff. I found ways to compensate and got through college and graduate school.

Before I went to visit Len Ochs, I had had a QEEG (quantitative EEG) done, because I was curious about my brain. The doctor who was there when we did the QEEG said, "Wow, look at this!" He showed me what he identified as the unmistakable signs on the map of an old injury.

I had never before thought that it might have had an effect on me and hadn't mentioned the old injury to anyone before this.

After my visit to Ochs I took the system home and started treating myself—and it wasn't easy, with the glasses and everything. And then, some time later, Len devised a way to do these cortical maps. So one of the very first maps done with his system was done on me. And Len's map showed similarities to the QEEG. So now I started doing the treatment differently, using his map, and following the site sort (the way all contemporary LENS treatment is done). In about three months of regular treatments I was able to function much more efficiently.

Now my memory is better in all ways. I no longer live with lists. I could not be doing what I am doing now if I hadn't done this work. And in retrospect I feel I owe Len Ochs a great deal. After a certain number of treatments I went over articles I had read and underlined previously and had absolutely no memory of what was in them, none whatsoever. And now I can read, and I can remember. It doesn't mean I don't have to reread the same thing sometimes, but I retain the most important information.

In 1998 when we started the Fibromyalgia Program at the Neurotherapy Center of Washington, a QEEG was done on me as practice for the staff. So I now had a post QEEG! Pre and post the disentrainment therapy! That's pretty good for evaluating a neurofeedback procedure. In the first QEEG, the EEG-slowing that had shown up in the delta (0–4 Hz), indicated the old injury. In the second QEEG, the EEG-slowing in delta was gone. We lined up both QEEGs and said, "Wow, look at this!" We readjusted the data to compensate the differences in the QEEG and made comparable copies. And there are the changes, right on the map. You know, I don't think we have many of those so far—a QEEG done pre and post the FNS treatment—it's really revealing.

Stephen: And how did you then begin to work clinically with the FNS?

Mary Lee: I began to use FNS with clients, some of whom were my regular "biofeedback along with psychotherapy" people. Some of them were people who just needed a lot of ongoing support. I would say, "You know, there's this new treatment procedure I'd like you to try. It's experimental but promising." And then I would give them a few of the FNS sessions. And amazing things started happening to people, people who had seemed forever stuck, changed.

Stephen: Do you have some treatment stories?

Mary Lee: The stories are wonderful. One person who comes to mind always called herself an "outlaw," which was a good description. She never had had a healthy relationship in her life. A risk-taker, she rather reveled in being different. This woman had been through the gamut of traditional therapies, without much benefit, and she seemed stuck with what I had been doing. Now, I didn't expect the changes that the FNS made in her. After about three months being treated with it, she was really changing in all kinds of ways; and, my goodness, she somehow got into a healthy relationship. Soon she threw herself into graduate studies, and got on with her life. I think she has probably finished her Ph.D. now. Interesting outlaw.

Then there was a fellow who had been hit by a car. Following the accident he had PTSD and migraine headaches, along with acute chronic pain. The pain in his head and face were so severe that Johns Hopkins Hospital surgeons had actually cut the trigeminal nerve (an irreversible operation on one of the ten cranial nerves, often done in cases of extreme pain). The surgery didn't do much more than all the medicines that he had tried. At the time we began seeing him, he was on morphine. When we started with the FNS, the pain levels went way down after just a few treatments. I mean, it was astonishing! A few seconds of actual treatment with "the lights," each week for several weeks and he was suddenly a lot better. And not only the pain, but many other things in his life were better—sleep, mood, energy.

Through other work I had done over the years, I knew Dr. Adrienne Fugh-Burman, who is one of the founders of the National Woman's Health Network. At that time she was doing some work at the (then) Office of Alternative Medicine. I thought, this treatment is something these folks really might be interested in. So I called Adrienne and told her what I was doing. She got me in touch with Dr. John Spencer, who was on the staff at Office of Alternative Medicine, and had a background in biofeedback—particularly EEG studies that had been done with rats at the University of Chicago. Dr. Spencer seemed interested at first and agreed to come out to see us. Then he got very crisp and said, "Well, I have exactly two hours I can stay, and I will arrive at such and such a time."

"Uh-oh," I thought.

So I set up patients who were willing to talk with him about their experiences. Dr. Spencer came at the appointed time, and I think watched three patients while we ran sessions. And then he would interview them. Well, he ended up staying four hours, and when he left, he said, "You know, we are supporting all kinds of research that people are calling alternative and new: homeopathy, yoga, massage, and acupuncture. Those things are ancient. This is the only truly new thing I have seen!"

A year passed and I was wondering if anything would ever come of it, when I got a call from Dr. Nancy Schoenberger from Kessler Rehabilitation Institute in New Jersey.

Stephen: Isn't that where Christopher Reeve was?

Mary Lee: Yes. They did a lot of work with him. Nancy asked, "Will you accept an NIH (National Institute of Health) grant to do a study with traumatic brain injury?" It seems Dr. Spencer had actually been working on this for a year. You know, there was a point at which the Office of Alternative Medicine had decided to set up clinical research centers around the country to specialize in certain things, and Kessler was the one designated for brain injury, stroke, and spinal cord.

So that became the study cited below, the results of which were really very good.

A Controlled Study Involving FNS and Traumatic Brain Injury

In 2001, a paper entitled "Flexyx Neurotherapy System in the Treatment of Traumatic Brain Injury: An Initial Evaluation" was published in the *Journal of Head Trauma Rehabilitation (16, no. 3 [2001]):260–374)*. The director of the project was Nancy E. Schoenberger, Ph.D., and included Samuel C. Siflett, Ph.D., Mary Lee Esty, L.C.S.W., Ph.D., Len Ochs, Ph.D., and Robert J. Matheis, M.A.

A summary of the paper says:

> *Objective:* To conduct a preliminary experimental evaluation of the potential efficacy of Flexyx Neurotherapy System, FNS, an innovative electroencephalography (EEG)-based therapy used clinically in the treatment of traumatic brain injury (TBI).

Participants: Twelve people aged 21 to 53 who had experienced mild to moderately severe closed head injury at least 12 months previously and who reported substantial cognitive difficulties after injury which interfered with their functioning.

Design: Participants were randomly assigned to an immediate treatment group or a wait-list control group and received 25 sessions of FNS treatment. They were assessed at pretreatment, posttreatment, and follow-up with standardized neuropsychological and mood measures.

Results: Comparison of the two groups on outcome measures indicated improvement after treatment for participants' reports of depression, fatigue, and other problematic symptoms, as well as for some measures of cognitive functioning. Most participants experienced meaningful improvement in occupational and social functioning.

Conclusion: On the basis of these results, FNS appears to be a promising new therapy for TBI and merits more extensive evaluation.

While the researchers describe this study as "preliminary" they conclude that the results are promising enough to warrant further research involving larger groups, placebo, and double-blind controls. They mention something that has occurred to many other clinicians: That FNS, by virtue of the fact that the subject sits with closed eyes, and that voluntary or aware behaviors are not involved in the treatment, lends itself exquisitely to this type of research design—unlike other form of biofeedback in which subjects very quickly figure out whether they are in the experimental or control group—that is, whether their efforts are producing any immediate result whatever. Further, since most clinicians are in the business of helping people rather than justifying the validity of the method, they have tended to focus on treatment rather than experimentation. (Most clinicians have absolutely no doubt the method works, the only questions are "how soon" and "how well"—there being a sizable gamut of individual reactions to the treatment.)

Brain and Spinal Cord Injuries at Stone Mountain

I had been skeptical whether or not FNS would or could work with spinal cord injury as well as closed head injury. Then I encountered Sharon, Peter, and Jim. Their cases were first presented in a paper I wrote on traumatic brain injury, presented at the Winter Brain Conference in Miami, Florida in 2002.

Sharon Overcomes Her Head Injuries

When I first met Sharon, about twelve years ago, she was a returning student in her late twenties at the college where I was teaching. After her first semester of psychology, I thought, "This is the most highly motivated, most ADD, adult student I have ever had." Intelligent and clearly of a good heart, she nonetheless misplaced all homework assignments, had to be given them again, forgot to do term papers, showed up at the wrong time for the final, etc. And yet she seemed very motivated—a paradox.

What I did not know then, was that Sharon had had three terrible head injuries before that time. In the first, just after high school, at age seventeen, she had been mugged with a baseball bat while walking through a "safe" part of San Francisco. She had been unconscious for a while, found by strangers, and taken to the hospital where she was deemed to have a concussion.

Sharon wasn't "quite herself" after that and noticed that her daily skills and her ability "to keep track of things" had withered. A couple of years later, she was in an auto accident where her head smashed into the windshield. After that, Sharon was riding a bicycle when she was hit by a car from behind. Bystanders were certain she must have been killed, so bad was the accident in which she sustained a number of fractures and injured her head and spinal cord again. (All these accidents had predated the time that she was my student.)

Unfortunately, Sharon was now to have a fourth head injury, the one that resulted in her coming to us for clinical treatment. And while this injury was the one that seemed to put her "over the line" in some way, it was the only one in which she had had some measure of control. She was driving on a winding country road and either dozed off or spaced out, for the next thing she knew her car was rolling over and over through a field and some woods. Though she ended up hanging in her seat belt, she hit her head on the roof during the pinwheeling. When she finally got out of the straps, she wandered off through the dark November woods without the vaguest idea of where she was going, or even who she was.

Of course the local hospital did some kind of cursory evaluation, said they couldn't find anything wrong, and told her that she could go home—which she still didn't know how to find. A friend had to come and pick her up.

A terrible time began for Sharon then. She was separated from her husband, and trying to raise a ten-year-old boy by herself. She had had a successful massage practice with a good clientele and many friends. Within months she lost it all. She could not keep track of appointments, in fact literally "disappointing" many of her clients and friends. Even her most ordinary coping skills seemed to have gone by the wayside, and she ended up penniless and living on total disability; a small monthly stipend from Social Security.

Sharon had been in that condition for a couple of years when she thought about returning to school. She had been given an "incomplete" in her Psychology of Consciousness course, which automatically turned to an "F" after one semester. (I knew she had taken the course some time ago.) She hated having the F on her record and asked if she could complete the course, which I agreed to. I looked up her records and then called Sharon and told her that hers would be the longest "incomplete" duration that I had ever turned into a grade (ten years).

By this time, I had already retired from the college to focus on my private practice and writing projects (but as Professor Emeritus, I still retained a few academic duties, including the ability to change grades). The reason for Sharon's "incomplete" was that she had failed to complete a requisite psychological journal, so I told her that she would have to turn in the missing journal, or come and see me for biofeedback work and thus recreate the journal, which she agreed to.

A map of Sharon's brain (see page four of the color insert) showed areas of frontal delta and very high occipital alpha consistent with some head and spinal cord injuries. The amplitudes were in the 20–40μv range, with high standard deviations, implying serious cortical instability. In making the maps in those days there were four seconds of observation with one second of stimulation—the evoked potential—built in. As we hit her F4 brain site (the right frontal region) she cried aloud as the one second of stimulation came on. "What's the matter?" I asked.

"I'm hanging upside down in my seat belt! I've just hit my head," she replied. *She was reliving her most recent accident,* of which she had previously had no conscious memory!

This site can be seen as a little "bulls-eye" or hot spot in the delta range on map #1. This constituted the focal area of her main frontal problem, and as we can see on map #2, after about seven months of treatment, it had completely disappeared.

Sharon proved, unlike many multiple head-injured patients, to be very robust and able to tolerate higher levels of treatment, so in twice-weekly sessions we were able to accomplish quite a bit. Slower to yield, however, was the high amplitude alpha, which seemed to originate occipitally as is typical, but perfused or spread over the parietal and into the central and frontal areas in Sharon's case. This may show a familial ADD—which her son also has—but in these high amplitudes may be indicative of spinal cord injury also. Indeed, when treatment began, Sharon had been in extreme pain, which was localized in the neck and shoulders.

Several times, to the astonishment of both Sharon and myself, as we treated one of her sites with just a few seconds of stimulation, her neck would "adjust itself" with a little clicking sound, as if an invisible chiropractor were in attendance, and then she would "feel much better." Sometimes incipient headaches were averted by the treatments.

One of the first areas to regulate itself with Sharon was sleep disturbance. Before treatment, her circadian cycle seemed all "messed up." As she said, she was half-asleep all day and awake all night. Now it was also "readjusting" itself. Her mood improved and she no longer felt suicidal; her energy began to come back. Friends noticed her improvement and told her so. She found she was able to remember more and more things and pulled an "A" in one of her college courses.

Sharon had always had abilities some people would describe as "paranormal." She would see or know things before they happened. As a masseuse, she could zero right in on a patient's problem area, and then tell the patient accurate information about the psychic wound or problem associated with it. When she was at her worst, after her last injury, these faculties had turned bad. She felt "spells" were being put on her, and she was suspicious of people. She had several encounters with entities that felt to her like evil spirits. She said she could hear other's thoughts, but they would be jumbled, intrusive, or malevolent.

With the FNS treatment, Sharon's psychic abilities "settled down" and became more sedate—and, she felt, accurate once more. Her dreams became less turbulent and seemed to include wisdom or guidance dreams. She made good progress in both psychotherapy and also as a valued member of a dream group at our center. She accompanied a tour to Guatemala to work with shamans and indigenous healers, and at times showed abilities rivaling or eclipsing those of the shamans. Without speaking Spanish, she did some independent traveling all over the country and seemed to get along quite well.

This past year Sharon was able to help her learning-disabled son improve his scores in college classes and help him with his research papers. She feels that her cognitive abilities, short-term memory, and focus have all improved.

"There is a room," she said in a videotaped interview, "where people who have had head injuries go. The real world seems very shadowy, very remote, and unreal. When you meet someone else who has been there, you recognize them. I am so glad I'm not in that room anymore!"

Peter: The Wounded Warrior
(Original version of this story presented at 1998 Winter Brain Conference, Palm Springs)[10]
One of our earliest patients at Stone Mountain Center, in 1996, after we began with the Flexyx equipment, was a Vietnam Vet whose worst injury was actually a postwar industrial accident—a thirty foot fall to a concrete floor that shattered his heel and broke his spine in several places. Though he was on about a dozen painkillers and antidepressants, Peter had been in excruciating pain for nine years before he came to our center. He had become a local legend.

After nine years of pain Peter had finally decided to do himself in with a shotgun and, to avert this, his desperate wife called the police. When they arrived, Peter ran out the back door of the trailer into the woods, where he easily eluded police. Finally realizing that a chase was pointless, he decided to give himself up but asked the officers not to restrain him because of his traumatic wartime experience. At first the police seemed to honor Peter's request, but then they pounced on him—

which turned out to have been a bad idea! So, in short order, there were five or six policemen in the emergency room along with Peter. The event made the papers, once more bringing the precarious fate of Vietnam Vets home to the local community.

When Peter came to see us a few months after that event, he arrived on crutches, driven by his wife (and wearing his green beret!). Within two months of twice-weekly treatments, the foot and spinal pain had abated, and he was walking with a cane. Within three months, he was able to drive himself the twelve miles to the therapy center, and travel places alone. His mood swings had also stabilized. He dug in more deeply to the process of psychotherapy and let out some of his pain. His marriage came out of crisis.

Soon Peter was walking unassisted, and contemplating a more active lifestyle, and maybe even taking on some part-time work (after a decade of total disability). Even his stolid neurologist allowed himself a little bit of awe.

The Case of Jim: Climbing Higher

Jim was a skilled rock-climbing guide with an excellent reputation who, while off duty and putting in a difficult "new route," had taken a "leader fall" and fractured his lumbar spine. With the injury he lost the use of, and feeling in, his legs. He had to be catheterized to urinate and never knew when a bowel movement was looming. Jim was told he would never walk again. He was essentially paraplegic.

The neurofeedback map showed the high and spiky occipital alpha that we sometimes see in spinal injuries. Early sessions seemed to work quickly to stabilize Jim's mood swings and eased the awful depression that had gotten steadily worse since the accident. (Jim had felt an overwhelming loss of personal power and mobility.) He began to get a little more energy.

On the thirteenth session, Jim jumped visibly in his chair as the stimulation was applied to what turned out to be one of his key sites. When asked what had happened, Jim said, "It felt like a bolt shot up my spine!—like electricity, or energy of some kind!" That very week, feeling began to come back into Jim's legs. After two more treatments (1 per week) he was getting the sensation that he needed to urinate, and in a few more sessions he began to redevelop urinary and bowel control; he could bear down and urinate. Hence, the catheter was used less often.

On his last day of treatment (under twenty sessions), Jim was able to walk down the hall and into the session unassisted and without crutches. Three years after his treatments had ended, I asked Jim to guide me, along with a half-dozen "youth at risk," on a rock climb. He hiked the half-mile or so in to the cliff with a heavy pack, climbed up to fix ropes, rappelled all over the rock, and expertly guided the young people. Jim had recovered about three-quarters of his original prowess.

Neurologists have tended to pooh-pooh these kind of results, claiming they must have been due to placebo or suggestion or are "not really possible," as one neurologist told me at a national conference where I presented the case. (So I told him I would order Jim immediately to begin catheterizing himself again, and get back on those crutches.) But all one has to do is talk to the clients to verify the reality of these stories.

A Dialogue with Len Ochs on TBI, November 2000

So from my point of view, most of these problems are relatively insignificant, that is, insignificant in terms of what is actually causing the problem. And yet a person's life may be destroyed by such an "insignificant" problem. It is almost like at rush-hour when traffic is leaving the city. If a car in a major intersection has a flat tire, that whole quadrant of the city can become paralyzed completely. That is an example of an insignificant problem causing widespread consequences. . . .

Len Ochs, Ph.D.

Stephen: I'm puzzled about TBI. Before I had worked with it clinically, I thought it was a dead end, a one way street, "Lights out!" But from you I've learned it may be one of the most responsive syndromes to work with.

Len: It depends on how functional people were before their injury. If they were previously high-functioning, it makes them easiest to work with, because they have the most resources. If someone has had a chronic problem all their life and never really functioned that well, and they come in showing the behaviors that they have lived with their entire life, that is different from someone who was functioning well, and all of a sudden suffered a severe degradation in functioning.

But it is true sometimes these folks seem *so bad*, and sometimes they have almost nothing, no memory of ever having functioned any better. I remember one woman who was referred to me, by a head injury specialist, as being a "borderline"* patient. Before becoming a head injury specialist, this referring doctor had been a psychiatrist—and he was pretty sure about his diagnosis.

The woman Madge (who had been referred to us) was hypersensitive, hyperreactive, and had this irritating way about her that people couldn't take. She drove her husband crazy and was driving people crazy at work as well. Everyone was walking on eggshells around her, afraid of offending her, or getting into fights with each other due to things she had done or said to each of them. Madge's behavior was typical of a borderline personality.

I treated her pretty steadily for about a week, and at the end of that time, strangely, she had a brief period of hypersexuality. She was chasing her husband all around the house! "Well, *that* wasn't happening before!" Both she and her husband were rather delighted with this side effect—or whatever you want to call it. But strangely, all that other irritating interpersonal stuff had stopped—pretty suddenly.

I said to her: "You know, you have shown progress that is very unlike progress shown by other borderline patients. They don't change as rapidly and dramatically as you did. Did you ever have a head injury?"

"Nope," she said. "I used to break horses when I was an adolescent, and I was thrown many times, and I broke my collarbone several times, but no, I never had a head injury."

And I said, "Can you tell me how you broke your collarbone falling from a horse and did not hit your head?"

"Oh," she said. "I guess I can't say that, can I?"

So *my* guess is that even her doctor, head-injury specialist though he was, saw her through his psychiatrist's glasses, and never changed his view of her as having had potential head injuries in the background

---

*"Borderline" is known in the literature as being associated with dissociated ideas, emotional manipulation, and brief, intense attachments. Halfway between psychosis and character disorder, it has a treatment-resistant reputation.

that could bear on her symptoms. So here we have a patient who was diagnosed psychiatrically but who, in fact, was actually a head-injured patient.

Stephen: What an instructive case! Can you say more about how head injuries seem to come across as character disorders?

Len: Well, it is incredible to me they don't all do that, but they don't. While we know enormously more about the brain than we used to, even with PET and SPEC scans and MRIs, *what we know is a drop in the bucket compared to what there is to be known.* I think that people can have dysfunctions in any and every domain, with a head injury. Or even from a brain virus.

Once some idiosyncratic kind of trauma happens to the brain and/ or spinal cord, any conceivable set of symptoms is possible. They tend to cluster around short-term memory problems, cognitive dysfunctions and mood instability, explosiveness and depression, but I have even seen immunological problems that are due to head injury. The key thing here is that very few clinicians have systematic accurate ways of probing the presence or absence of a head injury in a case history. They'll ask, "Did you ever have a head injury?" Invariably the answer will be "No."

Few probe much further: "Well, then, did you ever have a bump on the head?"

I remember one sixteen-year-old boy whose mother called me up. She was kind of halting in her speech and seemed almost embarrassed: "My son ran into a tree and broke his collarbone while skiing in the Sierras. He's been working with a psychiatrist for several years, and I just signed up for him to do psychotherapy for two more years, and two more years of medication, and he has got these symptoms. . . ."

And I said, "Wait a minute, don't say any more. Let me go down a list of symptoms." So I went down a list of about eight symptoms, and she was astonished: "How did you know?" Then she said: "Can you do anything about it?"

I said, "We do this work every day."

She said, "Well, how can it be that no one knew about you, and no one else knew about these problems (as a cluster)?"

I said, "I don't know."

She was conflicted about what to do, because she had just signed up for a two-year plan with the medication and all, and she didn't want to go against the psychiatrist.

So I said, "Well, you let me know when you make up your mind."

Well, she did finally bring her son in. The chief complaint was that, while he had always had a temper problem, now when he became violent, he was no longer responsive to his parents. His eyes would not focus, and he would just hammer at them and at anything around him. Actually it was like he went into some kind of seizure problem from which he could not withdraw until things quieted down.

He was young and still functioning fairly well in school, no outstanding scholar, but he was doing okay. I said, "For someone who has been functioning well, it generally takes six sessions to set things right, but in this case, maybe fourteen or fifteen sessions are required."

Well, time went on, but he was not changing and was not changing and was not changing. The parents brought him in every day. They traveled two hours each day to get to me. Then it was on into the third week—come to think of it, probably the fourteenth or fifteenth session—and everything clicked into place.

He was just much better, in most ways. I later got reports that his aunts and uncles would see him at a party, and say, "What happened to him?" He is much better now than he ever was. His temper is nowhere near what it was after the head injury, and possibly even less than he had before the problem, and his academics have improved as well.

Stephen: How would you account for the fact that it doesn't work and doesn't work and then wow!—it works?

Len: In this case it was probably due to this young man's temper problem. In other words, he had a preexisting violent streak that was amplified by the head injury. In treating the injury, the underlying physiology was also apparently treated.

Stephen: In a generic sense then, when people fail to improve, are we possibly talking about the existence of an underlying endogenous problem of some kind?

Len: Probably, or we could just be using the wrong approach, or it could be the approach is being used in an incorrect way. Even though, at this point, we have eleven years of experience with the LENS—it is still clear that it's not for everyone. *It really works best with the clusters of symptoms that show the whole CNS is disorganized.* And it really can address *pervasive subtle problems.* Because the more problems and subproblems a person has, the more things are probably wrong in the brain; and the easier it is to effect them globally. On the other hand, a single problem may not respond at all.

I wanted to say something about things going wrong in the brain, and the whole idea of brain damage. When some very knowledgeable people heard me talk about some of these results, and really let it in, they said, in one way or another, "Gee, maybe everything I know about head injury and brain damage is wrong." Most people physiologize brain damage, they structuralize it and say there is a problem with the *hardware* of the brain. So when we get these results, they start thinking: "Can this *procedure* resurrect dead brain tissue? What is going on here?"

The medical community especially sees brain damage as hard damage, *structural* damage. But obviously from some of the results we've been getting, there are many cases where the problem is *functional.* When problems seem to resolve themselves in a couple of days or a week, I think something else is happening.

Let me propose a question: "How do the signals (of the LENS treatment) know where to go in the brain, and how do they know what to fix?" And the answer is something like "Drano" being put into a drain. It doesn't know, in advance, where the block is. It goes through whatever channel is there, until it runs into a block, and then it works on the block to remove it. And I see this process operating in the same way. I see the energy of the treatment activating the channels over which impulses travel in the brain; and when this energy from the system encounters a neurochemical defense or a block, it basically goes through or gets rid of that block.

Postscript on TBI, pathology, and the anomalous: Given the multitudinous behavioral observations of people with lesions, chemical insults, etc., or those who have suffered a stroke, there can be absolutely no doubt that psychology and neurology are all tangled up in the human condition. Traumatic brain injury is indeed the "chameleon" of psychopathologies and can masquerade as fatigue, depression, anxiety, cognitive decline, mania, even character disorders. The fact must now be faced, even as it often was in the early days of psychiatry, that to psychoanalyze, or even undertake behavior-modification with people who are organically injured, may be not only "beside the point" but downright unethical, as it can distract people from the real underlying problem. Furthermore, prescription medications or such procedures as ECT can cloud and muddy the picture, making it almost impossible to ferret out the original cause of a problem, and discern where a cure may lie.

The cases presented by Ochs and Esty show that a mixture of a TBI and therapeutic or psychiatric fundamentalism can lead people down some very nasty cul-de-sacs. Head injuries need to be included in our diagnostic lexicon, and their chameleon-like nature studied further. A future time may come when it will be considered unethical practice *not* to probe skillfully for a history of TBI, nor do a QEEG or other form of brain map, as well as other neurodiagnostics before beginning a regimen of medication—or of psychotherapy.

5

HEALING THE MIND OF CHILDHOOD

Cerebral Palsy, Reactive Attachment Disorder,
Autism, Asperger's Syndrome, ADD/ADHD,
and Learning Disabilities

Sarah Franek, M.T.P., Stephen Larsen, Ph.D., Theresa Yonker, M.D.,
Curtis Cripe, Ph.D., Mary Lee Esty, L.C.S.W., Ph.D.,
and Len Ochs, Ph.D.

Why does my brain come in colors?

FOUR-YEAR-OLD PAUL (ON FIRST SEEING
HIS BRAIN MAP)

I write these words with goose bumps at the changes the FNS
(the LENS) has made in a little girl's life!

SARAH FRANEK, M.T.P.,
NEUROFEEDBACK PRACTITIONER

This chapter explores one of the most rewarding aspects of neurofeedback: working with children. In it, we discuss treatment with children
as young as six months, all the way through childhood and puberty to
the later teenage years. Conventional biofeedback and neurofeedback
practitioners have often reported that "children are our best clients."
Not only do they have more "neural plasticity" and are less habituated
in their ways, they do love pac-man; and the idea of "playing a computer
with my mind" is especially appealing to today's generation of young-
sters who took in science fiction with their mother's milk.

We have found that children respond beautifully, and artlessly, to the
LENS. To be sure, with seriously autistic, pervasively delayed, or wildly

oppositional children, it may be hard to get them to sit still in a chair for a few minutes and have the sensors attached. Small children can sometimes sit in their parents' lap and be gently held while the wires are attached. The offset, however, where they must sit still with eyes closed for ten minutes, is much too much for some children, including older or impulsive ones with attention deficit and/or hyperactivity. In these cases, we just automatically go to an offset of +20, the most gentle, and start with just a single brain site or two at one second of stimulation per site.

Time and time again, we have found that these kids are more compliant by the second or third treatment. Sometimes we can't get an autistic child to shut their eyes (as required for most treatments to have a quieter, more uniform brain wave to work with) for even a second at a time. And yet, the treatment seems to work even with the patient's eyes open and their limbs flailing. (I have trained my clinicians to do these kinds of treatments manually, so that the second of stim is delivered when the raw EEG is the cleanest—that is, free from the gross artifacts of muscular movement or eye-blinking.) By the third or fourth treatment we have often found a hyperactive kid who was virtually upside-down and wiggling furiously in the first session, to be sitting up politely for us to attach the sensors, like a proper little man, and evincing intelligent curiosity about the treatment and just what is going on.

Diagnostic categories included in this chapter on children include:

- The Autistic Spectrum, in which children seem locked into a private reality. This section also includes Asperger's Syndrome, a highly functioning type of Autism sometimes called the "little professor" syndrome.
- ADD or Attention Deficit Disorder, which may include several sub-categories such as the Hyperactive type (ADHD) or the Inattentive type.
- Cerebral Palsy, which often involves some kind of perinatal pre-birth damage that effects the nervous system, and may involve many levels of cognitive, neuromuscular, behavioral retardation that is also associated with:
- Pervasive Developmental Disorder or PDD, in which children fail to reach developmental milestones or to keep up with their peers in the ordinary stages of psychomotor development.

- The Abused, Abandoned, or Neglected Child. In its more extreme form, with young children, this goes by the name of Reactive Attachment Disorder (RAD).

These categories may also overlap with:

- The Traumatized Child due to war, flooding, 9/11 type events, which may have serious symptoms such as recurrent nightmares or night terrors, or dissociation.
- The Anxious Child, including those displaying panic attacks and OCD (Obsessive-Compulsive Disorder), where the child can only feel okay with compulsively repeated rituals, done seemingly to avoid something bad from happening.
- Oppositional Defiance, in which there may be great difficulty in finding out what the child wants, but it is decidedly the opposite of what the parent—or any adult—wants. This may shade into:
- Explosive children, with or without seizure disorders. (See the case of Alex in this chapter). This may be not infrequently mingled with other problems such as attentional problems or:
- Learning Disabilities, including dyslexia, aphasias, or nonverbal learning disorders. (While there are not so many examples of these in this chapter, this category of problems responds very well to the LENS.)

We usually tell parents that we do not hold out a *cure* for their child's problem. We may, however, help their children to become more flexible, adaptable, and to learn better. When the LENS technique is fully explained to parents, they usually like the idea that we do not try to "micromanage" their child's brain, and neither drug nor brainwash them. Unlike protocols that either deliberately attempt to speed up or slow down the EEG, the LENS lets the child's brain itself do its own regulating—and both parents and children are usually happy with the outcome. After all, it's really nice *just to be yourself*, more gracefully, and more easily.

The LENS is uniquely suited to infants and very young children because of its passive nature. There is nothing that needs to be understood, or even communicated verbally to the child, no "training protocol." In fact, it is quite wonderful to be able to say that there is *no activity for the child to either succeed or fail at*. This makes it the neurofeedback *par excellence* for these very young patients whose diagnostic categories normally have been thought of as being very difficult to treat, but which have what is clearly a neurological basis, such as in the case of Autism or Cerebral Palsy.

Also, as you will see in some of the cases presented, over a complete course of treatment, the LENS can be combined with traditional neuro-feedback, HeartMath, Interactive Metronome, a technique which helps children and adults fine tune their CNS sense of timing, expressive arts such as clay, painting or sandplay, as well as other cognitive and behavioral approaches.

Sarah Franek's Work With Cerebral Palsy and TBI

Sarah Franek, M.T.P., is a twenty-eight-year-old clinician who was trained by Len Ochs, Stephen Larsen, and Jim Giorgi. For over three years Sarah was the main clinician at Stone Mountain's satellite office in New York City.

The following is a general report that Sarah wrote in March of 2001 on her work with four children, which spanned a period of about a year from 2000–2001.

Sarah's Report
SARAH FRANEK, M.T.P.

I am currently treating four children under four years of age who have varying degrees of Cerebral Palsy or Cerebral Palsy-like symptoms. The cases of George and Jessica, in particular, will be discussed in detail. All four children are thriving with FNS (precursor of the LENS). To be sure, the children are, with the support and guidance of their parents, doing other things like speech and physical therapy, acupuncture, and Felden-krais, which uses gentle muscular movements to reprogram the brain and CNS, so it is hard to know to which treatment modality to attribute some of their truly remarkable gains. Most parents and the other practitioners seemed to feel that the progress was due to a combination of the healing modalities, but that the FNS had definite effects—accelerating their child's progress toward their developmental milestones.

Three out of the four were "difficult eaters," and were underweight before we began. They have all experienced significant increases in their appetites and are gaining weight. Reported changes in general are:

increased energy, more core strength, increased motor coordination, improved speech, the ability to pick up new skills more quickly, more responsiveness and interaction with the family, eyes less convergent or "cross-eyed," and calmer behavior. Those who, in the beginning, were not sitting are now sitting for five to ten minutes at a time. Those who were not walking are now "couch-cruising." Those who were not crawling are now crawling a little bit.

It is interesting to note how the various holistic practitioners have responded to the introduction of FNS to their treatment regimens. All therapists report that the FNS gives them "more to work with," that is, the children are more amenable to their particular form of therapy and the learnings associated with them. A few occupational therapists were so struck by the changes in their child patients that they videotaped them. Even pediatricians remarked that some of the children were markedly improved, while reserving judgment as to the cause. One school official added the designation "gifted" to what had previously been simply "developmentally delayed," after FNS elicited what seemed like a sudden learning burst in one child.

The Case of George: Brain Injured at Birth
SARAH FRANEK, M.T.P.

Little George was first brought in for treatment in December of 2000 at two years of age. During a long and difficult labor, an overly enthusiastic obstetrician had fractured his skull in two places in an attempted high forceps delivery—before a Caesarian-section was finally done on the exhausted mother. But George appeared to have died in the ordeal and had to be resuscitated. The heart rate on the fetal monitor had shown only 54 beats per minute during the botched delivery—very slow for a healthy fetus, which should have been twice that at times—and George was deemed to probably have brain anoxia (damage caused by oxygen deprivation).

George was in the Intensive Care Unit (ICU) of the hospital for thirty days. The clumsy obstetrician was subsequently fired, and his license to practice revoked—but that didn't help George a bit; he had emerged from the difficult birth massively developmentally disabled.

At the time he was brought in to our New York office, two-year-old George was passive. His muscle coordination was poor. At times he was stiff and rigid. He could neither stand, nor sit, nor walk. His eyes were convergent. The right side of his body was more inert than the left side and he was rarely able to use his right hand. His feet and legs were turned out. George had been doing Feldenkrais for a year and had undergone speech therapy, acupuncture, and cranio-sacral stimulation. His personality was generally positive and upbeat, although he suffered terrible separation anxiety when his parents would leave the room.

The first brain map was done over two sessions so as to not overdose or strain the child. (There was not yet a no-stimulation map available.) Eight regular treatment sessions were then conducted, following the site sort, and then George was mapped again. This time the map was done over four sessions, as he seemed increasingly sensitive to the process. (The mapping procedure itself can have lo-stim treatment effects in the very sensitive client.)

The mapping was done with the J&J C-2 EEG processor, no glasses, and using only the RF stim. (The reader will remember from chapter 3 how the Livermore Lab showed that radio frequencies (RF) not light, was the probable agency of treatment.) All leads were wrapped with radio frequency filters. (We did not have the "offset protocol" at our office at that time, so the treatment was done at two leading frequencies: +5 and +10. We typically accessed four brain sites a session, with six seconds at each leading frequency. Then we dropped to four seconds at the same offsets, then dropped again to two seconds twice at +5—because of the sensitivity factor.

Following this regimen of FNS treatments, the following changes were noted by George's mother and some of the other practitioners that worked with him: He began to make longer and louder vocalizations. His diaphragm was noted to be stronger. He was able to cross his arms, and hold and manipulate a ball with some dexterity. He had improved energy and became more capable of sitting up by himself; finally he could sit for about five minutes. Muscularly he was not as stiff and rigid. His appetite improved and he gained weight.

Over time, George's feet seemed less turned out, and he used his tongue more. He began to use his right hand with greater dexterity. His separation anxiety diminished and George was able to interact and engage with other children and his family at a birthday party in a way that he never had before.

Unfolding Jessica: Cerebral Palsy in a Four-Year-Old
SARAH FRANEK, M.T.P.

As I write these words, I marvel at the changes that FNS has made in a little girl's life. Jessica is three years old and diagnosed with moderate Cerebral Palsy (CP). The origins of her problem are unknown, but when she was perinatal, there had been a heavy crop spraying where her parents lived. She was born with a rotated brain stem, the left portion of which was shrunken but not totally missing, and a very small left cerebellar lobe. She was a late birth with a disintegrated placenta, and a thick white film present over her whole body.

Although beautiful, with delicate features and blond hair, when Jessica was brought to the office, she showed a severe right hemiplegia; her head was skewed to the right, as in tortocollis, the right eye seemed permanently shut, and her right hand was stiff and spastic, used as a claw, when used at all. She had low energy for a three-year-old and woke frequently at night. She was able to crawl with assistance. She did not have language, and with the help of a weekly speech therapist had been able to speak in one-word utterances, which were accompanied by finger pointing. Her disabilities were thought to be permanent and irremediable, but the family had been doing Feldenkrais exercises with her since about six months of age. We are pretty sure this gentle muscular and neural stimulation paved the way for the amazing results that began with the FNS.

We did not do an intro or offset—just a map with glasses unplugged. (This means that Jessica *did* receive a full second of RF stimulation at each site, while the machine read the site for four seconds total.)

After doing the map, which, as noted earlier, can have treatment effects in the sensitive client, Jessica's mother reported that when Jessica spilled yogurt on her right hand, she licked the fingers of that hand—something never seen before. Her right eye seemed more open, and she slept better.

Sessions were begun twice a week, the parents having been warned to look for the signs of overdose—i.e., tired or wired behavior. Jessica was treated at four sites per session, moving along the Total Amplitude site sort, stimulated at +5 for six seconds, a twelve-second pause, and then a stimulation at +10 for six seconds (for a total of twelve seconds per site = forty-eight seconds total).

After session one, Jessica's mother reported that she started speaking in two to three word—but complete—sentences, for the first time ever: "I wan' dat!" "Dat bear mine!" Her sleep improved, and she began exploring new ways of using her right hand.

After session two she was reported sleeping very well—best ever.

After session three she was noticed picking things up with her right hand. She had much more energy. Her grandparents noticed that she was more alert—they said it was "a striking difference."

After session four, Jessica began doing somersaults. She crawled over to an ottoman, pulled herself up and walked around it; after that breakthrough, she began regular "couch cruising." Now she was often speaking in three-word utterances. Her speech therapist was thrilled. Jessica sang "Twinkle, Twinkle Little Star" completely unassisted (the first time ever). To her parents' astonishment and mild shock, she pulled herself up the facade of the TV and turned it off with her *right* index finger manipulating the knob (she seemed to already know just where the device was to be turned off!). Her parents reported that, at this point, Jessica's energy seemed a little daunting—she was becoming just like any other three-year-old!

Jessica had undergone just a few sessions but, over subsequent sessions, her improvements continued. It seemed that Jessica had "developmental milestones" still unachieved and, with subsequent sessions, she was achieving them at a considerable pace. They followed a normal developmental course, with language, cognitive, and motor areas all actively showing change and improvement.

Her mother reported that, whereas prior to the FNS treatment, Jessica seemed clearly in the "developmentally disabled" category in terms of her ability to learn new skills, after FNS her ability had gone from 25 percent (that of a "normal" child of her age) to about 50 percent. The Feldenkrais work began to be *much* more effective, and Jessica displayed a smoothness and versatility in her functioning that, prior to treatment, had only been a much hoped-for-potential.

Postscript: Just recently I was delighted to see Jessica, brought in by her mother for a "touch-up." By now she was a bright, verbal, shy eight-year-old, with an absolutely endearing smile. She needed braces on her legs but walked unassisted and spoke and interacted like any normal eight-year-old!

The Case of Damon: Reactive Attachment Disorder

I don't believe in none of that demonism stuff, but that kid had that whole place in pandemonium in a few minutes. If we let him touch an animal, soon they were howling or screeching.

GEORGE, DAMON'S FATHER

REACTIVE ATTACHMENT DISORDER (RAD)

Reactive attachment disorder exists where an infant has been abandoned, neglected, maltreated, or combinations of the above. Such children often have pervasive developmental delays, as well as an inability to relate appropriately to peers or adults. There is a general consensus that children who have experienced reactive attachment disorder are more likely than "normals" to engage in pathological behaviors such as animal torture, or suddenly hurting other children, throughout childhood, and on into teenage years, and then into adulthood, providing the world with one more sociopath or antisocial criminal.

Damon's mother Daphne, in her early twenties, was addicted to crack cocaine and heroin during the time that Damon was carried in the womb. She also drank alcohol enthusiastically during her pregnancy (making it impossible to rule out the effects of Fetal Alcohol Syndrome on Damon, as well as other perinatal toxicities from drugs).

Astonishingly, however, Damon's was a fairly normal birth and, although he was small and delicate, he was without gross visible impairments. Both Damon's father George and Daphne continued to drink pretty heavily subsequent to Damon's birth, but apparently only Daphne continued with the crack. Not surprisingly, their marriage split up a few months after Damon was born. George left the state (they lived in Michigan), and Daphne set about to raise her child *and* keep her habit—not an easy thing to do.

There were strange men in Daphne's house all the time, and we don't know what Damon saw or didn't see, but there was certainly plenty of sex—it was how Daphne made her living for a while—and probably also lots of violence. Damon lay in wet diapers a lot, and when he looked into his mom's eyes, he probably saw little "lovelight," but rather the black pinwheels of Mom's addiction. They ate junk food (when there was any food), and inconsistency was the only constant. Daphne, when attentive, was probably screaming or sitting in a depressed stupor, staring at the wall.

When she was arrested for a minor felony, the Child Protective services got involved. Daphne was examined by psychiatrists as well as probation officers, and a law guardian was appointed for Damon. Daphne was ruled unfit, and Damon was headed for foster care when George was finally reached out of state, and notified of what was happening with his ex-wife and son.

George, who was quite a bit older than Daphne, had undergone a real reformation after splitting up with her. He had become sober through "Twelve-Step" and settled down in a new relationship with a woman named Annie whom he had met in AA. Annie was George's age—early forties—had raised children of her own, and was well equipped with motherly skills and instincts. George petitioned the court for the return of his son, and after he and Annie were screened and evaluated, he was awarded custody of Damon.

When the family arrived at our center, Damon, now three and a half years old, was immediately oppositional to the new situation. Anything that anyone wanted him to do, he did not want to do. His parents gave a frightening litany of complaints: wild tantrums, violent play, abuse directed at other children. He would "become" an animal for long periods of time, only responding with whines and growls, and it proved impossible to get him out of that state. But what immediately got my attention was his extreme cruelty to animals (this is a known precursor to even worse antisocial behavior, if not checked). Whenever he caught frogs or toads, he had a deft little mauling maneuver that was infallibly lethal.

On one occasion, George and Annie had made the mistake of bringing Damon to a pet store. Reflecting on this, George told me, "I don't believe in none of that demonism stuff, but that kid had that whole place (the pet store) in pandemonium in a few minutes. If we let him touch an animal, soon they were howling or screeching." Damon was also suddenly and unexpectedly violent with playmates, especially Annie's four-year-old grandson, who frequently would run out of the play-room, crying. Damon's father also warned me that he had an interesting way—being at just the right height—of hitting adults squarely in the genitals. Damon also masturbated and touched or flaunted his genitals frequently.

With some trepidation, I introduced Damon to the sandplay environment. Suddenly there were dozens of toys all over the floor and he was running over them, breaking them as he went. He shouted at me (the therapist), "I don't like you!" He ran into different rooms of the therapy center and hid.

When I had evaluated Damon and read the report from social workers and psychologists, I felt that not only was he developmentally and emotionally arrested, he was profoundly neurologically immature. He had missed many important milestones. I decided to try neurofeedback on his second visit. It would not be easy, for I knew this child would never sit still long enough for an offset or a map to be done.

George and Annie had never heard of neurofeedback, but they were desperate. So on the second visit we went to the room across the hall from the sandplay room to see if we could get Damon to sit still long enough for a treatment. Yelling and screaming, he refused. Sometimes, with very small autistic or PDD kids, we have a parent hold the child in his or her lap and restrain the child so that the electrodes can be attached to the head and the treatment administered. But we didn't even have time to try this with Damon, because he went immediately into a fierce tantrum. (He would have broken furniture if he'd been strong enough.) He hit and kicked with pretty good aim and with a clear intent to do damage.

I counseled using no restraint on him but just letting him expend his wild energy. The parents and I moved back to the sandplay room and invited him to come but he just screamed "no!" then "NO!" louder and louder. After about a half an hour he seemed exhausted and tearful.

At just the right moment I looked at him, smiled, and patted my lap. He came over and climbed into it. "Let's do biofeedback," I said. Damon was too exhausted to resist. He moved to his dad's lap in the treatment chair and I was able to attach the electrode to site CZ at the top of his head. He wouldn't close his eyes, but I was able to get in one second of stimulation.

That one site, which is sometimes used as a kind of "summary" of the whole cortex, had, of course, huge delta spikes, along with theta and alpha. There were also dense little spindles of high beta that are associated with anger and hypervigilance. It looked like a storm instead of a "symphony" in Damon's brain. Although he seemed quieter when leaving the session, it was hard to say whether this was due to the neurotherapy or the fact that he was exhausted.

The next week the report was amazing. There were a few small tantrum displays, but nothing like we had seen in the office the week prior. He seemed more cuddly and had begun displaying affection (without the sexual aspect). This affectionate behavior George and Annie had never seen before. They were truly astonished and pleased.

When Damon came back for more treatment, he seemed much calmer, and when I invited him in to the biofeedback room, he came willingly, ordered his dad into the treatment seat, and then climbed into his lap. Puckishly, Damon pointed to his head and indicated the biofeedback machine. At that session, we were able to do two seconds, one each at the FPZ and OZ sites.

Damon's play in the sandbox that day was a little less frantic and, although he dumped a lot of toys on the floor, it was not quite the chaotic scene that we had witnessed the week before.

The following couple of weeks were astonishing. Damon had begun to bedwet with a vengeance again, something he had done when his dad had initially taken over Damon's care from Daphne. "Good," I said. It seemed like a developmental stage surfacing, asking to be integrated. "Don't punish him," I told his parents. "It will probably go away again."

Sure enough, the bedwetting behavior persisted for about a week and a half, during which time the family's washing machine was very busy! Suddenly, the bedwetting stopped. (By the time of Damon's fifth treatment, he wet the bed only one night, the rest of the nights he did not.)

The second week of treatment, Damon had asked to sit in Annie's lap during the treatment, and the third week he asked for his dad again. On the fourth week he came in and sat in the chair all by himself. He looked at me. "Put the things on my head!" he ordered crisply. I obliged with alacrity. He still wouldn't close his eyes for the treatment (which is recommended in most cases to keep the blinking artifact from interfering with the brain waves).

However, I watched the raw brain wave carefully and only gave him stimulation where there was no artifact—the only way one can be sure that the stimulation, the brief burst of radio frequency waves, correspond to the brain waves, and thus have a chance of working. Given all of this, the proof, nevertheless, is in the "pudding," that is in the week-to-week clinical reports.

Now Damon's sandplay sessions were getting much more interesting. At one session the toys he selected, to the exclusion of all others, were sailboats; he wanted his mom to help him race them through the sand. In another session, he selected tools, rakes, hoes, and shovels and began a little "work project." He began doing that outside the sessions, too. When his father, an electrician, was working, Damon would try to work alongside him—without live wires of course—and with suitable warnings about the dangers of electricity!

In the family therapy sessions, George had voiced concerns about the violence of Damon's play and wouldn't engage with him physically. I asked George: "Who's bigger?" and encouraged him to give Damon lots and lots of wild romps on the floor. Hitting was discouraged, but wrestling, pouncing, and pulling were allowed. Damon seemed to crave these sessions, then, after he'd had enough, he would turn cuddly and be affectionate. He now was beginning to say things like, "I love you, Dad," and "I love you, Mom."

Initially, not knowing how else to control Damon, his parents had been using corporal punishment, but I encouraged them to try "time-outs" and penalties rather than resorting to physical punishment, which was capable of stimulating more violence in their son. This "time-out" method seemed to work and soon the need to punish Damon diminished.

His preoccupation with sexuality remained, but the sadistic overtones seemed to be less. Somewhere along the line, Damon had learned to swear like a Longshoreman, and now instead of a full-out tantrum, this cherubic little boy, when frustrated, would let out a string of curses that could curl the hair of day-care staff. At this point, Damon had less overt aggression, but there was a definite increase in fiendish attempts to manipulate. The boy was quite intelligent and was learning how to get his way in clever new ways—an unmistakable sign of cognitive development!

However, given all this progress, eventually Damon's bedwetting returned as the child became more relaxed with treatment—a not uncommon phase for abused children to go through as they relax their vigilance. Unfortunately, Damon's renewed bedwetting, coupled with "financial hardship," caused this working-class family to discontinue their son's treatment.

We don't know how many permanent scars from Damon's first three and a half years of life he will carry into adulthood, however, what does seem remarkable is how quickly, and with what little stimulation, Damon's developmental sequence was restored, and his innate health began to reassert itself. The neurofeedback cannot claim sole credit for these changes. A safe, loving, and secure home environment, and parents willing to be patient, calm, and consistent are key requirements. Good nutrition, and being kept away from lots of sugar, also played a part in Damon's improved state. (These recommendations had been made in the initial intake interview with Damon.)

A follow-up with this family two and a half years later indicated that Damon's more extreme behaviors had not returned and by this time, the bedwetting had been resolved. Unfortunately, George's new marriage failed, and Damon continued living with his dad. He had "personality traits" that were problematic, especially his manipulation of people and events, but his grosser behavioral manifestations, the tantrums and the violence, did not return. (Damon had undergone a total of seven visits to our office, and six LENS treatments, along with play therapy in each session.)

Alex's Journey Back: Injury to the Very Young Brain and Its Amelioration

THERESA YONKER, M.D.

Alexander is a bright, blue-eyed, curly blonde-haired boy whose journey through life has been an uphill battle. He was born to a forty-year-old professional mother (me); my career was that of a psychiatrist to children and adolescents. Little did I know that the most difficult case of my career was going to involve my own child!

Alex, a second child, was finally born after a difficult pregnancy and traumatic delivery. He was born with a condition called craniosynostosis, a total fusion of the suture lines of his skull plates. Translated, this means his head could not mold at birth, because the plates were fused. There was no soft spot, nor opportunity for the brain to grow and develop. This opening in the skull plate is necessary to allow the brain to grow for about a year and a half until fusion occurs.

Even getting a proper diagnosis was a nightmare for me, a physician who could not get my colleagues to listen to my concerns. Alexander had a malformed skull, lowset ears, a concave occipital region, and an extremely broad and tall forehead. At four months of age, he underwent a total skull reconstructive surgery, which required two blood transfusions and the care of a team of a pediatric neurosurgeon, a pediatric plastic surgeon, and a pediatric anesthesiologist. The goal of the surgery was to remove long sections of bone plate—requiring fracture of the occipital bone—and the insertion of resorbable plates.

Six months after the surgery, Alex was in an auto accident in which the car he was riding in was T-boned by a large SUV, along the side where Alexander sat in his car seat. The impact missed his head by inches.

This was the beginning of the journey's difficult part: Alexander suffered from night terrors and would awaken in the middle of the night wide-eyed with fear, crying and screaming. He would run around the house and try to hide in corners, away from the inner demons frightening him. He was inconsolable.

Alex suffered a grand-mal seizure, underwent numerous MRIs, CAT scans, and QEEGs but could not be assigned a definitive diagnosis. Upon entering day care, at the age of two, his behaviors escalated until he was asked to leave. We were told he would have to have an Early Intervention evaluation. He had sensory-integration issues, and extreme sensitivity, so that even the sound of a cricket chirping, a toilet flushing, motorcycles, a coffee grinder, or a vacuum running would result in his falling to the ground screaming and covering his ears. It was difficult to change his diapers; he would kick and scream through the process.

Alex finally became aggressive to those around him, reacting with a "fight or flight" type of response every time he perceived a threat to himself. He would lash out, kicking and screaming, and could only be stopped by physical restraint. He was involved in an Early Intervention program where he received a variety of occupational therapies. But his behavior did not really improve. Well-intentioned therapists questioned my parenting skills, as if that was where the blame lay. (When I think of what I went through from mental health practitioners, I pity the average parent with a head-injured or somehow otherwise defective child, as people are so quick to rush to judgment.)

We took Alex to many specialists, were patted on the head, and told to give him medication. I was resistant, but he was now four and nearing kindergarten age, and we had run out of options. Alex was tried on a trial of Clonidine. This put him to sleep very nicely but did not address the ongoing problems. More medications were tried: Trileptal, Depakote, Seroquel. But no medication seemed able to change the explosive rages that would come out of the blue wherein he would attack and chase caregivers and parents, trying to bite, scratch, or kick them.

Nor did anything seem to be able to stop the terrible threats and swearwords that poured out of his small, cute mouth when he was in this kind of condition. In between, by contrast, he seemed bright, bubbly, and happy. Because he seemed so intelligent and to be a quick learner, Special Education classification and a smaller classroom was ruled out.

Thus medicated, Alex moved into kindergarten and was having difficulty by the third week of school. Multiple conferences, interventions, and therapies were tried, but he was suspended, time after time, for his behavior. I had to take a leave of absence from my job, because advocating for Alex had become a full-time job in itself.

One day I was given the best advice I ever received, from a respected colleague. Dr. Richard Brown told me to take Alex to Dr. Stephen Larsen, who was doing remarkable things with the LENS, a type of neurofeedback. (I had been very well trained "in the box" but had developed a secret fascination with the strange world that lay outside those boundaries.) Given this, however, Alex's father and I remained somewhat skeptical that anything could help our son at this point. We had sought help from a local brain injury support group who had told us that Alexander's difficulty was a "permanent and unchangeable condition," and that we had better get used to it. And while they would give us support in facing the grim reality of that conviction, they could not give us hope. The whole scenario felt incredibly fatalistic.

So we decided to take a chance. The initial intake interview with Dr. Larsen actually gave me a surge of hope! Someone finally "got it!"

Dr. Larsen asked questions about things that I had long ago stopped trying to communicate to professionals. He nodded his head sagely and said that Alex's behaviors were probably neurologically-driven. A brain map was done that confirmed serious dysregulation, and incipient seizure activity, probably due to the injuries of Alex's birth, the early operation, and the accident.

Together we developed a rating scale for five symptoms. In Alex's case, these symptoms were: 1) explosiveness; 2) inability to learn from experience; 3) the startle factor (a reaction to anything sudden); 4) obsessive, rigid behaviors; and 5) enuresis (bedwetting). Alex started at a straight "10" (the worst) across the board in all these categories. Because of his sensitivity, extremely brief treatments—a second or two a week—were begun. (Because of the seizure potential for this child, the method chosen was a brief *stim*—an antiseizure procedure—even though Alex's neurological sensitivity might have warranted the lower intensity *no-stim* treatment.)

Slowly progress began. Alex became more flexible, he was less rigid and dug-in. He gradually became less explosive and was beginning, for the first time ever, *to learn from experience.* He was becoming capable of thinking before acting, and understanding and retaining the idea of consequences. *Now* we could apply therapy and behavior modification and it would have an effect. (This result, that of being able to learn from experience, is not a small change but a big one, as it makes everything else possible.)

Alex was gradually taken off all medication but continued to make progress. He was placed in a very structured school program, fortunately working with professionals who not only understood brain injury but who could see beyond it—to the wonderful little boy who was trapped inside.

Not that there were no setbacks. As we moved around the map, we hit a "hot spot" (one of the seizure foci, at O1, SL) in the back of the head, and the rages came back, rigidity reared its head again, and the enuresis returned. Dr. Larsen (who was also treating me for my own auto-accident-induced head injury) said, "This too shall pass." It was not unlike the story of Pinocchio, where the "real boy" was trapped inside—he would come back. The protocol was resumed, and Dr. Larsen was proved right.

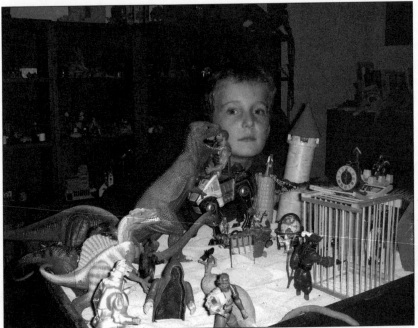

Fig. 5.1. January 2005: A child's disorganized mind . . .

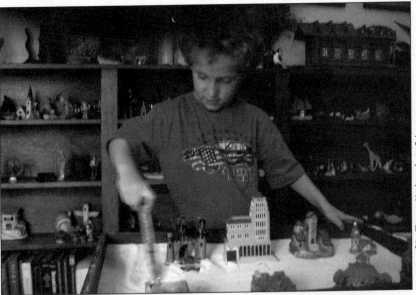

Fig. 5.2. . . . organizes itself as Alex positions a final piece in his latest sandplay (August 2005).

Over the ensuing weeks, Alexander slowly continued to emerge and improve.

Heretofore we had not been able to take a family vacation of any kind, because of Alex's blowups. We had stopped going to public places: fairs, restaurants, social gatherings, etc. Alex's older sister had been disappointed too many times, when we had had to suddenly leave a fun outing because of her brother's inability to stay in control.

All of this was changing, however. One day, on the way over to the neurofeedback center, we saw a secondhand camper for sale; it was in pretty good shape. We bought it and, in a few weeks, we were able, for the first time, to go on a family vacation, without any horrible blowups or the need to return home prematurely.

At the time of this writing (February 2005), we are approaching a year since we began the treatments at Stone Mountain. I, the psychiatrist mom, am definitely "out of the box!" I have become not just "a believer" in the LENS, I am in training to become a practitioner of it as well! I did not return to my job at the County Mental Hygiene department but instead am developing an integrative behavioral medicine practice that will incorporate the LENS neurofeedback with other modalities. The lesson for me was to follow my instincts as a mother, and to shelve the medical model of treatment for something unknown, not well understood, or (not yet) accepted.

I took a leap of faith and was rewarded with the rebirth of my son, the real Alexander!

The following incident was key in helping Alex's mother and I determine that we could discontinue the LENS treatment because, to our way of thinking, it proved that Alex had graduated from the LENS! A little over a year ago, the family had rented the movie *Ghostbusters*, a rather hilarious comedy starring Bill Murray. Alex became terrified by "Mr. Stay-Puff," the great "marshmallow-man" character who is as big as an apartment house but far more ridiculous than frightening.

While everyone in Alex's family was laughing at the movie, he was screaming with fear. Afterward, he insisted that all the ducts in the house be vacuumed, because there were ghosts in them. But this year, it was the whole family who was slightly apprehensive about seeing the movie again, given Alex's previous reaction to the film. Alex, however, insisted that they watch it. This time his hysteria was pure merriment and was echoed in the family's relief. Everyone laughed and laughed.

But there is one final postscript to this story. Dr. Theresa Yonker not only vacated her "box" entirely but has become a certified Lens practitioner. Though still licensed to medicate, she uses mostly nutraceuticals and neurofeedback to help her rapidly growing practice of children with CNS problems!

Softening the Inflexible Brain: The Autistic Spectrum and Asperger's Syndrome

What do you do when you can't get your child's attention, because it is raptly fixed on some (to your way of thinking) irrelevant stimulus, like an almanac, from which he proceeds to memorize the annual rainfall from Baghdad to Bangladesh? (His untouched homework is apparently of negligible interest to him.) Or when sent to retrieve something from the other room, his eyes light on a magazine and he picks it up and begins studiously reading it, ignoring his assigned chore. When rebuked for these attentional anomalies, he becomes teary-eyed and apologizes over and over again.

He swears he will never do it again, which is when he finds his little brother's *Gameboy* in the bathroom and doesn't come out for an hour. "I'll be out in just a minute," he says enthusiastically but echolalically (repetitively). And then he doesn't appear. For this autistic-spectrum child, his world of private preoccupations has once again triumphed over the social contract.

"The world is full of people who find fractal geometry easier than small talk," says a *Newsweek* article on Autism written in 2003. Four boys are afflicted for every girl, and some theorists believe Autism is an exacerbation of some "male" traits. For example, boys are often object-oriented rather than people-oriented. Epidemiologists have noted that the reported incidence of autistic spectrum disorders is growing exponentially.

Some of the "red flags" that alert parents are that their child does not acknowledge adults (or other children) when they come into what most of us consider "social space." These children do not meet people's eyes, or exchange smiles or nods. Some autistic children with normal hearing do not even respond to their own name when it is used to get their attention. Sometimes language development begins, and then, some time later, mysteriously ends. Parents accustomed to the "warm fuzzies" of anaclitic touch with infants or toddlers are surprised to find a wooden, unresponsive child in their arms. Many autistic spectrum children do not understand the normal human social gestures of touch, or are tactile-defensive.

In Asperger's Syndrome, sometimes called "high functioning Autism," the social impairment may not be as severe as in Autism. Still, there is the preoccupation with things instead of people. Ted, whom we treated at our center, could take apart a transistor radio and put it back together when he was five years old. When he was fourteen, he found his "niche," so to speak, and became one of the world's experts on water clocks. The report he gave to his class in an alternative school was "awesome" by all accounts. But he didn't get any social invitations from it because his manner was so, well, preoccupied. (Some kids in Ted's public school—where he had been very unhappy—even used the "G" word—"geek.")

Asperger's overlaps with what is also called "Savant Syndrome," which involves an incredible and detailed mastery of some body of intellectual knowledge, or facts. Psychology has elucidated a useful categorization of this difference, referring to *systematizers* versus *empathizers*. Not surprisingly, considering the preponderance of male autistic and Asperger's children, males tend toward the "systemizing" type of thinking. Females predominantly tend toward the empathic, or what Daniel Goleman calls "emotional intelligence," as discussed in his book of the same name on the subject.

Goleman, in fact, cites studies that show that emotional intelligence may be a far better predictor of success in life than intellectual intelligence or "IQ." Autism seems to prove the case—children who can do integral calculus but can't anticipate the needs or wishes of others. Some Asperger's children intellectually verge on what is thought of as genius, because of their mastery of some specific field of knowledge, but it always remains an open question, if that knowledge is usable, or useful, or interesting to anyone else.[1]

In the case we are next going to present, Asperger's Syndrome will also be seen as a heritable factor—if not the full-blown disorder, at least the temperamental traits that accompany it.

Aurora Makes It to Steamtown

Aurora was eleven when she was brought to our center. Pretty, with honey colored hair, she nonetheless carried herself hesitantly. As with many children in the autistic spectrum, she had been echolalic, repeating words and phrases again and again in an odd, insistent kind of tone, even when reassured that she was understood, or that her request would soon be granted.

This irritating mannerism alone made her less than socially desirable. She was extremely sensitive to loud noises and would have a reaction of almost seizurelike intensity to the sounds of slamming doors, noon whistles, loud motors, etc. This tendency of Aurora's also had a peculiar feature that hinted at subclinical seizure activity in her brain. Seeing flights of stairs could send her into a fit. When I probed for what the trigger might be, she couldn't say. Even the topic made her uneasy.

Aurora's mother thought that Aurora became agitated as her gaze followed the steps up. Suddenly she would begin making strange stereotyped movements with her hands and arms and whimpering. Needless to say, crowds, sudden commotions in the school environment, all had strong effects on Aurora, producing similar stereotyped or ritualistic behaviors.

Aurora had been a little slow in reaching her developmental milestones. Early on she had developed quite a good vocabulary—but then had failed to use it to communicate appropriately. She toe-walked for a couple of her developmental years and tended to avoid eye contact. At times she would become *extremely* emotional, though circumstances were only mildly frustrating. This is another sign of seizure disorder, or limbic-cortical kindling.

If she did something wrong, she would obsess about it and try endlessly to atone. She would have to change her clothes if she got the tiniest stain on them and she displayed allergies to molds, pollens, and dust mites. She was diagnosed as having Asperger's Syndrome by the Boston Children's Hospital, as well as Pervasive Developmental Disorder, NOS, (Not Otherwise Specified). For Aurora's parents, with their highly unusual and temperamental child, receiving a formal diagnosis was actually welcome.

Because of her tendency to get out of control in social situations, her dad made up stories about a very bad girl named Doris, who couldn't control herself. This story was very helpful for Aurora, as it gave her a way to handle the oppositional side of herself, and the actions she herself felt were unacceptable. She had a compulsive, clingy relationship with her mom, and a kind of scared, distant relationship with her dad—who was always telling her to "behave better."

Although we had seen Len Ochs do remarkable things with much younger autistic children, our full-scale neurofeedback services had only been in place for a couple of years, and we were very unsure of ourselves in regard to treating an older child with serious problems, already ingrained. We didn't promise much of anything, but the parents were determined to try anything that might help their daughter. And all the medical establishment had offered so far was medication.

The symptoms we chose to track were her extreme sensitivity to stimuli, her echolalic and stereotyped behaviors, and her inability to change from one activity to another. Aurora's mother was diligent about tracking, even counting and keeping notes of these behaviors, which was very helpful. Her dad, an engineer, was usually at work when Aurora came to sessions at the center and we learned that he was initially rather skeptical about this odd form of treatment. Nonetheless, he hadn't liked the way that medication had impacted on his daughter.

When we mapped Aurora's brain, as expected, we saw EEG-slowing, high amplitude theta waves over much of the cortex. Her first reaction to treatment was to get sleepy, then giddy and wired. (We generally think of autistic-spectrum children as "hardy" in that they can take fairly long and intense treatments. Dr. Curtis Cripe, whose work is described next, gives minutes-long sessions of EEG-driven stimulation, rather than seconds.) We were giving Aurora about six seconds per site at four sites, or about 24 seconds of total stimulation. After a few sessions she would become very emotional and irritable right after the session. At times she was very spacey.

We were getting worried about failure, but at approximately the sixth or seventh treatment—compressed into two weeks, so motivated were these parents—suddenly Aurora seemed more "even" to both of her parents. She began using a highlighter when doing school homework, and her concentration levels were better. By the third week, her teacher had noticed the changes, using the words "a leap of abilities" to describe Aurora's improved condition.

As we went along, however, it was apparent that this would not be just an easy, smooth course of treatment for, at times, all of Aurora's fears seemed to recapitulate after treatment sessions. These fears included a fear of the dark, or a fear of being left alone—panic set in when her mother would leave or go shopping. At one point, an earlier childhood fear of ghosts returned.

However, these regressions were soon offset by gains. When Aurora threw a (familiar) emotional scene in a restaurant, she got over it more quickly than before. Her sleep was steadily improving, and she was showing surprising initiative in new situations.

By the time two months had passed, Aurora's parents reported that she was more consistently "chipper," showing a good affect much more of the time. When "fits" interrupted this pleasant mood, they seemed acute but short of duration. She got a one hundred on a spelling test. She didn't need to have reassurances each time she got on the bus. At one point she commented soberly to her mom: "You know, I don't think I have a very severe disability anymore."

By the sixth month, her mother met with her daughter's teachers. All agreed she had made "excellent progress." She was more socialized, less agitated. In formal testing situations she needed less constant help and could be seen figuring things out for herself.

One teacher even recommended her for an "inclusionary" or mainstreamed program. A real milestone was that Aurora went on a five-day class trip without parental accompaniment and without freaking out.

Aurora's father, initially skeptical, was now firmly won over. He and Aurora had spent a week together while Aurora's mother was away. Aurora was much less panicky and nervous than she had ever been. (Before, the feeling had been that her mother *could not go away* because of the intensity of Aurora's panic.) Somewhere along the line, during treatment, she began to read silently. Before, she had had to read aloud. (Developmentally, this is a very large, not a small leap forward, because up until a century or so ago, very few people in the civilized world could read silently. Those who could do it were thought of as geniuses or freaks.) Aurora was showing herself more assertive with peers, and more independent. Math was still a problem for her, but on the whole she was keeping up with homework.

A little over a year had passed, and about fifty treatments had been completed. Aurora was still recognizable as "herself," but she was using her intelligence in really interesting ways. Her mother noticed her watching other children relate, and then adopting some of those relationship strategies herself. Her behavior seemed more appropriate in most circumstances. Over the Christmas holidays she was really even. She said to her mother: "You know, I'm really Aurora now—not Doris anymore."

Because the family traveled an hour each way to our center, we suggested a rest from the neurofeedback. During the spring semester, Aurora held her improvements; and then over the summer we held one of our "Open Houses," which Aurora and her entire family attended.

They told an amazing story: Aurora's father had a special hobby he had always wanted to share with his children—locomotives. For years he had wanted to take his family to "Steam Town," Pennsylvania, but Aurora would be far too sensitive to go anywhere near such a snorting, chugging, whistling place! But now that she was so much improved, they decided to give it a try!

The massive train yard/museum, presenting a complete history of railroading, was *very noisy indeed*. Every locomotive whistled, every diesel brayed mightily, as they chugged and roared along. Aurora weathered it all. The whole family was beaming! On the way home, they had stopped in to eat in a noisy pizza parlor, with trays dropped and shouting conversations. Partway through the meal, her parents grinned at each other. "We could never, ever, have taken her into a place like that (prior to her LENS treatment). She would have had to eat her pizza in the car!"

And that was the story they told. Aurora's father said, "You know, I study hydroelectric power plants and I am also a railroading scholar. I think I was a little like Aurora when I was younger, but I trained myself to be sociable and channeled my funny interests into making a living."

I thanked him for his honesty and his insight. He thanked us for "giving him his daughter." When Aurora heard this, she smiled and hugged her father. "That's my dad!" she said.

A two and a three-year follow-up have shown that Aurora is continuing to adapt to her environment more readily. She continues to do well in school, and her parents shared that she manned (or womaned) a booth at the Dutchess County Fair, where she did a credible job of meeting the public and selling raffle tickets.

To summarize this case, we do not feel we "cured" Aurora's

Asperger's Syndrome, but we helped Aurora's nervous system become so flexible that she could handle most of the demands for adaptation that her environment put upon her. She occasionally would panic or "have her moments" but they passed relatively quickly. She was able to control the socially dysfunctional echolalias and constant need for reassurance under most social circumstances; occasionally they would slip out when she was in the presence of her family. Aurora was still Aurora, but she had maximized her strengths and diminished her weaknesses.

Combining Modalities: Disentrainment Therapy with Other Developmental Approaches— Curtis Cripe's Work

Dr. Curtis Cripe is a handsome, bearded man who often wears jeans and a buckskin jacket. Sometimes he can be found in council with Native American Elders, or out in the desert on a hike or a vision quest near his Arizona home. Curtis's soft-spoken ways often lead people to underestimate his razor-sharp mind. He has a background in the physical sciences as well as psychology and has worked in the aerospace program.

But Curtis has a passion that guides his life now: he wants to help kids—all kinds of kids. His Crossroads Institute in Cave Creek, Arizona treats almost a hundred children a week. These children have serious disorders, ranging from the autistic spectrum to PDD (Pervasive Developmental Disorder), to ADHD, Tourette's, Shaken Baby Syndrome, seizure disorders, and Obsessive-Compulsive and Oppositional-Defiant disorders.

Dr. Cripe's success rate is phenomenal and explains why his office—in the middle of the Arizona desert—is always packed with people: families flying in from both coasts and the Midwest for evaluation and treatment. He does use a variety of evaluation and treatment methods, but at the core of his treatment, he says, is the Flexyx (FNS) approach that he learned from Dr. Len Ochs.

"It was a revelation for me," he said, "to train with Ochs. It took me a while to really 'get it'—what he was doing, but then I started really seeing it work, and it fit right in with the stuff I had learned from Glenn Doman." (Glenn Doman is a specialist in physical and cognitive rehabilitation who runs The Institute for the Human Potential in Pennsylvania. He is the author of *What to Do about Your Brain Injured Child*, and *How to Teach Your Baby to Be Physically Superb*.)[2]

Dr. Cripe explains his evaluation method this way:

Define through assessment where this person or population is on the neurodevelopmental spectrum with regard to: receptive and expressive abilities; auditory and visual processing; motor processing; overall integrative processing.

"What we have found," he says "is that FNS (LENS) aids tremendously in the acceleration of neurodevelopment, or allowing development to happen where it couldn't/didn't before. Our premise is that the brain has become disorganized through head trauma or other childhood issues involving illness, chronic ear infections, fevers, birth traumas, and/or allergies. In some cases, there is a genetic weakness or pattern, which influences the type of response or symptom. We follow Ochs in saying that the brain, and its normal developmental pattern, has become interfered with by these traumas, and our treatment should be aimed at restoring what the trauma disrupted. Our results show that about 95% of our client population respond favorably with positive improvement, advancing toward age-appropriate development, while 75–80% of the children who actually do the full program successfully achieve the desired results."

The Case of Matt: Erasing Autism
CURTIS CRIPE, PH.D.

Matt came to Crossroads at eight years of age with a diagnosis of Autism. During the initial assessment, it was found that he had not completed several stages of neurodevelopment (developmental delays). The stage he was in should have been completed by the age of two and tends to correlate to incomplete development of the pons (a part of the brain) and the pain receptors (hypo condition) that lie in the muscles. Additionally, the trigeminal nerve around the head appeared to be hyperactive. His behavior and the psychophysical measures were correlated.

The brain map (QEEG) showed that he had processing problems, with severe, slow wave activity across the entire head in delta and theta ranges. There was a "hypo-alpha" condition. Communication between parts of the brain was underdeveloped. This would cause a slowdown in Matt's ability to process information clearly and quickly.

The combination of the developmental delays, the hypo-alpha condition, and the underdeveloped coherence were the cause of Matt's problems in the domains of attention, activity (hyperactive) memory disorders, mood instabilities, and autistic symptoms. In other words, the map explained the ADHD. We knew we had to break up areas of neurological inhibition and exercise and retrain the brain. A neurological program combined with FNS was designed to address the complete picture of Matt's situation.

The neurodevelopment training program included two parts: a home exercise program for peripheral nervous system development (the *peripheral nervous system* in this case means all the nerves outside the CNS or the bony enclosure of the skull and spinal column), and the EEG neurofeedback for central nervous system development. In other words, one approach worked from the periphery "up" the neural tree, and the other from the CNS "down." In this case, because of the severity of Matt's delays, both parts of the training program were indispensible.

The first sessions consisted of working with CZ, PZ, and FZ sites, (which are midline sites between the two hemispheres) to balance and normalize his cortical activity. After the first few sessions, I switched to working with multiple sites on the 10–20 map within each session. After a certain number of sessions it was seen that Matt no longer exhibited the autistic behaviors. After another ten, it was evident that he was visibly maturing. By session twenty, Matt was placed in a mainstream classroom setting with peers and was able to work within the parameters of that setting. By thirty sessions, his improving grades reflected his further maturation and development.

Today, after twelve months under this program's protocols, Matt's diagnosis of Autism has been removed. He is in mainstream fourth grade, with his grades in the As and Bs. He has developed and maintained school friendships and is included in school functions and extracurricular social functions. Matt will graduate with flying colors from our program after a total of fifty sessions.

Ongoing Discussion with Len Ochs and Stephen Larsen on Disentrainment Therapy with Autistic Children and Children with Asperger's Syndrome

Stephen: Can you relate to us some of your clinical experience with autistic children or children with Asperger's Syndrome?

Len: This mother brought two children, a boy and a girl. The girl was older than the boy, she was about six. They looked like children from *The Shining* (a surreal horror movie). They had this glow in their eyes, and these semifixed gleeful expressions, and their hands out in front of them as if they were all legs and fingers. They wanted to kind of, you know, touch, fold, spindle, rip, mutilate everything in my office.

My associate at the time was treating the girl, and I was treating the boy. A few weeks after she started treatment, the girl was showing worsening signs of autistic perseverative behavior (behavior wherein the same words or actions are repeated over and over, stereotypically). This young girl often hid behind the office couch counting: "one, two, three—" up to ninety-nine.

I said to the therapist: "You're overdosing her! Stop it!"

And the therapist said, "No!" (He blamed the girl's persevation on her Autism.)

At that point I took over the treatment, cutting it back to six seconds. The girl improved immediately—within 24 hours actually. This experience began shaping my ideas about how sensitive some people might be. Their thresholds are so low that they get triggered by almost everything (so this would be *reactive* oversensitivity). The little boy also did well on the minimum dose.

Stephen: In the early days I saw you do some amazing things with autistic children.

Len: I worked with a fourteen-year-old autistic boy, whom I shall call Ed, who had tubersclerosis sclerosis. He had a very characteristic autistic gait, and wild seizures. He was aggressive, but he was also really aware. Not long before he would go off, he would say, "I have my seizures again!"

With treatment, the gait began to straighten out—without even any physical therapy. His drawings went from primitive, violent, and bizarre, to really complex and interesting. The violent content was diminishing with treatment. As he improved, Ed took on tasks in motor coordination. He began to play ping pong and became devilishly good; his movements became more graceful and coordinated and eventually he turned out to be a ping pong champion at the Special Olympics.

Stephen: Wow! That's really a story about releasing the creative power clenched up inside this kid. What about older autistic children?

Len: I also worked with Zach, age nineteen, and Patty, twenty-two, both of whom beat or were a danger to their parents. Zach had rosy cheeks and beautiful blond curly hair and weighed about a hundred and ninety pounds. Under many circumstances he was very sweet. But one day I heard shouting that rang throughout the office building and went into the bathroom to find Zach on the floor, where his father had wrestled him. Zach was yelling and was banging his head against the tile wall.

I ran to the office to get some pillows to stuff behind his head. Then I ran to the other offices and told the people in the building that everything was okay; the police didn't need to be called. His father and I restrained him until the explosion ran its course. This was Zach's pattern, his cycle, the breathless father explained. Nothing extraordinary—only you never knew when one would hit! (The parents had warned me during the initial intake interview that this was how these episodes occurred and now I was seeing one firsthand!)

On the screen there was this huge delta that looked like it went with the explosive disorder. At that time we began doing five treatments a week. The parents were enthusiastic enough with the results that they bought a system and continued to use it at home for their son.

Patty was the twenty-two-year-old who battered her parents regularly. I did some treatments for a few weeks and then sent her home with a system. Her father e-mailed me that night: "I see no difference in her. If she does not get better, everyone will know. But if she does get better, everyone will know too!"

You know, I have to confess, I really felt bad. That night I wrote an explanatory, maybe defensive e-mail. But it just so happened that there was a glitch, and my mail program never sent my e-mail. This was fortunate, because the next e-mail I got from Patty's father a few days later said, "Sorry! I was out of line, I apologize. You know I *do* think she's getting better!"

The improvement continued, and soon Patty had a job. Then she took a plane ride, to the Carribean and by herself, with money that she had made.

Stephen: And what of Asperger's Syndrome?

Len: I worked with a nineteen-year-old-boy who had been really quite compliant and reclusive. His mother brought him in for treatments and he became surly and opinionated and blunt—almost cruel. He'd say to his classmates: "You are not contributing anything to my life, so go away!" (People with Asperger's sometimes are this way, they can be very socially assertive about their feelings.) But he was functioning better. He had been in high school, now he was taking classes at the community college. True, he would ridicule the teachers, but he was out there going to class and doing the work. His parents might have been terrified at the change from the affable recluse, but they couldn't deny how well their son was functioning in most respects. His treatment was about six seconds a month.

Attention Deficit Disorder, with and without Hyperactivity, and Learning Disabilities

There are approximately five million children who are considered to be hyperactive (ADHD) children in this country. . . . Now we have a situation . . . where a schoolteacher who has some children who might not be as interested, who may be a little bored with the classroom, can require the children to take a drug in order to stay in the classroom. I'm not sure that that is a very hopeful or helpful sign.

SENATOR EDWARD KENNEDY

Sitting in front of a box that alters brain wave activity and brain chemistry for hours at a time, drinking in over 20,000 carefully-crafted, high-impact messages a year—75% of which come exclusively from 100 of the world's largest corporations (who

> *also own the television networks and most of the broadcasting*
> *stations)—is now what we call "normal."*
>
> THOM HARTMANN

If it's true that naming something brings it into being, then that seems to be true for Attention Deficit Disorder in the second half of the twentieth-century and into the twenty-first. Did ADD exist before we had a name for it? History shows no lack of distractible people, but according to epidemiologists, the (now-labeled) problem is getting worse. Statistics show that ADD currently affects one out of every three or four American families. The obstreperous "Baby Huey" is turning into a monster indeed—consuming massive amounts of Ritalin, costing parents and teachers immense amounts of money in therapies, special tutors, and remediations—all with inconclusive results. (And statisticians have made the ominous estimate that a third to half the population of prisons is ADD, so you know where your kid could end up if you fail to help him!)

"Where does ADD come from?" ask the aggrieved parents of these difficult kids. Is it mostly genetic, or is it cultural? Or does it have to do with "too much TV?" Is it due to junk food, sugar, preservatives, dyes and additives to food? How about electrical fields, radio and television broadcasting—which our ancestors never had to contend with? There is one thing that the intellectual community generally agrees on, and that is that no one has the irrefutable answer.

As a child I looked at the mountainous pile of papers on my dad's desk (he was a teacher and had a second career caring for a parish as a minister) and wondered why it never got smaller. Then I looked at the smaller piles on my own and my brothers' desks—or, even worse, looked into our backpacks or lockers at school. I knew that at times, and when I "really tried," I was a straight A student. But when the subject didn't interest me, I just let the assignments slide. I daydreamed when that uninteresting subject came up in class, and the textbook remained unopened.

My cousin had a different problem. He was very bright and got mostly As. But he would compulsively read whatever you put in front of him. He had a prodigious amount of knowledge but my aunt didn't get much help with the household chores. My cousin could just as easily be found wallowing in his splendid comic book collection as his schoolbooks. This penchant is now referred to as "hyperfocusing" and appears in the autistic spectrum, as well as with ADD. Parents can't understand how the same child who can play Nintendo till the cows come home, oblivious to all outside stimuli, can't focus on homework for longer than thirty seconds without noticing that he is very hungry or without having to play with the dog.

Looking back, I now see that though we didn't have a name for it at the time, there was definitely ADD in our family. The human brain is smart enough to compensate for its own handicaps, however, and many adults acquire a modus operandi that helps them function despite their handicap. I myself completed graduate school and a successful twenty-eight year college teaching career and am the author of many books, as well as innumerable articles and papers.

Because I could recognize ADD in some of my students and empathize with their learning problems, for my college psychology courses I developed special techniques to keep the attention of my students. In this, I used storytelling, media stimulation, experiments, and "hands-on" experience with biofeedback equipment. Students gravitated toward these classes.

In addition to developing these special performance techniques designed to hold their attention, I used lists of "learning objectives," set up tutoring opportunities and study groups, gave ungraded "sample-tests," and also tried to respond to students' different cognitive styles—giving some the chance to take tests orally, or on the computer, if that suited them better. I also modeled for them how you do the "clean desk, and organized file-drawer thing." (If they were clutterholics, sometimes also called "pack-rats," I had them have a section on organization in their psychological journal, and work at keeping the journal itself well organized.) Cumulatively, these aids made a tremendous difference, and students who went on to successful professional lives have often come back to thank me for paying attention to *how* they were learning as well as *what* they were learning.

I made a major breakthrough to finding another way of thinking about attentional problems when I met a writer and lecturer on ADD, Thom Hartmann, who has graciously contributed a Foreword to this book. Hartmann, who claims that he, as well as certain of his children, have grappled with ADD, has written over a dozen books, performed humanitarian pilgrimages all over the world, and rubbed elbows with major political and religious figures. He believes that ADD is the result of a collision between genetic endowment and modern culture. ADD and ADHD kids are "hunters in a planter's world," as he puts it. At one time, under simpler, Paleolithic conditions of life, "distractibility" and impulsiveness may have been highly adaptive strategies.

Since Neolithic times, civilization has tended to favor settled communities and an agrarian lifestyle rather than the hunting and gathering activities and peripatetic lifestyle that characterized the Paleolithic existence. Farmers, as opposed to hunters, are less distractible, more organized, more cooperative (being also less individualistic or unconventional). Modern societies are "high-context" in that they tend to reward the "bean-counters" who can maintain routines, follow clocks and calendars, tolerate the inexorable boredom of routines, and save money.

Hartmann's ideas helped me to understand my own "largely hunter" family, and even to recontext their ADD style as something that "came with my (genetic) territory." I remember my tree-climbing, slingshot-wielding youth—and the fact that my siblings and I practiced archery, and later marksmanship with guns, for hours. (We also ran frequently, jumped and pole-vaulted over obstacles, wrestled, fought, and stalked each other for hours.) Hartmann, has in fact, helped a whole generation of people with ADD in their families change the *gestalt* or pattern just a little, to see being "a hunter" as a positive creative style as opposed to a pathological deficit. Recognizing the difference in style can help one— and one's relatives—more skillfully adapt both to culture and one's own "nature." We owe Thom Hartmann a debt for helping us see an old proclivity in a new way, and thereby freeing ourselves from a culture-bound judgmentalism in the process.[3]

How Do We Know If Someone Is ADD (Or Has "Hunter" Genes)?

DSM III and IV put forth the following criteria for ADHD:

1. When required to remain seated, a person has difficulty doing so;
2. Stimuli extraneous to the task at hand are easily distracting;

3. Holding attention to a single task or play activity is difficult;
4. Frequently will hop from one activity to another without completing the first;
5. Fidgets or squirms (or feels restless mentally);
6. Doesn't want to, or can't, wait for his or her turn in group activities;
7. Before a question is completely asked, will often interrupt the questioner;
8. Has problems with job or chore follow-through;
9. Can't play quietly without difficulty;
10. Impulsively jumps into physically dangerous activity.[4]

Hallowell and Ratey, in their well-established symptom scale, include: a search for stimulation, easily bored, creative, intuitive, highly intelligent, trouble going about things in a conventional way, low frustration tolerance, addictive behaviors, chronic problems with self-esteem, underachievement, or a sense of underachievement, disorganization.[5]

The following diagnostic categories can also be mistaken for ADD, although they may in some cases overlap it: Bipolar Disorder, Anxiety Disorder—including Obsessive-Compulsive Disorder—and Autism/Asperger's spectrum problems. In these situations, a careful clinical interview can ferret out the accurate diagnosis. One can also look into family history to see if any of these diagnostic categories is prevalent. (Until the middle of the last century, one would mainly hear that there was "a nervous condition" in the family, or that someone had to go away for frequent "recuperations" or that alcoholism existed.) In other instances, probably a dual diagnosis is the safest alternative. As in the earlier case of seven-year old Jacob cited in chapter 1, an overall CNS (Central Nervous System) dysregulation had hyperactive and inattentive features mixed with anxiety, obsessive-compulsive aspects, oppositionality and explosiveness (not to mention an atypical insomnia in a child so young.)

Some Cases of ADHD and ADD That Have Been Helped with Neurofeedback

Kiffer was about eight when he came to us. When he woke up every morning, every member of his family knew it. His behavior was described as a "bomb going off" or "a typhoon." Suffice it to say that his activities soon had *everyone* in the trailer—kids and adults—awake. He was a good-natured kid, but more like "a force of nature" than a civilized little man. We knew he was bright, but his scores in school were in the "just passing" range, and he was regularly written up for his impulsiveness, exuberantly pushing other kids, or just as joyfully scrapping. Sometimes he would just get up and walk around the classroom while other kids kept their seats.

The majority of our early progress was made with SMR training, occasionally mixed with beta sessions. Our American Biotch equipment at the time also trained EMG, so that at the same time as Kiffer trained theta down and SMR up, he did muscle relaxation. The family brought him in regularly, at first for bi-weekly, and then weekly sessions. After about twenty sessions, he was about 50 percent improved.

But the real transformation—including some startling personality changes—didn't occur until we began the EEG-driven stimulation treatments (FNS at that time). That was when his mother, eyes round with wonder, described Kiffer, one fine summer day, serving lemonade and cookies to her guests, something he never had done before. Other acts of thoughtfulness ensued, confirming that this was not just an anomaly. The FNS sessions were, in fact, so effective, on top of the earlier training, that we only did about six to eight of them. (The parents had some financial hardship, and paying for the sessions was a stretch for them.)

Later we were shown a report card by Kiffer's proud parents; it indicated that he was now getting As. About a year later we learned that he had won an academic prize in a statewide competition. (Part of the pleasure of living in a rural area with a relatively stable population is that we get to do informal longitudinal studies on some of our clients. Now, seven years later and most of the way through high school, Kiffer is a strapping young fellow who likes to help out with logging, and still gets straight As.)

Subsequently, with other ADD and ADHD children, we reversed the sequence with equally spectacular results: disentrainment first, followed by traditional SMR or beta training, or maybe even theta or alpha-theta for creativity. The results tend to support the theoretical position we have taken that it is the *flexibility*, rather than the "training-up" one particular range or other that does the trick. (However, it is also nice to know how to get into one of those useful states and prolong it when the situation warrants.)

The Case of Cynthia and ADHD

Eight-year-old Cynthia had been diagnosed with ADHD. This was unusual, since the disorder, like Autism, seems far more prevalent among boys. Bright-eyed and mischievous, the angelic-appearing little blonde waltzed boldly into the therapy room for the intake interview. She looked sweetly up at me and said, "I eat light bulbs!"

"Is that what makes you so bright?" I responded. Indeed, she was very bright, with an uncanny charisma that included the ability to get other children into all kinds of mischief—in and out of school. Her motor was running constantly, and Cynthia not infrequently flabbergasted adults who didn't know what to do with her. Her mother, though, couldn't stand the thought of occluding this sparkly, difficult, wonderful little selfhood with Ritalin—as school authorities and doctors had advised her. She wanted her little girl to "be herself" at the end of whatever therapy she underwent.

And this is just what happened. Neurofeedback and sandplay therapy were used as primary modalities. Cynthia was able to use the "free space" of the sandbox to express her creative imagination. In the process, the play itself became more coherent and less chaotic and wildly obsessive. The play mirrored the new self-imposed order that was emerging in her psyche. Soon complimentary reports were coming back from teachers and grandparents. Cynthia was just as impish, but somehow not so annoying. She seemed to be less intrusive and demanding, more appropriate. Now the positive side of her personality was emerging without the ragged edge of the hyperactivity.

As the weather changed, we began increasingly to take little walks around the farm adjacent to our therapy center. Cynthia had an insatiable thirst for nature and loved to study all the little creatures that lived in puddles, and under the roots of trees. As summer wore on, at Cynthia's request, we instituted hippotherapy (as we had with Jacob). Horses are wonderful cotherapists. Being large, strong, and furry, they naturally attract kids' attention. By being mostly placid and gentle, they teach, wordlessly. Cynthia's graduation session from therapy included (as it had with Jacob also) a (supervised) horseback ride. Her mother was immensely proud of this, and glad of the route she had taken.

I have always loved Freud's saying about psychoanalysis, that it "speeds up the process of maturation." I feel that neurofeedback does the same thing, only much better. Some of the young people that have been brought to our center try to meet the challenges of adapting to an (unbalanced) society with nervous systems that are immature. Social and educational structures pose challenges they just can't grow up fast enough to meet. In neurofeedback, and particularly in the LENS, because it "feeds-back" the person to him or herself, there is something almost like "cooking" going on. An "alchemical transformation," my Jungian colleagues would say. If we overdo the stimulation (turn up the heat) there is regression, and all the old bad behaviors can return. If we titrate our treatment just right, however, there is a slow, almost unnoticable maturation that takes place until something gets noticed—he serves lemonade, or she does all the dishes without being asked, etc.

Randy's Maturation

Randy was an explosive fifteen-year-old who had a low academic average and a history of head injuries along with his ADHD. He was placed on stimulant medication, but it only seemed to make him even more erratic and wild. A few months before he came to us, he had stolen the family van, driven without a license and, rushing into the school parking lot just as classes were letting out, then (inexpertly) rolled the van over—in front of everybody—to the dismay of the administration, and the glee of the students. (This event also got the attention of his parents, needless to say.)

Part of the problem with having Randy on meds was that he was erratic about taking them. Either he would trade or sell them to other kids, forget to take them, or having forgotten to take them, he would guiltily take a whole bunch at once. Ritalin inflamed his impulsivity, and in addition to the family van incident, he had punched a lot of holes in the plaster at home. Randy's brain map showed "hot-spots" corresponding to the injuries, with both dysregulated delta and theta.

At first Randy would only shrug his shoulders or say "I dunno" (when asked how he was feeling). But in treatment, he suddenly began remembering how he had gotten this injury or that one. He wanted his mother to confirm his memories: "Hey, do you remember when I was jumping up on the bed and bounced off and hit my head on the radiator?" Or "That one was that stupid bike accident!"

He became interested in looking at his brain map and seeing how the sites on it connected to his injuries. At this point, we began no longer to need the "second opinion" of one of his parents on the subjective rating scale. He would rate himself, even moving back up, or regressing on a particular symptom like irritability or procrastination, moving himself up or down a half point, rather than a whole, as if making fine distinctions.

At the last session Randy had brought all his 8s and 9s down to the 1–4 range. In addition to his behavior maturing and improving, Randy was maturing physically as well: his voice was deepening as he aged. Suddenly *voila!* a much more dignified and thoughtful young man was making his appearance. Maturation had caught up to Randy.

These are not isolated incidents. In the past year, satisfied parents have recommended our work to other parents who are seeking to help their troubled children and, as a result, we now have a whole population of young people who come to us to "get their maturation sped up." When the regular treatments give these children more energy, emotional and cognitive flexibility, and freedom from anxiety, they naturally start achieving the developmental milestones that are right there waiting for them.

What I especially like is seeing Thom Hartmann's "hunters" come into their own. Every negative trait that can be identified in kids who are neurologically dysfunctional can have a positive trait, or "surprise" awaiting them when self-regulation or inner balance is achieved. Hyperactivity can turn into high energy. Restlessness can turn into versatility. Pathological hyperfocusing can expand to include more activities than just video games. Poor self-image (because the kid has no self-control) can turn into a healthy self-image as that self-control is gained.

In his books *ADD Success Stories* and *Healing ADD,* Thom Hartmann has also developed useful strategies for living with ADD, and taking the "hunter" into account in one's self-appraisal. The following list is designed to help those afflicted with ADD and is applicable to children, older students, or adults:

1. Break schoolwork down into smaller units that are more manageable.
2. Sit in the front of the class.
3. Look for the most interesting teachers.
4. Color code everything, highlight and mark up books.

5. Keep reminders where the individual can see them.
6. Read summaries before chapters.
7. Double check everything for careless errors.[6]

Learning Disabilities

In the final section of this chapter, I discuss with Len Ochs what is meant by Learning Disabilities, and how the LENS can address them.

Stephen: I am very interested in how the LENS helps with learning disabilities. I'm quite convinced it does, but I don't know what the operative mechanism is.

Len: Well, first of all, consider that there are many, many, many different reasons for learning problems: from visual processing problems; to being able to associate sound with what you see and to make visual discriminations and auditory discriminations; to be able to take information in, and sort of know what you have done with it; to be able to recall it, sequence it and prioritize it, track it, and organize it. So there are many potential kinds of learning problems. They say that alcoholics are "not able to learn from experience." So is that a learning disability or what?

Stephen: There's a question on the CNS Questionnaire (see chapter 11) that relates to this issue of not being able to learn from experience. I think it's so important. It's real, and it's a dimension that ought to be recognized as such and monitored.

Len: It's possible to really track people's ability to do this. A damaged or disorganized brain can go round and round in the same track and never seem to get anywhere, and it has to do with a fundamental inability to utilize the data of experience. It's a neurological problem. In the sense that LENS treatment increases flexibility, and clarifies perception, it makes it easier to process sights and sounds, juxtapose them with memories and concepts, to organize and retrieve them, and to play with them in one's head. Yes, I would say LENS is quite extraordinary in its applicability to many kinds of learning difficulties.

Stephen: Is it best if it is combined with other cognitive kinds of approaches?

Len: Well, it all depends on the timing. If simultaneously, a person is utilizing four different therapeutic modalities, and something is going wrong, then there is the job of sifting out what approach is leading to the problems that are arising. So my preference is to do things in an iterative, sequential fashion. So you try one and you try another one, and you try the first one again, you try the second one again, and you try the third one, and then you try the first one again. I have seen LENS facilitate every other approach and I have seen every other approach facilitate LENS. So there is a real interactive kind of a symbiosis between different kinds of approaches.

So if you come back to using this treatment after using another one, the other approach will enhance the ability of this one to work. They are all different forms of stimulation, and by taking things in through one modality, or one kind of process, that will probably facilitate taking things in and organizing them through another process. I think, in so doing, we are probably opening up more channels in the brain. And each time a different approach is used, we are facilitating communication within the brain.

Stephen: I'm thinking of Howard Gardner's notion of multiple intelligences, and Dan Goleman's idea of emotional intelligence. You know Abraham Maslow said, "If the only tool you have is a hammer, everything begins to look like a nail!" In a sense, the adaptive, intelligent human has a whole toolbox, a whole bag of tricks: a hammer, a saw, a drill, etc.

Len: Right, and the adaptive, intelligent human is able to learn the appropriate use for each one, and switch back and forth flexibly as the job requires. You don't just stay there hammering.

Conclusion

Our work with children is immensely gratifying due, in part, to the fact that the younger the patient, the more likely the success of the intervention. The very immaturity that frustrates parents and teachers alike can be an ally for the neurotherapist. Always working *with* rather than *against* nature, we try to see the positive side of symptoms that may be seen by others with different outlooks as negative. Keeping our treatments always within the bounds of the comfort and sensitivity of the child, we find results becoming more durable and permanent with the treatment. The natural entelichal processes (energies in nature that aim at a goal) of child development that have become blocked or retarded resume.

As we have demonstrated, expressive arts such as sandplay, drawing, painting, sculpture, mask-making, dance, and acting can really help developmentally disabled or delayed children find their lost selfhood and resume a natural growth process. Combined with LENS, these therapies can offer awesome results in self-development and maturation, allowing a child to have a reasonable chance of attaining their natural potential to become a fully functioning adult.

6

THE TWILIGHT ZONE

Fibromyalgia, Lyme Disease, and Chronic Fatigue Syndrome

*Stephen Larsen, Ph.D., Len Ochs, Ph.D., and
Mary Lee Esty, L.C.S.W., Ph.D.*

The title for this chapter was drawn from an image or a metaphor we keep hearing from people who, in some way, suffer from one or more of these syndromes: "I feel like I'm in 'the twilight zone'" (after the TV series based on strange or anomalous experiences people have had). The metaphor suggests that there is a dimness and a faded quality about life, and that people become stuck in a kind of mental and emotional "twilight." In this murky realm, diagnoses are easily confused, depending on which cluster of symptoms predominates, but sufferers speak of fatigue, depression, anxiety, chronic pain, muscle stiffness and weakness, insomnia, cognitive cloudiness, disorganization, and procrastination. Some sufferers coined the term "fibro-fog" to describe the way this group of symptoms makes them feel.

In Epstein-Barr Syndrome, or Lyme disease, the presence of a causal micro-organism is diagnostic, and the medical treatment is varied accordingly. But even after the prescribed regimen of weeks of antibiotics, in the case of Lyme disease, for example, the CNS of the person may not fully recover, leading to the lingering syndrome called "neurological Lyme disease," for which the antibiotics seem to do nothing. Likewise the viral infection of Epstein-Barr leaves the victim perpetually fatigued, and often with muscular stiffness and pain.

Interestingly, all of these disorders emerged as clinical entities in the late 1970s and '80s, roughly around the same time as each other. But it takes a discerning diagnostician to ferret out which diagnosis to actually use, which makes a critical difference to the treatment chosen.

Post-Traumatic Fibromyalgia

There is one kind of fibromyalgia that follows serious accidents; it is sometimes called "Post-Traumatic Fibromyalgia."

Piedad Bernikow is a sufferer of this latter syndrome. About six months after her car was rear-ended in 1992, she developed a series of symptoms that were finally diagnosed as fibromyalgia syndrome or FMS. (There is also a related syndrome called MPS, myofascial pain syndrome.)

Noting the effects of this syndrome on herself, Bernikow began to research the intriguing statistic that women are far more likely to develop FMS than men, although some men definitely have it (as in the case of Jay described later in this chapter). Much of the reason for this, she says, is due to the different physiognomies of women. Women have poorer muscle tone than men, and more soft tissue, two factors that cause them to respond differently (than men) to impacts and injuries.

She describes some typical fibromyalgia patients at the Mayo clinic:

A woman who had been in a severe skiing accident;

A woman who had been thrown from a horse;

A woman who had undergone extensive spine surgery;

A man who had fallen backward into a hole at a construction site and was buried alive;[1]

A woman who had suffered a low impact rear-end car accident. (Some studies even show that serious injuries with fibromyalgic complications can be sustained in auto collisions of less than 15 mph.)[2]

An individual suffering from fibromyalgia can have traumatic global effects such as those caused by toxic chemicals, very high fevers, shock reactions to medications, vaccinations, or electrocution. (One of our first fibromyalgia patients was a man who had been hit by roughly 1500 volts from a high-tension line. He lived with ceaseless widespread pain, fatigue, and insomnia.)

To diagnose fibromyalgia, most medical doctors use a test of 11 out of 18 specific points of pain tenderness. This was used as one of the criteria of illness/relief in an important study entitled "Treatment of Fibromyalgia Incorporating EEG-Driven Stimulation: A Clinical Outcomes Study" conducted by Dr. Stuart Donaldson and others.[3] Donaldson is a major biofeedback researcher and fibromyalgia specialist, and developer of EMG, or muscle-based protocols to treat myofascial pain. (This study, which we will henceforth call the Mueller-Donaldson study, is key to our discussion and will be cited frequently throughout this chapter.)

The subtler symptom dimensions that accompany fibromyalgia, however, are often left out of these more simplistic kinds of diagnosis. As well, sometimes doctors will even say to their patients: "It's all in your head," and insurance companies sometimes send patients to their *own* psychiatrists to prove that the patients are malingering.

Bob Flaws, who has pioneered holistic approaches for fibromyalgia patients, has developed a much more extensive list of symptoms, below.

90–100% of Fibromyalgia Patients Have:

Generalized body pain affecting all four quadrants of the body
Fatigue
Muscular stiffness

70–90% of Fibromyalgia Patients Have:

Post-exertional malaise
Sleep disturbances
Headaches (migraine or tension)
Tenderness to pressure at specific points
Swollen feet
Numbness and/or tingling
Difficulty thinking and concentrating ("Fibro-fog")
Dizziness
Sensitivity to light, noise, and/or smells
Hypersensitivity to stress
Dysmennorrhea or painful menstruation
Dry mouth

50–70% of Fibromyalgia Patients Have:

Irritable Bowel Syndrome (IBS)
Blurred vision
Mood swings
Heart palpitations
Cold extremities
Feverish feelings
Allergies

15–50% of Fibromyalgia Patients Have:

Restless Leg Syndrome
Muscle twitches
Itchy skin
Hearing disturbances
Night sweats
Breathing problems
Proneness to infections
Skin rashes
Interstitial cystitis
Temporomandibular Joint Disorder (TMJ or jaw problems)
Multiple chemical sensitivities.[4]

This constitutes a much more comprehensive inventory than the usual medical catchall one of "tender points" and reflects the pervasiveness of this disorder and the fact that its effects cover a very broad spectrum. There is also a strong overlapping with the CNS distortions that we address with the LENS treatment.

When it comes to fibromyalgia, conventional medicine has pretty much bottomed-out. Painkillers, steroids, and antibiotics have all been tried. But these, in turn, wreak their usual side effects on delicate constitutions already damaged by a bout with the illness. And for the most part, "the efficacy of available treatments (e.g., pharmacologic, aerobic exercise, biofeedback, hypnosis, physical therapies, multi-modal/multidisciplinary, and so on) have typically demonstrated only moderate success, and large numbers of patients remain very impaired, even disabled."[5]

As mentioned, fibromyalgia is disproportionately found among women, although it is by no means an exclusively feminine disease. The

(Mueller-Donaldson) study quoted in the preceding paragraph tells us that 60 percent of people diagnosed with Chronic Fatigue Syndrome will also meet the criteria for fibromyalgia. Coderre, Katz, Vaccarino, and Melzack suggested a model in 1993 that has subsequently governed most of the CNS-focussed treatments. It is called the "central plasticity model of chronic pain." In this model, there is less of a focus on the muscles, fascia, and connective tissue that seem to be the locus of the pain, and more of a focus on the hyperaroused and irritable condition of the CNS, which amplifies and overreacts to peripheral proprioceptive signals.[6]

Stuart Donaldson found that among subjects with consistent CNS symptoms—including insomnia, hypervigilance, and cognitive cloudiness—the results from myofascial EMG biofeedback alone were not what had been hoped for, hinting at the probable presence of a centrally mediating factor.[7] The presence of such a factor would explain the global nature of some of the symptoms, and how they all seem to occur together.

Do you remember, from Psychology 101, that strange-looking anthropomorphic figure called the "homunculus," stretched out along the sensory and the motor cortex, the ugly guy with the huge lips, face, tongue, and hands, and dwarfish other parts? This zone of the physical representation of the body that is both receptive (sensory) and active (motor) is where we are consciously aware of ourselves as sensing and responding organisms in the world. If this site is neurologically hyper-reactive, it would distort the reception of signals from all over the body, cloud the external senses, and perhaps interfere with motor abilities.

Donaldson found that EEG-driven stimulation was highly effective in ameliorating the central-processing dimension of fibromyalgia. In the Mueller-Donaldson study, EDS (EEG-driven stimulation), an earlier version of the Ochs's protocol (using the I-400 and glasses with LEDs) was used. It was found that "vaguely diffuse" pain treated with the EEG-driven stimulation tended to reduce and morph into more specific areas of muscular pain, which could *then* be treated using EMG, physical therapy, and other modalities.[8]

The summarizing discussion of the Mueller-Donaldson paper is important enough to be included here:

These 30 Patients treated primarily with EDS (using LED glasses, in an earlier version of LENS) experienced significant reductions in a broad array of symptomatology associated with FMS (Fibromyalgia Syndrome) that also corresponded to changes in EEG patterns from the beginning to the completion of treatment. Notable improvements were seen not only in pain intensity but also in cognitive processing difficulties, mood, sleep, and (to a distinct though less marked extent) tiredness, and fatigue. Physical examination procedures including pressure algometry further verified physical improvements. Correspondingly, positive changes were highlighted by a general reduction in usage of a variety of prescription and nonprescription medications for pain control, although in some instances there was a self-reported increase in the use of alternative or complementary (e.g., herbal, vitamin, and so on) preparations. Employment and/or disability status remained unchanged in slightly more than half of the subjects, but in the remaining portion, major reengagement in employment and relinquishing of disability status were in evidence. Evidence from follow-up questionnaires pointed to benefits being maintained an average of approximately eight months after treatment termination.

These findings raise both clinical and basic science implications. Practically speaking, the clinical improvements were accomplished with a multi-modal treatment package but one that emphasized a specific brain wave-based treatment. EDS was typically the sole focus of treatment until those symptoms most distinctively reflective of CNS dysfunction improved sufficiently for other therapies to then be implemented more effectively. Most frequently, patients first reported significant improvement in mental clarity, such as the ability to focus and maintain concentration, as well as mood and restorative sleep. Self-reported pain then appeared to change in nature and quality to the extent that patients began to experience a reduction in their "all-over" body pain and an increase in specific localized aches and pains. In tandem with this change from a diffuse to more localized or regional type of pain experience, patients also seemed better able to describe their pain sensation in specific as opposed to vague terms.

This change in pain experience served as an indicator to begin physical therapies focused on reduction and management of the now more localized pains. In our clinical experience, this involved a combination of massage and myofascial release therapies, biomechanical and postural reeducation, muscle stretching and strengthening exercises, and EMG-guided neuromuscular retraining of identified myofascial pain syndromes and muscle imbalance patterns.

Prior to EDS, attempts by means of the more standard physical therapies to treat the diffusely represented pain and associated symptoms of FMS had failed. Following initial treatment with EDS, only a very modest amount of these other therapies was required to lead to successful outcomes. The overall cost-effectiveness of this approach with the patients reported in this series was apparent as well.

Given that a multi-modal treatment was employed, it might be argued that the role of EDS remains uncertain. Indeed, within the context of this preliminary investigation and due to the limitations of the design of a study conducted in a clinical practice setting without research funding, it is not possible to conclude with certainty that EDS is a beneficial therapy for FS. However, examination of the treatment session ratings for pain intensity, sleep quality, fatigue, cognitive clouding, depression, and anxiety provided some preliminary support for the central role of EDS in instigating the change process in this group of patients. Indeed, comparisons of these ratings from the beginning of treatment to just before any other therapies were instituted and to those obtained at the end of treatment suggested that the major significant differences in symptom ratings were largely accounted for in this first phase of treatment with EDS. Although the trend to continue improvements in all areas was manifested in further incremental positive changes on all symptom ratings, only the pain intensity rating showed further statistically significant change from this intermediate point in the treatment to the end of treatment.

Further, it should be noted that the incorporation of other therapies was typically at a low level of intensity, much lower than might typically be the case, and for which there has previously been reported modest (or hardly any) success under most circumstances. Hence, it would appear that EDS may have contributed a specific and necessary ingredient that was the prime initiator of therapeutic efficacy. Still, this is only a tentative conclusion.

Moreover, these findings do not suggest that EDS would necessarily be successful in isolation for the majority of cases, and a multi-modal perspective is likely still to be indicated. There were, though, four participants in this study who received solely EDS as an intervention and benefited substantially from this treatment alone. In the reality of the clinical practice setting in which all of the participants were treated, it is not possible to fully isolate all therapeutic components and their corresponding efficacy. Moreover, it is the clinically apparent success in alleviating symptoms that drives the treatment approach at any given stage.

Further research is justified to verify these suggestive findings in larger samples and in direct comparison with more standard therapies, including single and multi-modal interventions in randomized controlled designs. In future research, it will be important to examine the efficacy of EDS in patients randomly assigned to treatment under double-blinded conditions. It also will be important to assess the effects of EDS alone versus any other therapies.

For example, EDS alone could be compared with EDS plus other specific therapies in various combinations and in varying sequences of timing to yield component analyses of different effects. If there is an optimal timing for the institution of other therapies besides EDS, it will be important to identify reliable and quantifiable indicators of this shift, whether in terms of specific levels of symptom ratings, the change from diffuse to more localized pain, patterns of EEG activity, or other parameters. Moreover, given that there was considerable variability in the numbers of EDS sessions provided, it will be important to better identify the range of optimal number of treatment sessions.

Further, given the central role posited for change in the EEG as a function of EDS and presumably corresponding improvements in symptom reports, it will be necessary to more clearly demonstrate the link between changes in the EEG and various outcome measures. This may require more frequent monitoring and mapping of the EEG coinciding with measurements of various symptoms and functional outcomes.

The findings reported here also are provocative in contributing further to the basic scientific understanding of FMS. The improvements in symptoms potentially reflective of CNS dysfunction heralding subsequent amenability to other physically oriented therapies were matched by a corresponding change in brain wave patterns from pre- to post-treatment. The relative preponderance of low frequency (delta, theta, and low alpha) activity detected primarily from relatively anterior and central cortical recording sites that was in evidence at the outset of treatment normalized by the conclusion of treatment. This further underscores the potentially important role of CNS dysfunction in ongoing manifestations of FMS (fibromyalgia).

The extent to which this may lead to further developments in the understanding of the etiologic or maintaining factors in FMS remains for future research to determine. Investigations that utilize more quantitative EEG assessments, instead of the sequential single site recording of the present EDS procedures, as well as correlation with other measures of CNS functioning, would contribute to a broadened understanding of CNS processes and FMS. In general, then, this approach holds some promise for reducing the suffering of the many individuals debilitated with FMS by immediate clinical applications and future refinements in these techniques, and by contributing to a better understanding of the basic disease mechanisms of FMS. Future research under more highly controlled conditions will help to evaluate the fruits of this promise.[9]

A Discussion of the Mueller-Donaldson Paper, and Subsequent Fibromyalgia Studies

The above paper is useful in several regards. By utilizing and comparing "central" versus "peripheral" approaches for dealing with FMS, it opens a conceptual dialogue. At Stone Mountain Center we have treated far more patients on the LENS or its predecessors alone, without the supplemental therapies, than the sample in this paper. Our finding confirms that the treatment as a "stand-alone" treatment may lower subjective discomfort on a variety of clinical dimensions, and improve generic functioning.

However, we have also more recently begun to use supplemental approaches, such as the Bales Photonic Stimulator (see also chapter 12), that shines infrared light directly on the muscles, nerves, and fascia, thus treating the peripheral dimension. We also have a Feldenkrais worker on our staff and have used that approach with some patients, as well as referring these patients to massage therapists, acupuncturists, and Qi Gong and yoga practitioners. So we would agree with Mueller, Donaldson et al., in saying that, in our experience, attacking the problem "from both sides" (that is CNS based and neuromuscularly based) seems to offer the most potential.

A recent clinical experience was of Irene, a computer programmer who was always "on" and began to develop what seemed like repetitive strain injuries, along with carpal tunnel aspects. But the focus of the debilitating pain was in the neck and shoulders, which were inflamed and tender. She was also sleepless, fatigued, and "tired of fighting the pain." For the first five sessions, photonic stimulation seemed to "do the trick" giving her 50–60 percent relief. But after a while, she regressed, and the treatments even seemed to make her worse. Likewise, with the acupuncture, massage, and chiropractic that she tried. The pattern was fairly consistent: "a little better right after the treatment, then worse again." On the whole she was no more than about 20–25 percent better, and sometimes—with stimulation or stress—even worse than she was before.

Irene had read some of our literature on neurofeedback and asked to try it. Just the offset and the map produced a global improvement that nothing else had even come close to. By the third actual treatment, she was saying she was 95 percent better. Now the massages didn't hurt as much, the acupuncture seemed gentler, and she could accept infrared treatments at a medium level again. This single case seems to illustrate the importance of central factors, in the "neural plasticity" model.

As with most things living, there is not an "either/or" setup, where either this or that approach is the correct or only one. And it is intriguing how a few seconds of cortical treatment can make the subjectively perceived sensation of pain in the extremities lessen. But also, as in the above case of Irene, muscle spasms and inflammation, in other words "hypertonia," can go down. The only workable conclusion is that neither the brain nor the peripheral muscles and nerves should be considered in isolation. They form feedback loops with each other, and other parts of the anatomy. When the CNS is quieted, the muscles, as if in recognition, seem to lose that hypertonic or irritated condition.

However, sometimes the inverse is true, as I have seen when treating a large violent horse with a head injury, peripherally with the photon stimulator. After several minutes of treatment, accompanied by thrashing and eye-rolling, he heaved the biggest sigh and became still. After the treatment, he was nuzzling all the clinicians and his owner. Ochs believes that frequently in global pain and fatigue syndromes, the peripheral areas are bombarding and overwhelming the cortex, so it can't function normally. Then it gets irritated—or shuts off—which both have their consequences on the mental life and behavior of the patient.

Apropos of the Mueller-Donaldson Study, it should be noted that LENS equipment and procedures have progressed several generations since that study was done (primarily in 1998, 1999, and 2000). It is assumed that the current equipment offers a more penetrating effect on the cortex, through pulsed radio frequency stimulations (as opposed to flickering lights), and a refined and weaker feedback stimulus, allowing more control of the treatment level. This study, redone on the current equipment, might even show improvements.

The Case of Jay: An Early Encounter at Stone Mountain Center with Fibromyalgia and Its Effect on Mental Health

The supervising psychiatrist at the local county mental health center made a referral of a patient we shall call "Jay" to us. The doctor was not very hopeful or optimistic, but he and his patient had run out of options. Jay had contracted a viral infection some twenty years prior and had been suffering from terrible physical exhaustion and pain ever since. Jay's quality of life was so restricted and so poor that he was not only badly depressed but occasionally suicidal.

Although Jay's psychiatric diagnosis was Major Depression, severe, *he* believed his depression was an outcome of a debilitating battle with fibromyalgia. When the doctors tried to cure his depression with SSRI-type drugs, the result was disaster. He told us that, for him, Prozac triggered a psychotic episode that had landed him in the psych ward of the local hospital—upon his release he had been seeing a psychiatrist at the County Mental Health Center; said psychiatrist referred Jay to us.

Jay had done so many bouts of antibiotics, that his intestinal flora were permanently decimated, leading to all kinds of digestive problems. With Jay unable to work, the family's financial burden rested on his wife, who was stressed in about fifteen ways—raising the children, earning the money, watching over a sick husband, etc.

While we did not hold out much hope for Jay, Len Ochs told us of his success treating people with fibromyalgia and informed us of the Donaldson study. The improvements we would be looking for would be similar to any of the categories that we treated—improvements in flexibility, clarity, mood stabilization, energy. But twenty years of a degenerative-seeming condition is an awful lot to reverse. Jay's brain map showed a preponderance of lower frequencies, delta and theta, as well as alpha perfusion in the frontal areas.

Jay's Medicare, which we were able to accept in those days (around 2000), allowed him to come in for treatment twice a week. I did psychotherapy and helped him deal with the emotional fallout of his diminished life, while my colleague, Jim Giorgi, did the FNS treatments as a kind of an adjunct.

I think we all were astonished when, over a period of about two months, Jay actually began to improve at an undeniable rate. First his energy picked up, and he reported sleeping better. His mood improved slightly. He seemed less suicidal. He was able to taper off and then eliminate the low doses of SSRIs, drugs that he claimed were not helping him anyway.

After about three months, even Jay's skeptical psychiatrist allowed himself some amazement. Jay's newfound vitality was very apparent; he was able to take long walks, play more with his children, and help out around the house. By the time Jay finished treatment, he and his wife had realized a lifelong dream—they opened a successful bed and breakfast in their home. Five years after the discontinuation of Jay's treatment we are still sending them clients (who are among our patients who come up for longer courses of treatment, or who are professionals-in-training for our neurofeedback programs).

TBI and Fibromyalgia: The Rush Study
MARY LEE ESTY, L.C.S.W., PH.D.

Four people in our Traumatic Brain Injury (TBI) Study (from a field of twelve participants) had fibromyalgia as a result of their TBIs. After disentrainment treatment, they were all significantly improved for fibromyalgia. Their pain was gone except for one patient with a prior history of migraines, who improved in many ways but still had some migraines. Three of the four were able to return to work at their previous levels.

Deborah's Fibromyalgia

In March of 1998, I got a call from a seventy-year-old fibromyalgia patient who was being treated at the Rush-Presbyterian St. Luke's Medical Center in Chicago. She had heard of me through one of our study participants. I invited Dr. Stuart Donaldson and Dr. Len Ochs to the meeting. Fortuitously, the annual meeting of The Association for Applied Psychophysiology and Biofeedback (AAPB), which both men were attending, was in Florida near where this woman lived.

Now let me take a little detour here. I had read in *Biofeedback Magazine* about Stu Donaldson's work using EMG for carpal-tunnel syndrome, and how it had helped employees of the Ford Motor Company cope with overuse injuries. So I took a workshop of his, because I wanted to know what he was doing. It was very interesting, but one of the things that struck me was, at the end of the first day, he said that he couldn't understand why "We can help almost everybody with carpal tunnel and myofascial pain, but we haven't been able to help anybody with fibromyalgia, it doesn't last."

And so a little light bulb went off in my head; and I thought, "Well that's interesting!" Because I was treating people—often for other things, though some of them had fibromyalgia—and they were telling me that their pain was going away. So I went to Stu, whom I didn't really know at all, and I said, "I'm doing this weird stuff with Len Ochs, and people are telling me their pain is decreasing. What if you combined that with your EMG treatment, wouldn't that be an interesting thing?"

So then I went to Len Ochs and said, "You really ought to talk to Stu Donaldson." So they got together. Stu sent someone from his practice down to Len's to get trained. And that led to Stu's published article:

"Treatment of Fibromyalgia Incorporating EEG-Driven Stimulation, a Clinical Outcomes Study." Stu also wrote an article entitled "A Retrospective on 252 Referrals with Fibromyalgia"[10] that appeared in the *Canadian Journal of Clinical Medicine* in 1998. At the Palm Springs Futurehealth Conference (which was about the same time as the publication of Stu's article in 1998), Stu gave a workshop on how they had conducted the study. When I realized that I had the same capabilities in my office, we started the whole fibromyalgia project.

Flash forward to a little later that spring, when Deborah called me from Chicago and told me about her thirty years of fibromyalgia pain. She had just gotten out of the hospital recently, one of many she had attended to treat her condition. She said she had told her husband, "If I don't feel better soon, I am calling Dr. Kevorkian!"* And then she asked me, quite plaintively, "Can *you* help me?"

I said, "I don't know!" (But Ochs and Donaldson encouraged me.)

Deborah came in for treatment in May of '98, and I have to say, she was in terrible shape. At the beginning of treatment her gait was so unsteady that she needed help walking. Even in a short walk down the hallway, she would veer into the wall.

We did a brain map for her and followed the site sort (FNS treatment had come a long way by then). Deborah was treated at first with the I-400 machine, because she was so fragile, and I wanted to be as gentle as possible. However, she later was treated with the C-2 and did very well. (C-2 being the later generation machine that utilizes radio waves rather than lights.)

Deborah came for weekly treatments, then alternated with a week or two of no-treatment, followed by treatments again. She also received surface EMG (electromyographic muscle relaxation) treatments, following Dr. Donaldson's protocol, as well as myofascial treatment. The biofeedback training, including autonomic (GSR and temp training) was done by a colleague, Joan Nelson, L.C.S.W.-C. (In my opinion, physiological biofeedback and therapies are essential along with the brain stimulation for a full recovery from Fibromyalgia syndrome.)

Deborah's husband, who was quite wealthy, had told me when we started that if I could help her, he was interested in funding fibromyalgia research.

---

*Dr. Kevorkian was the medical doctor who practiced assisted suicide.

Within only a few months (July and August) Deborah was able to begin playing golf again, without any pain, for the first time in I don't know how many years. She wasn't completely well, but she was much improved.

The patient's physician, Dr. Jan Fawcett, wanted to invite me to come to Rush to explain what we had done, because they had had no expectation that her condition could ever improve. (Deborah had been documented as being ill for thirty years when she began treatment with us.) In September, I got a call from the head of Rush. He had just done a checkup on Deborah and he said to me: "Will you come out here and show us what you are doing?" Now this was a conscientious doctor who had known the patient for many years, and had had no reason to expect her sudden reversal of symptoms. "What is happening here?" he wondered.

So I went to Chicago in what would prove to be one of the more interesting experiences of my life. Facing me were about twelve male physicians, all of whom were skeptical, and I was trying to explain this—to say the least—rather unusual procedure to them. Of course, the first question they asked was, "Where are the animal studies?"

I managed not to laugh but was afflicted for a while by images of pigs running around wearing dark glasses, with LEDs (the early FNS equipment). But actually, the event went very well, and afterward the Rush team continued to follow Deborah's progress—and progress it was! The patient continued to improve in the ways we have learned to expect from this treatment: overall CNS improvement in sleep and energy, as well as freedom from pain. Over the next year, some awful things happened to her, things that I thought would set her way back; I mean some very tragic family things. At one point, however, her doctor called me and said, "You know, I am astounded and so grateful. I don't think Deborah would have survived these events if her health and resilience hadn't been so improved by your treatments."

In September of that year, her husband asked me to write a brief proposal of any research I would like to do. It couldn't be any longer than a page, or he wouldn't read it. He didn't mention any specific level of funding, so my initial proposal was low—about three hundred thousand dollars. When the donor pressed me as to whether this amount would be sufficient or not, I expanded it to approximately seven hundred fifty thousand dollars.

On June sixth of the following year (1999), Deborah handed me a handwritten note (which I keep over my desk at home) notifying me that on July 1 her husband would be depositing one million dollars to the Rush Institute for a study! She started referring to the Neurotherapy Center of Washington, DC (my office) as "the ultimate spa." Occasionally she will call and say, "I am ready for a tune-up!" I'm not even sure she needs it because she is doing so well, but of course we oblige. She is golfing, swimming, very active socially, and has been pain-free for over five years following her treatment.

Stephen Larsen Interviews Dr. Mary Lee Esty on TBI and Fibromyalgia

Stephen: So how is fibromyalgia related to TBI?

Mary Lee: Of the people in my TBI study, there were four who had post-traumatic fibromyalgia. I didn't know very much about fibromyalgia at the time, but they all had pain, and with the FNS treatments, they got well from the pain. I think only one of them was still taking medication, and all were back at work and had recovered their previous level of functioning. They had varied between five and ten years, as I remember, of being unable to work after their respective trauma.

Stephen: I think it is an amazing story how that tight little study, with Nancy Schoenberger et al., led to the much bigger fibromyalgia study.

Mary Lee: The setting for much of the new study was to be Rush-Presbyterian-St. Luke's Medical Center in Chicago, a huge thing that involved consent forms, protocol, coordination by sites, data collection, and processing. The whole thing had to go, of course, before their IRB, the Institutional Review Board, for the protection of human subjects. And it took a long time to get on the agenda because they had fifteen hundred research projects ongoing. They do a lot of research along with treatment. But it was chosen because Deborah had been a patient at Rush for thirty years and they saw her FMS symptoms rapidly disappearing, and her energy and clarity returning. We treated fifty-six people at my site and eight at Rush, because Rush had never done the procedure and it took some time for them to find and train the people to do the procedure.

Stephen: What did you learn from that much larger study?

Mary Lee: During the study, many of the complications that make the diagnosis and treatment of FMS so difficult became apparent. Treatment outcomes will always be adversely affected when chronic infections from Lyme disease, parasites, mycoplasmas and congenital conditions such as Ehlers-Danloss—a heritable connective tissue with joints that constantly dislocate—are misdiagnosed as FMS or coexist with FMS. There is no treatment likely to produce a reversal of symptoms. One positive result of simultaneously treating so many people diagnosed with FMS was the opportunity to compare the EEG maps of people who responded positively to those who did not. The data may give new insights for making better treatment plans and identifying those who need to be evaluated for infections and myofascial pain syndrome. The most important outcome of the study is that we have demonstrated that EEG-related stimulation is essential to recovery from FMS.

Coping with Ehlers-Danloss

The Ehlers-Danloss Syndrome (EDS) is a group of heritable systemic disorders of connective tissue manifesting joint hypermobility, skin extensibility, dislocations, subluxations, and tissue fragility.[11]

In ordinary terms, the victim of this genetically based disorder suffers continuous dislocations, or "falling out of joint." People with Type III of this illness take frequent falls as hips, knees, and ankles dislocate, sometimes with extreme pain. Down they go to the pavement, or even down stairs, suddenly compounding the pervasive pain with incessant injuries. For some, even turning over in bed can be a risky affair. Dislocations can be accompanied by acute pain.

For Sheila, who was referred to us by a local psychiatrist, the case was severe, with all of the above symptoms, plus constant fatigue and pain. In many respects it was just like fibromyalgia, but with this extra little glitch of the constant dislocation. She was insomniac and highly anxious. Sheila was also afflicted with Sjogren's Syndrome, an autoimmune problem of dry mucous membranes throughout the body.[12] This double affliction, which is known to occur a certain percentage of the time, had truly compromised the quality of her life. Amazingly enough, however, on the cognitive level, Sheila, a Ph.D. psychologist, was fine. She did not have "fibro-fog." She could read, solve problems, even perform public speaking.

She had had a very successful practice before the acute stage of the disease struck. Now her life was a solitary existence and she was in a great deal of pain. She was on disability insurance, was an insomniac, and was tired much of the time. However, she was also a relatively quick responder, much to our surprise. (We used photonic stimulation with Sheila because of her weak and atrophied limbs.)

One morning, subsequent to her having undergone treatment with us, she called our center in tears. "I turned over in bed without screaming for the first time in years," she said as we realized that her tears were "good" tears, expressing how much more hopeful she was feeling. Her dislocating shoulders were less painful. Not long after that she had enough stamina to go to the county fair as well as walk several miles. She had a great time that day, only to collapse the following one. She was in quite a bit of pain, but with a merry little defiant smirk. "Oh well," we said, "we hope you had fun!"

Soon she started a romantic relationship with a fellow that lasted for several months. It didn't work out, but it was the first such assay in a long time.

After about six months of treatment, Sheila's symptoms have stabilized. While she is not fully better, she is nowhere near as bad as she had been. The Sjogren's is still there, she still has dry eyes and mouth, but it's a little better with medication. The important thing is that, for this person with a terrible, complex affliction, enough of her symptoms ameliorated, without going away entirely, to enable her quality of life to improve dramatically.

Neurological Lyme Disease

Lyme disease was first discovered in the United States in 1975, near Lyme, Connecticut, after a mysterious outbreak of what seemed like arthritis. It wasn't until 1982 that the spirochete that causes it, *Borelia burgdorferi*, was identified. Sometimes called, "the Great Impostor," because its symptoms can be mistaken for those of other diseases, it hangs out with a couple of ugly companions, or co-infectors: *Babesia* and *Ehrlichia*.

Lyme has been mistakenly diagnosed as MS (multiple sclerosis), ALS (Lou Gehrig's disease), Alzheimer's, fibromyalgia, and Chronic Fatigue Syndrome. On the neuropsychiatric side, its effects have been diagnosed as "bipolar" or mood instability, depression, cognitive impairment or "brain-fog." It also causes headaches, affects vision, and can be implicated in cardiac problems.[13]

In the beginning, many organ-systems may be invaded while the patient shows no symptomatology. The springlike spirochete self-propels through the body, actually swimming better through tissues than through blood. But the sinister invader is also *pliomorphic*, a master of disguises, sometimes appearing spiral, sometimes round. It invades cells, and on leaving them, they collapse around it, forming an eldritch cloak for it to wear. Because of its pliomorphism, it is extremely hard to find and treat.

The classical bulls-eye rash (*Erythema migrans*) that is supposed to be a sign of the infection only occurs in about 30 percent of the victims; and most doctors consider tests such as QRIBb less than accurate. In fact, it is now accepted that deer ticks (*Ixodes dammini)* are only one of many avenues possible to Lyme proliferation. Fleas and gnats carry it, humans pass it to each other through an exchange of bodily fluids, or even through the nursing of babies. Infants may be born with Lyme, and some cases even are believed to have been passed on through *in-vitro* fertilization.

The only acceptable medical treatment is a round of antibiotics, usually administered for a minimum of three weeks or a month but often, in practice, for much longer periods of time. Or rounds of antibiotics are repeated, or different antibiotics are tried. These approaches frequently fail. There have also been numerous cases of doctors who were prosecuted or lost their licenses for prescribing treatments other than the officially acceptable one. "State medical boards seem to be trying to protect the medical insurance industry rather than the patients," writes Jeff Kamen in *Alternative Medicine*. The alternative medical routes are much more complicated, cost more, and take longer than the (inadequate) official treatment. And even when the symptoms that characterize the acute phase of Lyme Disease have been successfully diminished by an aggressive treatment of antibiotics, the metabolic and neurological residues remain.[14]

It is important to note at the outset of this discussion that *the author is in no way suggesting the LENS can have any curative effect on Lyme disease.* The neurological aftereffects, however: the fatigue, the joint pain and the sensation of tender points throughout the body, the dizziness, headaches, the "fibro-fog," and the debilitating depression that remain *even when the acute or infectious phase is over* do seem to respond to treatment with the LENS.

T. J. Tackles Lyme Disease

T. J. is blonde, attractive, late thirties and appears physically fit and athletic. She is interested in literature and the arts and, while at Bard College, was a talented apprentice to Robert Kelly, a distinguished American poet. But during the late summer and fall of 2002 she felt like she had begun falling apart. She had been having extreme anxiety and fatigue, and at night had dreams of "bugs in her blood."

When she started getting joint pain, she went to a lab for the standard tests: The Western Blot, and the QRIBb. When she brought the results to her doctor, he said, "I don't really believe in these tests very much, but if they work at all, you have Lyme disease." She also felt she probably had gotten multiple bites during this time (she owned both dogs and cats, had a garden beloved by deer, and liked to hike the extensive Shawangunk and Catskill mountain trails).

T. J. had slowly come down with a raft of anomalous symptoms—an eye problem that seemed like "pinkeye" in which her eyeballs felt sticky, and wherein there was "a cloud over everything." Rather abruptly she discovered that she couldn't read, whereas prior to this time she had been an avid reader. And when she listened to people talking, it was as if she couldn't process the words that they were saying. Her executive functions—the ability to plan, sequence, and organize, on which she had prided herself before—seemed fragmented.

T. J.'s wage-earning profession was health care, and she was caring for a quadriplegic who needed her sometimes for four nine-hour shifts in a row several days a week. It was very intense and very stressful work. T. J. said she had to give every ounce of her energy to her job and, on returning home at the end of the workday, she barely had energy to eat the nice, nutritious dinner prepared by her husband. Usually, she would be asleep by 7:00 P.M.

Having a serious work ethic, T. J. kept on in this way day in and day out. Her social life disappeared and she became a hermit. "I knew I still had all my parts," she said, "but they weren't working so well together." Her doctor, fortunately, had a holistic bias, so as he put her on the obligatory heavy doses of antibiotics, he also added acidophilus to compensate for the assault on her intestinal flora, and CoQ-10 to help her muscles and metabolism. T. J. kept on keeping on.

T. J. had been functioning in this debilitated, "twilight state" for three years when she came to us for LENS and photonic treatment (a gentle infrared light treatment described more fully in chapter 12.) After the first few sessions, she noticed that she was extremely irritable (a sure sign of overdose). Consequently, we cut her stimulation way back, down to the lowest possible "lo-stim" level with the neurofeedback, and minimum treatment with the photon stimulator, basically "painting," as they call it, moving a gentle infrared light over her fingertips and down her spine. At these levels, T. J.'s extreme irritability diminished, but she noticed some other things that had her troubled. (She was also seeing me for psychotherapy.)

"I'm really *confronting* people," she said. "What's happening to me? Am I this really mean, aggressive person inside?"

"No," I said, "That doesn't seem like you. Tell me about the situations."

In every instance there was a locked-up, loaded issue with the other person. Invariably, T. J. had been patronized by, or overwhelmed by, that other person and hadn't been able to hold her own. Frustrations began (somewhat volcanically) to reveal themselves. Much of her family of origin (ancient) stuff came up, mingling with problems with her current family that needed to be addressed. In this "outbreak of symptoms," T. J. was learning to find her balance between gentleness and firmness; to stand her ground while dancing with others.

Then, with ongoing treatment, things subtly began to shift. Here we switch to her own narrative so that we may better understand what was happening to T. J.:

From "mostly cloudy" days, my days became "partly cloudy" and then, "partly sunny." There was a sense of fear, before a pivotal crescendo. At that point, there was a kind of death and rebirth inside me and I was seeing a lot of things. (Luckily, I have a really wonderful, patient husband who nurtures me, and I don't drink or smoke.)

Week by week, I experienced subtle improvements. I didn't have to go to bed at 7:00 P.M. every night. I could feel energy moving in my chakras (in Hindu metaphysiology, subtle energy centers). I had more muscular strength, and then more core strength. I can read again, deeply and with feeling, digesting things that are profound. My job is less stressful now (I still care for the elderly and dying), however, in this space I find "room" to heal myself.

Now, after some months of the LENS treatment, I feel more integrated, as if all of my various parts have become my best friends. (Initially, I had felt that I still had my parts but they weren't working well together—as if my whole physical being had arrhythmia. Now I'm feeling much better—like a well-tuned piano.) And I don't feel like I'm going to sink into a pit. I'm more hopeful. My potential has returned; I feel I have access to it again.

One day I was swimming (I love water, and I love to swim). While swimming, I noticed that my previous limitations were gone. As I was doing the crawl, my "strait-jacket"—a previous sense of physical confinement—dropped away. I relaxed into an ease that felt like it contained a boundless potential.

I am so thankful that I hadn't given up, that I didn't settle for feeling only "half-okay"—a "half-baked rutabaga." When I was very ill, everything within me was fragmented, even the genesis of a thought. It was like my soul was trapped in a storm inside me. Now I can formulate, and think something out clearly; now I can actualize my thought or inspiration.

You can say what you want, but for me that is the pinnacle of being human.

At one point during the "evaluation" portion of a session, T. J. looked at me and asked, "What's better than 'improved,' 'good,' or even 'excellent?'" Before I could reply, she answered her own question by saying, "Wonder Woman!" She flexed her bicep and laughed merrily.

Summary on "The Twilight Zone"

In Epstein-Barr and Lyme disease, at least the culprit that causes these diseases—a wicked micro-organism in each case—has been identified and named. (Epstein-Barr is named for the men who discovered the causative micro-organism associated with that disease, while Lyme disease—caused by a spirochete inside of a tick—was named after its place of discovery near Lyme, Connecticut.)

However, with fibromyalgia, or Chronic Fatigue Syndrome, the jury is still out with regard to the disease's "causal aetiology"—in effect, where it comes from. So while we can't devote much time or effort to sleuthing, we can work to balance and ameliorate the oftentimes damaging neurological consequences of these syndromes or diseases. While we cannot propose any *cures* for these deep-seated debilitating conditions, we can and do, through our work with the LENS, improve the flexibility and efficiency with which we function!

7

HIGH ANXIETY, DEEP DEPRESSION

Panic, Obsessive-Compulsive Disorder, Anxiety,
Phobia, Depression, and Bipolar Disorder

*Stephen Larsen, Ph.D., Len Ochs, Ph.D., Karen Schultheis, Ph.D.,
Evelyn Soehner, M.A., Thomas E. Fink, Ph.D., and Lynn Brayton, Psy.D.*

*Alpha works in the same fashion as an injection of epinephrine
might work. The person not only feels energized, but the wheels
begin to spin in the head. And they begin to get obsessive and
ruminative, and they begin to explain and find reasons in their
environment for their obsessing, when actually it is coming from
within. It escalates and becomes intrusive in the processes of
the brain. It is too much energy, energy that the brain does not
know what to do with, or the mind does not know what to do
with, so you get all this restless behavior.*

LEN OCHS

This chapter takes on two of the most common symptom domains in the
DSM IV-r: anxiety disorders, and depressive or mood disorders. Though
they are not the same, there are indeed relationships between them, and
in the clinical setting one hears about "anxious depressions" and "anxiety-driven depression." Both anxiety and depression give a characteristic emotional "coloring" to experience and may appear separately or
together.

The approach we take in this book is that both anxiety and depression are based on CNS dysregulation, although of different kinds. Anxiety tends to appear (though not always) with higher frequency brain waves, from alpha (8–12 Hz) all the way up to hi-beta (22–28 Hz). Anxiety is often associated with energy, indeed too much energy—although it is also punctuated by bouts of exhaustion or depletion and often appears comorbidly with insomnia, hypervigilance, and irritability. In these conditions, alpha often transgresses its usual brain locus (in the occipital and parietal lobes) and perfuses forward through central and frontal regions, sometimes in surprisingly high amplitudes (10mv and up).

Depression is more likely to manifest in delta (0–4 Hz) or theta (4–8 Hz) and is usually identified with "EEG slowing" in a waking brain wave. Delta/theta may appear anywhere in the cortex but has been identified by Davidson and Rosenfeld as particularly problematical in the frontal areas, and appearing asymmetrically between the hemispheres.

However, the maps presented by each human being represent a unique configuration. Sometimes bad depressions are accompanied by alpha abundance, and without much delta or theta. Conceptually at least, these seem to represent personality types that drive themselves to a kind of desperate exhaustion by seemingly draining all of their resources all of the time.

Although the difference between these types might be highly significant for traditional neurofeedback practitioners, because they have to set up "reward" and "inhibit" protocols to begin training (say "reward beta, inhibit theta," common in ADD treatment), in the LENS work the difference is less significant. This is because *whatever the signature* of the condition, say elevated theta and inadequate beta, and *whatever the dominant symptom complex,* be it anxiety or depression, the protocol is the same: Make a map, and follow the sequence it provides by treating the patient at the offset predetermined by the Offset Procedure. Keep the frequency and level of treatment within the bounds of sensitivity or reactivity of the patient, being careful neither to overstimulate them nor exhaust their resources. If this is done, then the brain will *normalize itself,* with low frequencies increasing and high ones decreasing; amplitudes will also lower and normalize.

Though slow, high amplitude delta and theta waves are often considered the signature of brain damage, as well as serious depression, they often yield rather quickly to treatment. It is the pervasive or monolithic alpha coherence that often proves most stubborn and resistant to treatment. In general, it may be harder to quiet a brain that is constitutionally "over-revved" than speed up one that has become lethargic. Difficult, also, are the bipolar types where we see both low and high frequencies simultaneously, and depression and mania alter on some hidden time-table not fully understood by either the clinician or the patient.

Dialogue between Stephen Larsen, Len Ochs, and Karen Schultheis Regarding Alpha and Delta/Theta

Stephen: Would you talk a little bit about the two ranges, the one more related to the delta-theta complex and the other more related to the alpha complex?

Len: When delta and theta are more prominent in the EEG, I see this as basically as a brain injury from some "external" source, even if it occurred *in utero*, from drug addiction, or mechanical trauma, or viral or environ-mental toxicity. When we see alpha becoming more frontal in the EEG record, it is as if the alpha itself is the trauma that can evoke delta and theta. This is where you get "depressions that are secondary to anxiety" situations (alpha in these amplitudes being the anxiety system activity, or energy system activity). And alpha works in the same fashion as an injec-tion of epinephrine might work. The person not only feels energized, but the wheels begin to spin in the head. And they begin to get obsessive and ruminative, and they begin to explain and find reasons in their environ-ment for their obsessing, when actually it is coming from within. It esca-lates and becomes intrusive in the processes of the brain. It is too much energy, energy that the brain does not know what to do with, or the mind does not know what to do with, so you get all this restless behavior.

Stephen: But there could be depression at the same time?

Len: Yeah, the depression comes in as a reaction to this restless energy that won't settle down.

Stephen: So this would be an "agitated depression."

Len: Only the agitation may be internal. It may not be obvious, but they may be spinning their wheels inside their heads. When I see frontal alpha, I say "restless soul." Only one patient I have so confronted has ever denied that.

Karen: I've definitely seen the same thing.

Stephen: And the cognitive effects of that would be?

Len: Cognitive manifestations, or cognitive effects? They think and think and think. They are noisy in their heads. They may actually be stimulation-seekers, they may throw themselves into work or keep themselves preoccupied visually and auditorially.

Stephen: So how does that match with the "old" attribution of alpha as the absence of thought, or idling?

Len: Who knows? But there is a difference between the observation that someone has a lot of alpha and giving them feedback for alpha activity, in which you are basically evoking a change in the brain by fiddling with alpha as a variable. That is not to say that you have more and more alpha activity in daily life just because it is becoming more prominent, under reinforcement (classical reward neurofeedback) conditions.

Stephen: It is a different kind of alpha too, isn't it? It may appear different on the raw EEG?

Len: It can be, and also it depends on where you are reinforcing it, too.

High Anxiety

Anxiety is one of the most bruited about, discussed, and feared (if you can fear fear itself) of human sensations. The evolutionary roots of anxiety are not hard to find. Those predecessors of ours who, in the Pleistocene era, developed an acute warning system to alert them to danger survived, while those who lounged about in the marshes or on the savannahs did not. Anxiety, like depression, can eclipse all other states in its onslaught. And yet, at its best, anxiety gets us moving like nothing else can.

Anxiety seems able to take many forms, from panic attacks, to phobia, to dissociation, to the rituals of compulsion and the endless thought-loops of obsession. As mentioned, anxiety tends to manifest in the EEG toward the higher brain-wave frequencies—alpha, (SMR), beta, and hi-beta. The higher frequency brain waves galvanize us into action and keep our attention (mostly) on the subject at hand. But we've also seen the inverse: anxiety so intense that it paralyzes us. (There we are, up in front of all the other students in that awful public speaking class, and we're paralyzed. We mix up our words, forget our carefully prepared thoughts, grimace, and then blush furiously as the autonomic nervous system chimes in.)

Anxiety can make us uptight, spastic almost (*angst* means "constriction" in both German and Greek). We respond rigidly to life's events with such behaviors as obsessive-compulsive rituals, fears focused on an object or situation (phobias), or fears that are seemingly focused on nothing at all, which is sometimes the same as "everything," as illustrated by a *Peanuts* cartoon in which Lucy is giving five-cent psychiatric diagnoses to Charlie Brown. He obligingly and neurotically recites everything he is afraid of. Her final diagnosis of Charlie is that he has a *pantophobia*, or a "fear of everything." This is commonly called "generalized anxiety disorder," "free-floating anxiety," or sometimes "agoraphobia," which is a fear of going out of the house.

Traditional biofeedback has a good track record of working with performance and sports-oriented neuroses. Athletes from Eastern European and the Soviet Bloc countries have, for years, used psychological strategies such as relaxation and positive visualization to perform in a consistently outstanding fashion at the Olympics. Biofeedback seems an obvious enhancement to these activities in that it teaches self-awareness and self-regulation wherein one can participate in one's own level of arousal and the psychosomatic attitude with which performance is approached. Activity in the beta to hi-beta ranges can indicate a limbically driven cortex, and even muscle tension, as EMG has a hi-beta like frequency. Traditionally the remedy has been sought in the alpha range, which sometimes produces a "neutral" more physically relaxed state. It also is clear that "visualizations," of activity in a deeply relaxed state could be accomplished in theta —as in Budzynski's "twilight learning"—and theta is known to be effective in some aspects of memory formation.

The opposite of performance anxiety is to achieve an "effortless," neutral state, as you perform whatever skill or art, as in Mihaly Csikszentmihalyi's "Flow experience."[1] (There will be more on this subject of "optimal performance" in chapter 15.) What we can say at this juncture is that the LENS offers a unique, and rather painless, way to help overcome all kinds of anxiety—through a more flexibly functioning CNS.

Let's look at some of the ways in which the more acute forms of anxiety can interfere with people's functioning—and their lives.

Evelyn Soehner, M.A., and
Thomas E. Fink, Ph.D., on Anxiety

Evelyn Soehner and Tom Fink run the Acorn Health Associates in Millersburg, Pennsylvania. Tom is a clinical psychologist, and Evelyn a Biofeedback/Neurofeedback clinician. Working together as professional partners, they are also husband and wife. When Evelyn began working with FNS and getting great results with it, she naturally shared this with Tom. But her husband, an experienced clinician who, in addition to running a private practice is also a consultant for schools and industry, is from Missouri. "You'll have to show me," he said, and he referred some of his more difficult cases to his wife for neurofeedback while he continued to do psychotherapeutic work with them. Some of the outcomes of these collaborations are given below, following an excellent essay on anxiety written by Tom.

What, Me Worry?
Thomas E. Fink, Ph.D.

Who hasn't been anxious? Confronted by a growling Rotweiler, playing the part of Hans in your third-grade play, driving home from college in a winter snowstorm, or meeting with the IRS auditor to review the "questionable donation deductions" on your last three years' income tax returns—all produce heightened states of physiological and emotional arousal that we call anxiety.

Threats to our well-being, whether symbolic or real, arouse our senses and produce physiological changes such as increased heartbeat, shallow breathing, sweaty palms, shaky hands, increased alertness, and other adrenaline-mediated responses. Or our thinking may speed up or become rigidly fixated. Attention may be highly focused, or outwardly focused and hypervigilant. These "fight or flight" responses may or may not be beneficial, depending on the nature of the situation and the response required to deal with it. In any event, this uncomfortable anxiety should subside after the dog has been leashed, the school play is over, you arrive safely at your destination, or the audit is complete and your Visa/Master Card credit limit is sufficient to cover the additional federal taxes, fines, and interest imposed.

The so-called anxiety disorders occur when heightened arousal *persists*, however, in spite of the absence of appropriate stressors (e.g., Generalized Anxiety Disorder), or when arousal occurs in an exaggerated manner, perhaps even to a heightened awareness of one's own fear responses (e.g., Panic Disorder). Maladaptive emotional and avoidant behavioral patterns may develop in response to stimuli associated with these anxiety states (e.g., phobias). And a person may develop elaborate behavioral and cognitive rituals to avoid or reduce overarousal (e.g., Obsessive-Compulsive Disorder).

The variants of anxiety disorders are multiple, involving emergent syndromal behavioral/cognitive/emotional patterns that the psychiatric DSM system has attempted to capture as though each is a distinct mental disease. The latest version (IV-r) of the DSM describes eleven distinct types of anxiety disorders. These include Panic Disorder with or without agoraphobia; phobias, including specific phobias (e.g., fear of flying) and social phobias; acute and post-traumatic stress disorders; generalized anxiety disorder; and anxiety disorders due to several distinct physiological influences, including substance-induced disorders and anxiety conditions that are caused by medical conditions.

In actual situations, persons with maladaptive anxiety remain idiosyncratically stuck, although there may be emergent patterns that bear family resemblances to one another. It is useful to identify these emergent patterns by name, both to be able to communicate with one's colleagues about them, and/or perhaps to share treatment strategies that work optimally for one or another "type" of condition.

What appears common among all anxiety disorders is the characteristics they share: (1) Central Nervous System (CNS) overarousal and (2) recurrent and "stuck" response patterns that interfere with flexible and adaptive person-environment interaction. CNS hyperarousal can take many forms that, as we shall see, are reflected both behaviorally and on FFT analysis* of the EEG. Similarly, a person's "stuck" patterns are reflected in recurrent and maladaptive behavioral, cognitive, and emotional styles, as well as a distinctive lack of variability on EEG analysis.

---

*Fast-Fourier Transforms that break the raw brain waves into "bandwidths."

Acorn Health Associates—The Evaluation Process
THOMAS E. FINK, PH.D.

In our practice, the referral of a person for FNS treatment begins with a standard, one-hour psychological interview, during which social and medical history is collected, as well as information on current symptom presentation, and expectations about treatment. For the three cases described below, such an interview was only necessary for one, (Nick), since the other two patients had been patients of mine in a standard psychological practice for several years. (Having worked with two of the three individuals prior to using FNS on them provided me with a small and informal "waiting list" type of a control group that enabled me to witness, first-hand, the effectiveness of FNS. It was this experience with FNS that contributed to my current degree of enthusiasm about its effectiveness.)

For the assessment of anxiety, a number of standardized self-report inventories are available to aid the collection of baseline symptom severity. The reader is encouraged to look at a number of these, including The Beck Anxiety Index (BAI). Also see Antony, Orsillo, and Roemer (2001) for a comprehensive list and discussion of currently available anxiety measures. Although not critical for successful treatment, such measures are useful in documenting improvement, both for clients who often forget just how much they have changed, and for therapists who may need to justify treatment to third party sources.

Nick Learns about Coping with Panic and Depersonalization

Nick was a sixteen-year-old high school sophomore, the oldest of two children born to caring but anxious parents. His mother had a history of panic attacks and his father, an accountant, was described by his wife as a "Type A" personality. Nick, however, appeared to be an average teenager, with generally normal adaptation to his social environment. He had male and female friends as well as a girlfriend, and he participated in a range of age-appropriate social and recreational activities. He was an average student.

His mother had noticed, however, that beginning at about the age of four, Nick had begun to express fears about his parents dying and had to be periodically reassured. But otherwise he appeared to be functioning normally until a precipitant event occurred while he was working part-time after school as a dishwasher at a local eatery. It was here that he developed the first of what an evaluating psychiatrist would eventually describe as a "de-realization event."

While washing dishes, Nick became aware of himself washing dishes. He described this as an "out of body" type of experience during which, he reported, he no longer "felt like himself." He found this experience very unpleasant and disturbing, and over the course of the next several months, several similar ones were to follow. He kept these experiences to himself but he regularly worried about his "normalcy."

Eventually, Nick mentioned his situation to his mother. She took him to their family physician, who referred him to a psychiatrist. The psychiatrist began a course of SSRI medications, eventually finding a dosage of Prozac that was beneficial, and Nick reported he began to feel "pretty good." Shortly after that, however, his girlfriend was killed in an automobile accident. He was extremely upset by this event, became depressed, and then began to experience anxiety attacks, sometimes as often as three or four a day. His concerns about school became exaggerated and there were days he was too anxious to attend school or, if he did, he experienced anxiety attacks and had to leave.

He was referred to a psychologist, who saw him a few times and appeared to carry out some nonspecific counseling without noticeable positive effect. Nick was never psychiatrically hospitalized, but he was involved for a time in a partial hospitalization program. Concurrently, he began a course of increasing medication use that, by the time he was seen in our practice, consisted of 60mg of Prozac per day, 20mg of BusPar per day, and 1.5mg of Klonipin in the morning and 1mg of it at bedtime.

Nick was reporting ongoing difficulties, by this time, with lethargy, weight gain, and decreased memory and general cognitive abilities. His grades suffered and he was becoming increasingly socially withdrawn. His mother reported that he was afraid he would never be "normal" again. In a phone consultation, his psychiatrist described him as the most difficult case of anxiety she had ever treated.

At this point, Nick came to my attention. I referred him to my partner, Evelyn Soehner, for neurofeedback, while I prepared to undertake the psychotherapeutic part—a "double-team act"—for this highly anxious patient.

After treating Nick for a little while, the first thing I noticed was that his psychotherapeutic sessions were becoming more productive; I wondered why this was. Eventually I came up with the answer: Nick's anxiety was less, could it be that funny neurofeedback stuff Evelyn was doing? My clinical eye had seen his convoluted defense mechanisms and affect-dysregulation dwindling. Because of *this*, his self-insight and coping strategies were better. I was kind of astonished, but after the neurofeedback work with Evelyn, I began working with Nick's referring psychiatrist to reduce his medication. Before long, Nick was able to eliminate the BusPar (a potent drug that addresses cojoined anxiety and depression), and reduce the Prozac to 20mg (or one third of what he had been taking). Soon he was able to come off the daytime Klonopin, and use it only at night for sleep.

Nick might have been willing or able to come off his meds entirely, but his family was too anxious, as they felt that the meds kept rekindling him as well. (Although Nick's parents were fearful of his abandoning the meds entirely, they *did* agree that, in general, their son was becoming very much improved!) As Nick's panic attacks abated, I taught him "cognitive-behavioral" management skills, which would have been ineffective prior to the "neurological storm" of his anxiety subsiding.

Nick was able to enroll in college. He was in and out of treatment over the next couple of years, when a truly horrible *deja-vu* happened: another close female friend of his was killed in a car accident. He came back to treatment in earnest; wherein I noticed that Nick was now really able to *process,* and to delve deeply, into the suffering that he was experiencing.

Shortly thereafter, something truly amazing began happening! Nick had been quite close to the father of the young woman who was killed. Evidently my patient had learned some things during his *prior* bereavement and suffering because, at this time, he began to support the bereaved parents. "It was so interesting to see this shift in him," I remember thinking at the time, "from being this total *victim,* to a substantial *helper.* In effect, he became so empathic and concerned about *others,* that he forgot about *himself.*"

David Works through Obsessive-Compulsive Disorder
David was a married, practicing family physician, whose life and career were increasingly and negatively shaped by recurrent fears, intrusive and

obsessive thoughts, heightened and generalized anxiety, and compulsive, checking behaviors. He harbored irrational fears about contracting infections such as AIDS from his patients. His between-patient hand-washing assumed such intensity that it was interfering with patient flow. The checking behavior that had begun when he would have to rush home to make sure that he had turned off an appliance, one *that he knew he had unplugged*, now became evident in his practice. (Where and when had this careful, attentive physician regressed into a neurotic OCD ritualist?)

When conducting physical exams on his patients, David often had to repeat them, because he doubted the veracity of his touch. (Severe anxiety trumps "reality" every time.) He could not leave his car without repeatedly putting the emergency brake on and off. He had A.M. rituals and P.M. rituals.

Each night David looked forward to drinking two or three cocktails, and sometimes several large glasses of wine, with his wife, since this was the only activity that allowed him to truly relax. He had been in and out of psychological and psychiatric care since the beginning of medical school. He was also using a large dose of an SSRI (Zoloft, reputed to help with OCD), without significant benefit. He was depressed and miserable when he again sought psychological treatment to help improve the quality of his life.

David was referred to Evelyn for neurofeedback while I conducted the psychotherapy. Conventional cognitive/behavioral therapy teaches people, however reluctantly, to intervene in their own compulsive behaviors or obsessive thoughts. *Stop what you are doing and take a deep breath. Count a few breaths. Now take a more constructive appropriate behavioral approach.* It all sounds very good, but once the impulse has arisen, OCD usually has a fierce, almost demonic power of its own.

What I began to notice was that as David's neurofeedback progressed, it was becoming easier for him to make use of the cognitive-behavioral strategies. (What had not worked for the neurologically aroused and driven person seemed more possible to the quiet, more balanced person David was becoming.) First he noticed that his A.M. rituals were becoming shorter—and he was getting to work on time. Then the P.M. rituals decreased, because he was actually looking forward to getting home. The alcohol consumption also moderated.

Occasionally, David still has intrusive thoughts. He hasn't needed or done neurofeedback for about two years, although he still comes in every six months for a catch up—an "existential" session as I like to call them.

Jim Masters His Rage

Jim, another physician and surgeon, suffered from bouts of rage. He was in his second marriage. His first one had ended rather suddenly when his then-wife abruptly left town without telling Jim where she and their young daughter were going, even though he could have guessed the reason. People found him to be narcissistic and arrogant, as well as angry.

His second marriage was currently in trouble. He had a poor relationship, not only with his wife, but with his two children. He recently had been reprimanded by his hospital's board for unprofessional behavior in the operating room. He was known to rage, and berate fellow physicians and other health care staff, often in front of patients and their families. He had few friends and little respect, in spite of his good clinical knowledge and surgical skill.

While Jim was outwardly angry and critical, inwardly he was anxious and worried about his own abilities, concerned about the outcome of his efforts, and prone to catastrophizing, exaggeration, and feelings of dread. As well, he had an aggressive psychological defensive style that led him to attack and blame others without assuming any responsibility for his own behavior.

This was the point at which Jim began neurofeedback, already having tried psychotherapy for a while. Within about a month he began to be less defensive and guarded, and in therapy sessions he began really contacting his own internal feelings of inadequacy. He was able to experience firsthand the anxiety that lay inside the aggression, which masked it. As both his neurofeedback and psychotherapy progressed, Jim became more humble and more empathic.

Jim's listening skills emerged, and he often could be found simply listening to a family member or a staff member, and empathizing with them. His relationship with his children improved enormously, and he began indulging in activities with them that he "didn't have time for" before. His marriage was improving. He was becoming more philosophical, and manifesting more of that touted "emotional intelligence" that

Daniel Goleman writes about so well.[2] (Jim's is also a perfect example of Goleman's point that an individual's intellectual and professional intelligence are not enough; the emotional kind of intelligence is what tells the tale!)

Imagine everyone's surprise when Jim won the Doctor of the Year award! The nurses had actually grown quite fond of him and had voted for him. He was nominated for the same award a second year—and this is telling—but he declined the nomination so that one of his colleagues could be honored with it instead!

Tackling Agoraphobia

During the mid-1970s, I had two jobs: college professor and psychotherapist; both seemingly separate. In my biofeedback program, I showed students about their autonomic nervous systems and their brain waves, then I drove over to the Counseling Center in Kingston and did talk-therapy and dreamwork with my clients. (I suppose this is an example of how "compartmentalized" our thinking can be. It was only gradually, and with cases like the one next presented, that I realized how important it could be to integrate these two disciplines.)

In the mid-1970s I began psychotherapy with Violet, a department store clerk who had only a high school education. Violet had agoraphobia, terrible anxiety attacks with panic, and continuous sleep disturbance, as well as stomach problems. Violet remained adamant about not wanting to take medication for the anxiety, as similar medication had once made her terribly sick.

All through her Roman-Catholic youth, her mother had filled Violet with anxiety-producing stories about abductions and men taking sexual advantage of women. Thus, Violet had never left Ulster County in her thirty-five years of life. After an unsuccessful marriage that lasted only six months, she went to work for the department store, ate lunch apart from all the other employees (because she was so anxious), and lived at home with her two elderly parents (one of whom was the neurotic mother).

In over four years of psychotherapy, I had helped Violet feel validated and supported, and to gain more insight into her family situation. But the psychotherapy did not do much to alleviate the terrible anxiety that plagued this patient, making her seem rigid and shaky, always on the edge of panic, frightened by her own shadow. Anxiety seemed to have been ingested by her *cum lacte* as they say, "along with her mother's milk."

Some insights developed with Violet during her course of psychotherapy helped to improve her relations with her co-workers, and her ability to set boundaries with her very needy parents, but her crippling anxiety persisted. Bioenergetic exercises proved only mildly beneficial, as Violet did her share of pillow pounding, "stress-postures," and abreactive screaming at the mother (in absentia, of course).

But one day I felt inspired to bring an EMG machine (for muscle tension) over from the college lab to the clinic. Violet and I began to do muscle relaxation biofeedback, coupled with autogenic training for relaxation, and the results of this combination were impressive: Violet began to sleep better and was a little more relaxed during the day.

But still the pervasive anxiety dogged her. We went on for a while with "deep relaxation," with very mild improvements. But then I got another inspiration—and did my first clinical EEG biofeedback! I brought the cumbersome stand-alone Autogenics 120 machine from the "biofeedback lab" at the college. (The instrument was used as an adjunct to my course in consciousness.) At first I tried a simple alpha protocol, because Violet's main occipital production was high amplitude hi-beta (22–28 Hz). Within only a few sessions, Violet's anxious hypervigilance began to wane as she learned to produce more of the modulated alpha (about 10 Hz) the equipment rewarded with a pleasant tone.

Her family and parents were now to be astonished at the personality transformation that began in Violet. She became more outspoken and assertive (less "wallflower"-like). Several times at home and around relatives, where her doormatlike compliance had been accepted as a given, she would sense she was being teased or railroaded, set her feet, frown, and give forth an impressive "No!" or "Back off!" A younger sister who had always bulldozed Violet suddenly found the "doormat" standing up and glaring right back at her. (This was such a frightening experience for the extroverted sister, that she began to defer to Violet in ways she never would have dreamt of, before. Gradually, she became more respectful of Violet—even at times asking her older sister for advice about her love life.)

Violet began to show a talent for finding things no one else could find and this soon blossomed into an ESP-like intuition whereby she could guess what people would say before they said it. She probably had always had this talent, but now she was giving it expression, and really "calling things like she saw them" in the family context. She not only participated in the family's annual Thanksgiving football game (which she had never done), but she executed a decisive tackle on her brother-in-law, a sturdy man who was amazed as he went down, and then laughed uproariously about it.

Soon Violet began dating and having an affair with a romantic Latin fellow who picked her up from work in a snazzy sports car. She moved out of her parents home and got her own apartment (nearby, so she could visit them, while keeping her independence). Eventually Violet was able to behold, in all its urban splendor, New York City—which she had never done in thirty-five years—see the Statue of Liberty, and go up to the top of the Empire State Building. She traveled to other states and took a Caribbean cruise with her sister. (Boy, did those two, now more like peers, get into mischief!) As we were concluding our therapy, Violet was practicing for her driver's license (just the idea of that would have had her in tremors in her pretreatment condition).

What seemed to have broken the tyranny of anxiety for this young woman was finding a "place" or a state inside herself where her anxiety was inoperative. When she found it, she was freed-up. She became less rigid and more flexible. The agoraphobia dissipated with the anxiety, and Violet became assertive enough to stand up for herself.

More Learning About Anxiety

In another early instance, however, I found the alpha solution that had worked so well for Violet, to be totally ineffectual for an older man with serious panic attacks. He too had hi-beta, insomnia, and hypervigilance. There was no precipitating incident that we could discover, but his anxiety seemed to be deepening. (By this time, we had a full American Biotech EEG setup attached to the therapy office and were seeing a lot of ADD kids, and using a variety of EEG protocols: SMR and beta training, as well as alpha and alpha-theta.)

We tried alpha training twice a week for a couple of months on this patient, but he only got worse. Eventually he had to be hospitalized and medicated. I made a mental note of this failure, and only later, when I had studied the LENS approach, did I understand it better. (More on this shortly.)

Over the (approximately ten) years since then, I have had a chance to use the disentrainment approach on a variety of anxiety disorders. The ensuing positive results have been similar to Violet's, whereby we were simply lucky that alpha training was good for her. But in some cases, the "good idea" of the therapist might be just the wrong thing (as I had discovered in the aforementioned case of this panic-attack victim).

When I initially met Len Ochs, my entire training had been to see "alpha" as the gateway to inner peace; it was the panacea, the *antidote to anxiety*. I also believed it contained the key to optimal functioning, and possibly the development of ESP, based on some studies I had read. Beta was "good," (for the ADD kids), while theta was "bad." For people with too much anxiety, beta was definitely "bad," alpha or theta was "good."

However, in the LENS type of mapping and evaluation as developed by Len Ochs, we have come to see that an abundance of alpha, and wrongly placed high-amplitude alpha, is indicative of "anxiety system" activity. In fact, to reward alpha in a traditional protocol might sometimes not only be counterproductive, it might actually *exacerbate* a patient's symptoms. Upon realizing this, I could no longer view alpha as the panacea I had earlier believed it to be.

For the experienced practitioner, it is possible to discern the type of problem the "alpha" may be carrying, based on the look of the waveforms and their location in the brain. It is not unusual or problematical to find a certain amount of occipital alpha in many "normal" people when they have their eyes closed but frontal alpha above 5µv (5 microvolts) can signal cognitive cloudiness, memory problems, ADD, anxiety or certain pain syndromes. Contrarily, in the literature, some studies exist that insist that frontal alpha can be benign, even opening the doorway to intuition. (At least, however, it's better regarded than frontal delta or theta, which is implicated in everything from depression to sociopathy.)

So it was that we began to look at the whole spectrum of brain wave ranges in a new way as we began to wonder whether the operative variable in some cases was not the "desired" brain wave range being "achieved," but rather the *flexibility* acquired in the achieving of it? In the case of Violet, could the effective therapeutic factor have been something different from moving out of "bad" hi-beta into "good" alpha, but rather the ability to *move neurologically* between the possible states? As a matter of fact, upon serious reflection, I saw in no other way than flexibility is "optimal functioning" possible.[3]

Hence my "deprogramming" as a brain wave fundamentalist at the hands of Len Ochs. All of the rules one can learn may be true 75 or 80 percent of the time, but be *very* untrue for the rest. I have seen alpha be a carrier of (or present when there is also) terrible depression and lethargy, and I have seen delta be a carrier of anxiety. Sometimes also, it is possible, with certain computer screens, to watch a patient's brain waves morph in and out of each other. You suppress a hi-beta with a brief stim, and it does go down, but alpha pops up. Or you suppress alpha and delta pops up. (And this is also an argument for the disentrainment/flexibility approach as opposed to *protocolus desiderata:* someone's good idea of what your brain ought to be doing!) Please see the accompanying box for further commentary on this.

Sometimes the therapist's "good idea" may ask the brain to do something that it can't do. As I discussed in this book's Introduction, when I was still living with the aftereffects of old head injuries, I would try to do beta training to enhance my mental energy. I would almost instantly doze off in the chair, and enter a vivid hypnagogic theta state. I was asking my brain to do *beta,* but even a small effort overdosed me and threw me into *theta.* (After a year of the LENS type training, when I would ask for beta, up came the beta, and no drowsiness! But theta also did not seem hard to access.)

Several years ago, at the invitation of Rob Kall, I presented a paper at the Winter Brain Conference on FNS and Optimal Performance. (Chapter 15 is an evolution of this paper.) I originally used "Tao" in the paper's title, because the Oriental concept seemed so right-on in describing this concept of brain flexibility—"playing ball on running water, riding clouds." It's not that obsessives, after training, will never think another obsessive thought, it's just that they don't, er, well, obsess about it! But in their newer, healthier state *they just slide away from the obsession* because it's not really useful, and they have better things to do. (This would be the opposite of "redoubling your effort when you've

LEN OCHS "ON THE MEANING OF THE EEG" (SEPT. 2005)

There are several problems with attempting to standardize interpretation of the EEG. First, while I used to see good functioning only when the EEG was low in amplitude, I have lately seen good functioning with high amplitudes in each and every band. Here are some examples: (1) EEG amplitudes can be too low, and occur with poor functioning. (2) EEG amplitudes can be very high and yet the person may function well, even brilliantly. (3) EEG amplitudes may be "normal" and yet occur in the presence of poor functioning. The problem is that we don't know when one situation is at hand, or when one of the others is.

Second, when one looks at the EEG, it is difficult to tell if it will drop, or if it will rise. We have a reasonable degree of confidence that when a site has low variability (as measured by too low a standard deviation) then we can expect that amplitude to rise with treatment. However, in some instances the amplitude will fall after it rises; while in other instances, the amplitude will remain high. When I first started seeing these rises, I was alarmed because I thought that functioning was about to deteriorate. Now that I have this happen enough times, and realize that high amplitudes can happen with high functioning, I'm less concerned about it.

There are further problems linking various types of EEG, such as Delta, Theta, Alpha, Low Beta, Beta, and High Beta, with subjective states. First, rarely is the location of such brain waves stated; that is, whether they are observed at the front, back, sides, or top of the head. In some places, specific types of activity are normal and even good, while in others they may be pathological. Second, rarely if ever is the amplitude of the observed activity mentioned. In some instances low amplitude activity can be a sign of good functioning, while high amplitudes may be signs of pathology—except, as noted above, when they are signs of exceptionally good functioning.

Here are some examples:

- High-amplitude alpha, when observed at the front of the head, can be indicative of attention-deficit disorder, alcoholism, fibromyalgia, and depression. But when very low in amplitude, and dispersed all across the head, it can be a sign of relaxed attention.
- Delta, under some waking conditions, can imply depression and impairment when observed in the front of the head. Yet it can also be a sign of great creativity when awake.

To summarize: the meaning of various kinds of brain wave bands cannot be generalized into simple catchphrases. It is the subjective state of the person, and his or her functioning, that are more important than the EEG readings as indicators of functioning levels.

forgotten your aim" or the neurotic who, when he discovers a strategy that *doesn't* work, keeps doing it.)

The neurological flexibility gives one more internal freedom whereby new cognitive strategies and habits may be built. In fact, for more advanced practitioners, we could posit a *metacognitve* flexibility. It feels as if you have the reins in your hands instead of (yourself) trudging in the traces, pulling the cart.

The eminent mythologist Joseph Campbell once met a one-hundred-fifteen year old man in India and asked him the secret of his amazing vitality and positive attitude. "Anxieties don't eat at me. I eat anxiety!" The old gent replied, astonishing and edifying Campbell. With anxiety, it is always a good question to ask, "Who has the upper hand?!"

Myrna Breaks Free from Anxiety's Prison

The following case shows how effective the LENS treatment can be in treating high anxiety. At the beginning of this story, Myrna was a twenty-two-year-old woman who had been an honor student through eighth grade. Her IQ was approximately 120, well into the "superior" category. But in high school she seemed in danger of "falling through the cracks." She had a bad time in junior college because of her phobias about germs, and she had compulsive little thoughts, did compulsive little rituals, and had periodic panic attacks. She felt socially inept, and ill-equiped to deal with life as a young adult. In this regard, she was not unlike many young people with an anxiety disorder.

Myrna's OCD had gotten far worse when she found her grand-mother, who had died suddenly, on the basement floor. Then shortly afterward, Myrna's mother had to enter the hospital for an unexpected gall-bladder operation. At this point, Myrna seemed to need "constant reassurances." She was afraid of everything. Her OCD rituals got much worse.

Then September 11 struck, and Myrna went into a serious panic. As the news of Anthrax spiraled out of control, her phobias about germs and infection kept her paralyzed at home. She became agoraphobic and housebound, spending her days hiding behind venetian blinds, shaking with panic. She feared the world would end, that terrorists would come to our sleepy town, and that the local post office was already riddled with germs. Her social life, a little shaky anyway, withered away, as her friends could never get a "yes" answer to an invitation they had extended to her.

Inside Myrna was a smoldering rage that would erupt, from time to time, at her mother. The family medical doctor put her on Ritalin, which slightly improved the rage attacks, but she hated how it otherwise made her feel: wired and irritable. Then the doctor tried Prozac, which was a little better, but her basic anxiety persisted.

Given all of her constant anxiety, it would have been nice for Myrna to be able to sleep at night, but invariably she would not be able to do so. Awake in bed, her thoughts would jump desperately from strategy to strategy about what she could do, if anything, to improve her condition. Sometimes she thought about ending her life.

To make matters worse, Myrna had another neurological symptom that rounded out her misery: restless leg syndrome, in which her legs were full of a jumpy, restless energy all night long. It is something you have to have experienced, as have I, to know how nasty a symptom "restless leg" is. At the very beginning of Myrna's life, this smart, attractive, young woman felt desperate and trapped.

As we began treatment, we worked together to identify five areas that we could track from week to week to see how she was progressing: anxiety, panic attacks, sleep disturbance, restless leg syndrome, and cognitive cloudiness—including "feeling stupid."

Over the first few weeks of treatment, the first symptom to show signs of relenting was the sleep disturbance. At first I had suggested melatonin along with the neurofeedback, and this worked very well. At least this enabled Myrna to get to sleep, but then she would awaken a few times due to her restless leg syndrome. However, soon Myrna was sleeping most nights, and the restless leg syndrome had begun to diminish. By the sixth session, both the restless leg syndrome and the insomnia were gone. Around the same time, she had begun to forget to take her melatonin. However, she still seemed to be getting a good night's rest.

One day Myrna came in to tell me that she had gone to the mall with her mother. (This may seem like nothing for a young woman in her twenties, but for Myrna, it was earthshaking for her to be able to go out in public again.) Over the next couple of weeks, Myrna went over to a girlfriend's house for the evening—and even ventured so far as to go to the movies with friends. Her rituals and obsessive thoughts were in decline.

In the early spring of 2002, Myrna went to New York City and made a solemn visit to Ground Zero with her father. "Wow!" we all said.

Myrna's big breakthrough, though, and one that really showed how much better she was getting, was a blind date that she went on. The young man, a Marine, spent most of the evening in a kind of braggadocio about his "corps," and the "wimps" from the other branches. He also exhibited behavior that could be called "male chauvinist."

Myrna locked eyes with the woman friend who had introduced them. The woman's eyes had a knowing look that said: "Sorry!" Myrna stood up and said, "I want to go home." When the date acted smugly cajoling, then coercive, she said. "Thanks very much, I don't really want to spend any more time with you!" And the evening was over.

Myrna sat in my office in astonishment as she told me this story. "What are you doing to me? I never ever could have done that before! I would have suffered that boring *#@&*!!! till the end of the evening, and probably gone out with him again if he had asked—to please *him*, not *me*!" She looked at me almost accusatively.

I said: "Well, which way would *you* rather be? I'm not sure I can do the reverse transformation!"

She registered what I was saying, and a defiant look flitted across her face: "I'll never go back!" she said.

"Well, then," I said, "it sounds to me like you're getting more real, becoming who you really are."

She shook her head and again uttered the sacred mantra, "Wow!"

When I had asked Myrna at the beginning of treatment if she had any intention of going on with school, she had shown a defeated look. "I don't think so," she had said. "I had a really bad experience. I don't think I'm cut out for school. I'll just get married."

In a recent session, two months after the above, Myrna informed me that she had set up an appointment with the local college to arrange to begin classes in the fall.

"I thought you had given up on that," I said.

"I just thought I'd give it another try," she replied. "I feel smart again."

The following week Myrna applied for a job in a local day-care center and got it. Then she told me she had another blind date. This time it had been set up by, of all people, her biker dad.

"Oh wow!" (I was the one to say the mantra this time.) "Go for it!" I said. "But if he's a male chauvinist, you know the drill!" She laughed.

To our mutual astonishment, the date was a success, and her relationship with this man seems to have turned into a steady thing. Myrna now has a whole new circle of friends, more mature than the old circle, and she has come to feel a little more mature herself. Above all, she feels *normal*.

In a recent session, she acknowledged that she had not told her new boyfriend that she had been, well . . . "that way." I looked up quizzically from my notes. "You mean anxious?"

"Yes!" she replied emphatically.

"You don't seem that way to him now, do you?"

"No."

"Then you could be the one to decide to make that disclosure, and when. You could pick and choose your time to do so, if you did."

Myrna nodded. She knew the choice was hers.

(See the color insert, page 3 for an illustration of Myrna's Subjective Symptom Ratings Chart.)

Deep Depression

I think of it as the "La Brea Tar Pits," a place where you and everything around you is in frozen stuckness, and it seems like it could last a million years.

A DEPRESSED CLIENT

"Affective," or "mood disorders" were not understood as a clinically inclusive entity until relatively recently, when DSM III and IV placed categories heretofore separate into this new metacategory. These disorders imply that people's mood fluctuations have a global effect on their functioning. (They do!) Think of a continuum from "mildly blue" (dysthymia) to serious "clinical" depression, or the gentle undulations of mood called "cyclothymia," on up to the high peaks and deep vales of bipolar, or "manic-depressive" disorder.

The reframing is probably useful, because it is based on neurology. The overall problem shows how dependent the cerebral cortex, the most evolved part of the brain, is upon the subcortical regions, notably the limbic system. There they are, these organs that have found names even as their roles were discovered: the *thalamus* and *hypothalamus, hippocampus, amygdala, geniculate nucleus.* Further, there is the now expanding role of the *cerebellum*, particularly the *cerebellar vermis*, upon the subtle levels of our functioning, including our ability to read and our ability to communicate emotion. And then there is the *cingulate gyrus,* actually the inner fold of the cortex, which is highly implicated in OCD.

Emotions hover closer to the existential threshold than thoughts. *They tell us what is important.* That's why urgent issues of life and death are always attended by strong emotion. Emotions, present in milder forms, color thoughts and are sometimes presented as feelings and sentiments. We don't like to see feeling romp roughshod over thought, but neither do we relate well to human beings whose thought is detached from feeling, or who show no feeling whatsoever.

When the cerebral cortex is damaged, raw limbic emotion rages freely through human words and deeds, as we have seen in the literature on TBI. The frontal lobes keep our inner "animal" in check. There is, in fact very convincing evidence that sociopaths and recidivist criminals have a shrunken or impaired frontal lobe. Lacking this "buffer" of social evaluation and inner control, the sociopath is said to be "capable of anything." (Additional evidence suggests that one of the primary causes of frontal lobe underdevelopment is a lack of primary nurturance and a "normal" family life.)

Dr. Maurice Sterman has theorized that the presence of slow, high amplitude waves in any area of the brain signals a failure of the cortex, at that area, to inhibit subcortical influences. There is a kind of "hole" in the cortex. This is consistent with the fact that we know that the rhythm generators themselves are limbic, thalamic, and reticular nuclei. The presence of this slow wave activity during waking consciousness signals that the cortex has failed to contain its biological understory. The primitive, "old mammalian brain" wins out again. We see "mood swings," and emotional instability, which seems to have no inner defense—or containment. Frontal delta, for example, may not only indicate depression, but an inability to plan for the future, to think clearly, and to take the needs of others into account.

The LENS therapist never heads for such an area directly with his/her treatment, for that would be to challenge the cortex where it is the weakest. The site sort, in fact, is designed in such a way so as to treat the entire brain before touching *that most damaged* site. Now bear in mind that the map *reads* the brain at each site, either in a *stim* or *no-stim* condition. (However, it's usually the case that the most sensitive patients have a *no-stim* map done.) LENS therapists say that the presence of localized foci of delta or theta often predicts a relatively short course of treatment. An example is a local woman whose mother had been bipolar. (In the old days they called it "Manic-Depressive.")

Isabel's Story: My Brain Is Mush

In those same old days, the mood-stabilizing effects of Lithium carbonate had not yet been discovered, so Isabel's mother had frequent absences and hospitalizations, leaving Isabel alone with nurses and *au pairs*. Isabel's own depression only came on in midlife, after a failed marriage to an alcoholic husband, and later, a giddy but—ultimately—failed love affair with a much younger man. This affair was, for Isabel, a wicked emotional merry-go-round, but after Isabel got off of it, she was despondent and enervated.

Isabel had lost all joy in life, it seemed. She was indifferent to her grown children and young grandchildren. Earlier in her life, she had taken great pleasure from reading long gothic novels. Now she would put a book down after reading a few pages of it. She found herself making futile lists of tasks that she never carried out. Her memory seemed shot, for she would find the lists days and weeks later, and realize she had done nothing about them. She was insomniac and irritable.

Isabel's brain waves showed high amplitude frontal delta in two foci but spread across the entire region. This explained her fogginess, and her poor planning, sequencing, and organizing skills. The rest of the cortex looked relatively okay. Her "premorbid history" was relatively good, despite her absent and volatile mother. (Isabel had actually proven to be a much better mother herself.)

I assigned a medium prognosis to Isabel, believing that she would require approximately 30–40 sessions. However, from the first few sessions, Isabel began to show improvement. Her insomnia diminished and she began dreaming—which gave her abundant material for psychotherapy—and her energy improved.

Isabel had been staying with family nearby when she first came to us. Her stay with them had been temporary, however; she presently lived a hundred and fifty miles away from our center. However, she was so motivated to get better that she faithfully made the six-hour round trip commute to our offices every week.

As Isabel's course of treatment progressed and her energy continued to improve, she told me that she was jogging daily on the beach with her dog, and kayaking in the open ocean. In sequence, Isabel noticed that she was able to remember her lists without checking them, read and remember magazine articles, and conduct the routine bookkeeping that her business required, in a clear-headed fashion.

After about three and a half months, Isabel reported feeling extremely functional in managing her business, and being much more involved, once again, with her family. Soon she was able to play a leading role in the family confrontation and eventual rehabilitation of one of her daughters who was becoming alcoholic.

By the time she had completed the thirty sessions we had originally projected for her, she was not only "recovered," she had become the highly functioning woman she had previously been at her best. Overcoming obstacles and winning, Isabel felt she was now functioning optimally.

After a hiatus of about nine months, Isabel came back for a few neurofeedback sessions. She reported that she was still functioning pretty well, and had solved a lot of family problems by "preventive intervention"—bringing things up, and working on them while they were still little problems instead of big ones. I noticed that she had a plump, seven-hundred-page gothic novel with her. "Reading?" I asked with a slightly raised eyebrow.

Her look told me she remembered how she had been when we started: "I couldn't even read *Donald Duck*," she said. We laughed.

Jeremy Experiences Thanatophilia: *An Obsession with Death*

Jeremy was twenty-six years old when his younger brother killed himself. Through Jeremy's long university career, at which he did well, Jeremy was somehow haunted by the idea of doing the same thing to himself. He and his brother had inherited not only the same affective disorder—depression—but the same flawed upbringing, with parents who were alternately withdrawn and abusive.

His doctorate led to a university position, a social-science teaching appointment at a good university. Despite psychotherapy and a variety of medications, Jeremy's thoughts of committing suicide continued without abatement. Depression, of course, was a part of it and governed the ebb and flow of the urge, or its intensity. Jeremy eventually decided to give up academia; it just didn't meet his needs any more. He needed a more intense grappling with life—or none at all.

When I first met him, he had come East to attend law school. Referred by a respected psychiatrist, he seemed bright, earnest, but troubled. While I was doubtful we could do anything to help him, given the many excellent physicians who had tried and failed, I told him that we were, nonetheless, willing to do our best.

My misgivings turned out to be unfounded. From the beginning, Jeremy's subjective rating scale showed mild but steady improvement. In fact, this is exactly what we look for in a lasting cure, as the nervous system improves at its own rate, and in its own fashion. (As the cortex gets more robust, the effects of the treatment seem to reach into the subcortical, limbic governors of affect. We see mood instability decrease, sleep improve, and anxiety diminish—usually in an organic way unique to the individual.) Week by week Jeremy's subjective rating scale showed a decrease in suicidality.

Our Stone Mountain clinician, Carrie Chapman, had been doing most of Jeremy's treatments at our New York City satellite office. Carrie had told me, in our frequent supervision meetings, that Jeremy was doing "well," but I wasn't prepared for what I found when I came down for a clinical interview with him. After our convivial "catching up on the professional and personal levels, I remembered the serious issue of his suicidality. His score on the subjective rating scale was down to "0."

"You're kidding," I said.

"Nope," he replied, "I just don't think of it. It's a thing of the past."

Just recently, after a two-year hiatus during which his law school career progressed considerably, Jeremy came back for "a touch-up," as he said. I met with him on a Spring day.

"How's the suicidality?" I asked.

"I haven't really thought much about it," he said, "until I had a big disappointment with a love affair about a week ago."

"That's pretty good," I said, "considering how bad it had been for a while. I think it should probably clear up in a few sessions."

"That's what I think too," he concurred.

We both were right. I saw Jeremy last month. "How's graduate school?" I asked.

"I graduate this June," he replied, with a pleased look.

"No!" I said. "Has it been that long?"

We slapped a high-five. "I'm so glad you're still around!"

The Divine Fire, Bipolar Disorder

Kay Jamison has written a marvelous book, *Touched by Divine Fire*, on the creative yet disturbing legacy of bipolar illness, or as it used to be called, Manic-Depressive Disorder. The book is made richer by the fact that Jamison herself suffered from the disorder.

By definition bipolarity is unstable. When we look at its EEG power spectrum, we see the humps betokening depression (delta/theta) and those reflecting hyperactivity or hypervigilance (hi-beta). In between, there may be a trough where there is not much energy, in the alpha/SMR/beta range.

This means that neurologically, this is a brain of extremes; it is either bottomed out in a kind of torpor, or alternatively, as Jamison put it, "touched by divine fire." In the latter phase, especially its extreme form, the mind and metabolism seem driven by a demonic intensity that is "otherworldly." Normal practical considerations vanish, and the soul may be seized by a religious or creative zeal that can seem monomanical or "insanely driven" to other people.

The LENS Helps, But Does Not Cure, a Case of Psychotic Depression

One sixty-five-year-old woman, whom we shall call Rachel, was diagnosed with a chronic case of severe psychotic depression. For years, she had not only "heard" a voice, but the voice, clearly male, spoke outloud, *through her*, in a gruff and bombastic manner. He said he was God, but his main business seemed to be to rebuke her constantly.

The sins that evidently earned her the rebuke (and it all must have been true, because God said so) were mostly sexual sins that Rachel had committed when she was thirteen years old. An older cousin had groped her in front of the fish tank, and she had just stood there, not knowing what to do, but secretly enjoying it. But God wouldn't let her forget her lustful enjoyment. (And no plethora of Freudian analysis or interpretations seemed to matter "one jot or tittle"; in fact God told her psychiatrist in no uncertain terms, that he didn't like Freud at all, because *he was an atheist!*)

He had first come to Rachel in the shower some twenty years ago, asking her, as she stood naked before him, to declare him "her God " by a ritual of turning around three times and repeating the oath of loyalty that he spoke to her. Ever since this (evidently rather perilous) Faustian bargain, the Voice had been with her, but mostly in a negative, hostile, and threatening way.

Over the course of Rachel's thirteen psychiatric hospitalizations before she came to us, she had already received thirty-nine ECT's (electroconvulsive treatments that are considered for severe clinical depressions). She had been plied with every antipsychotic and anticonvulsive medication known to psychopharmacology—many of which backfired. Still, she was on nine different medicines at one time when we first saw her. (Hers was the classic case of taking medicines to control the side-effects of medicines—neuroleptics, anticonvulsants, tricyclics, SSRIs, benzodiazepines, stomach tranquilizers, and heavy-duty sleeping medications.)

Rachel had previously earned a Master's degree, but with the medication and shock treatments she had received, her demeanor was now very strange. She walked with a shuffle, occasionally freezing catatonically. She spoke in a slurred, mumbling fashion, except when the Voice came out, which was powerful and guttural, ordering her around and berating her. Often she would argue back in a futile fashion, accompanied by wild-eyed, distorted facial expressions.

Over the years, Rachel had been diagnosed by various psychiatrists and institutions as being Manic-Depressive (the old name for bipolar), Schizo-Affective, Schizophrenic, and/or having Dissociative Identity Disorder (previously called Multiple Personality Disorder), and/or Obsessive-Compulsive Disorder. (We see how impeccable the diagnostic categories of modern psychiatry can be!)

Rachel's first arrival at our center was dramatic. She arrived in a thunder and lightning storm, accompanied by her husband, Pete, a steady, very devoted man, and her son, Tom, who had made the referral. Her son, after all the psychiatric failures, was certain that she really needed something like an "exorcism" and wanted me to do one immediately. Pete, on the other hand, just shook his head. But there was a desperate pleading in his eyes. Both men sat in on the initial session.

Almost immediately I found myself engaging "God" or as we later came to call him, "the Voice." The Voice told me—in no uncertain terms—that he didn't think much of me as a therapist, and that I had better not try to "cure" Rachel, or he would have our center struck by lightning and burned to the ground. Lightning was, in fact, crashing around us in an ominous way, and the Voice seemed to be exploiting its presence in his grandiose manner. He rebuked Rachel for her (actually rather innocent) sexuality, and for actually trying to "kill him" one day while he had systematically driven her into an insane frenzy, with a broom. (Rachel had darted hysterically around the house brandishing the broom and screaming at the Voice to get away from her.) Vocal outbursts like this, Pete assured us, had not helped their relationships with the neighbors in nearby apartments, or upstairs.

Though at the outset I was extremely skeptical that we could accomplish much of anything in such a severe and complicated case, we agreed to try. On the second session we did a brain map, which showed an actual storm in her brain. Even with the unholy cocktail of medications, her amplitudes were over 40μv of delta and theta, twenty of hi-beta spindles (very high) and seizurelike spikes that reached close to 100μv.

Because of the acuteness of the case, supportive Pete agreed to drive the hundred mile round trip to our center three times a week for the first four months. Within the first few months of treatment, Len Ochs, who had come East to train our staff, evaluated her brain map and met her in person.

"Oh, my God," he said to me after meeting, ". . . *them.*"

"No, it's *her* God that's the problem," I replied. "I am reminded why I never did like that Old Testament *Jahweh* guy very well!"

"Well, that's who you've got!" he said. Then he grew more serious. "Stephen, this is going to be a long haul—if you can do anything at all."

Three times a week we got to see quite a lot of Rachel. Other clients would be astonished to hear a loud argument between a punitive male voice and a plaintive or hysterical female one emanating from behind the closed doors of the bathroom—and then watch, astonished, as *only one small woman emerged.*

Soon, however, Rachel noticed that she was sleeping a little better. Her husband hated his wife's medications, both in terms of cost and in terms of what they seemed to be doing to her. He asked the doctor to start withdrawing her from the most potent of them. As she came off one medication after another, soon she began to walk and speak more normally. The awful *tardive dyskinesia* (in which patients are condemned to neuromuscular movements such as writhing, or tics, that they can't stop) was present, but diminished.

Soon Rachel tried bolder excursions to shopping malls, then bus trips for seniors, during which time she was able to appear more normal, or at least keep the "conversations with God" internal.

Rachel had always loved to dance but hadn't done so for years. Soon she and her husband were going out to nightclubs around Monticello and Liberty. She became the belle of the dance floor, and Pete loved dancing with her. She wrote an articulate and eloquent letter to President Clinton, supporting him in his time of woe, and received a personal reply, which she proudly showed to everyone. She spoke publicly at her local chamber of commerce, B'nai B'rith, and to some seniors groups and, apparently, was quite eloquent. Pete said he was "in awe" of her intelligence, her command of language, and her passionate liberal beliefs.

But as much as we celebrated these improvements, and her increasingly normal appearance and manner, the depressing daily "voice of God" continued to blight Rachel's life. (I think of Monty Python: "He wasn't a nice God, you know!") Some joy came into her life when she and her husband became grandparents again when their closest son and his wife had a baby. Watching Rachel play with her cherubic grandson, you would never catch a glimpse of that bad old Jehovah guy.

Postscript: Three years ago, on returning from a day spent visiting their new grandson, she and Pete had a head-on collision with a school bus. The long-suffering Pete was killed instantly, but Rachel survived—and with a new head injury. Strangely enough, during the months of her hospitalization, the Voice seemed to have disappeared. Unfortunately, as she seemed mostly to have gotten better, it made its indefatigable return. Rachel was remanded to the psychiatric ward of the hospital, where once again medications were applied with reckless enthusiasm. But "God" remained stronger than anything that we—or anyone else—could do!

Rachel is now ensconced in a fairly pleasant residential treatment facility for seniors. I saw her at a festival, a little less than a year ago, and she remembered me and greeted me warmly.

Thomas: A Case of Bipolar Disorder
LYNN BRAYTON, PSY.D.

Thomas came into my practice when his therapist became very ill. Because her return was anticipated in a few months, our therapy was primarily supportive in nature. Thomas had been in treatment for many years with a diagnosis of bipolar disorder. Eight years prior, he was employed as a professional and a supervisor. He had an excellent work record but began having major problems when a new and highly critical administrator took over his division. Thomas's job, which had been secure for twenty-six years, suddenly seemed threatened when many of his peers were fired.

The stress of this situation precipitated a great deal of explosive anger and eventually catatonic depression in Thomas. His wife was a nurse and cared for him during his depression; her care prevented his being hospitalized. He attempted to return to work but was unsuccessful and was placed on long-term disability.

Thomas's response to medication was relatively poor. Medication changes seemed to be frequent and he was unable to find a medication dosage or combination that did not leave him drowsy or agitated. The meds would be changed cyclically when he became hostile and explosive, for example, and then there would be another change several weeks later when he experienced side effects or became lethargic.

Personally he was generous and kindhearted, a people-pleaser and a gift-giver. However, except for his family, he was very socially isolated. He seemed prone to being misinterpreted in social situations and was somewhat unskilled at responding to them. His loneliness drove him to be more attentive and affectionate than was appropriate, and this was viewed by women as flirtatious. Any conflict, however slight, was viewed as an attack and his response was defensive and hostile and often escalated the situation. His frustration tolerance was poor and he was easily irritated by relatively benign situations. In therapy he was honest but tended to discuss subjects that would earn my approval.

He reported having had a very happy childhood within a supportive, tight-knit community. Any discussion of his past conflict at work left him highly agitated and bitter. After weeks turned into months and it was becoming increasingly clear that his therapist would not be able to resume treating Thomas (due to her progressed physical illness), I began to look at different ways of approaching his treatment. We had one EMDR (The Eye Movement Desensitization and Reprocessing discovered by Francine Shapiro) session regarding his job situation and his response was remarkably positive. And while his bitterness about his job improved, his overall irritability did not.

We began using the LENS and his response was immediately positive. His wife was also very impressed with this treatment for about one month until Thomas underwent a session in which he was overstimulated and, as a result, he became highly agitated. At that point his wife did not want him to continue with the LENS treatment and actively opposed it. Thomas continued in spite of her objections, and after fifteen treatments his changes were remarkable.

He began to use less of the Ativan that he was on. He also was sleeping less and doing more household chores. His wife was pleasantly surprised when he planned an anniversary trip that turned into a second honeymoon. He was complaining of muscle soreness, which seemed to be the result of his increased activity level. His appearance, which was always good, but casual, changed more to business attire, and he made a point of showing up at his wife's office with lunch plans or flowers. His psychiatrist noted that Thomas was the most relaxed he had ever seen him.

After Thomas assumed most of the household chores on a daily basis, painted the house, cleaned the baseboards and ceiling fans, his wife finally had a change of heart about the LENS treatment. Thomas wanted to continue weekly LENS treatment even though he was maintaining his therapeutic gains for several weeks during the holidays and vacations.

A Postscript on Anxiety and Depression: In conclusion, both anxiety and depression are states that distort our normalcy. Anxiety makes us hypervigilant and overaroused, depression is its underaroused sibling. Because the two distortions frequently intermingle, it is hard both for psychopharmacologists to know what drugs to use, and for conventional neurofeedback practitioners to pick their protocol.

The LENS procedure threads the opposites and helps to disentangle the variables. As people become more neurologically stable and quiet, their neuroses and defense mechanisms also wane. They become more amenable to psychotherapeutic interventions. Their self-image improves, and they are able to meet life's challenges with more grace.

We have presented some rather serious cases in this chapter, people for whom we attempted therapeutically to quell the excesses of anxiety and gently lift the depths of depression; and we have acknowledged our failures along with our successes. I hope that these may have communicated both the amazing powers—as well as the limitations—of the neurofeedback method that is the subject of this book.

THE DIVINE MADNESS

Epilepsy, Explosive Disorders, Tourette's Syndrome, and Tics

Stephen Larsen, Ph.D., Karen Schultheis, Ph.D.,
and Len Ochs, Ph.D.

How'd you like to find yourself as the Frankenstein Monster?
MICHAEL, WHO HAS EPILEPTIC
"POST-ICTAL PSYCHOSIS"

Since the times of the ancient shamans, people have interpreted a seizure as being "taken over" by something else: as the visitation of a god—or a demon. Early religions called seizures "divine madness" and sometimes incorporated them into rituals, such as are still practiced over much of the third world today. Examples of this are the possession rituals of Brazilian *Umbanda*, or even the idea of a state trance medium such as the *Sungmas* of Tibet, whose pronouncements were the basis for major political decisions. But if the possessing spirit was an intrusive and intransigent demon, instead of a god, the perilous course for the shaman—or later, priest—would be *exorcism*.

Explosive disorders that in their intensity rival seizures have been channeled into the service of the community, so to speak, in traditions such as the Norse *Berserkers*. These were warriors who fought in a state of frenzy, possessed by "bear spirits" (and wearing their "bear shirts," hence the word "berserk"). They were thought to be invincible. There is also the Indonesian "amok." When in this condition, the person who is "amok" is in such a frenzied state that they are not held responsible for their actions, whatever those actions may be.

What is certain is that we are invited to take a look at our own

223

reality-system as we contemplate these powerful and disturbing human behaviors. Moving from the demon-haunted European Middle Ages, where having a seizure could mean taking a trip to the stake, we pass through later centuries with their "ducking stools" and literal pits of serpents (sudden shock or fear was thought to frighten off possessing spirits). The nineteenth century's "moral treatments" were slightly more "humane" but still included straitjackets and padded cells to restrain the "frenzies" of patients.

Only in the twentieth century did medical and pharmacological approaches gradually come into their own, after hypnosis and pycho-analysis had shown their powerlessness over seizures. It was Hans Berger's 1924 discovery of brain waves, though, that gradually opened the way to the modern perspective that epilepsy is primarily a neurological disorder—a malfunctioning of the brain characterized by giant spikes and waves. Soon thereafter, pharmaceutical treatments for epilepsy were evaluated by their effectiveness in quelling the kindling of large cortical potentials.

In some of the personal stories that you will encounter in this chapter, you will see the agony of seizure disorders, the harm caused by crude and primitive attempts to control them, and how neurotherapy can sometimes "save the day." The author hopes that the twenty-first century will see the problem of seizure disorders effectively addressed, with the widespread implementation of neurofeedback as the most therapeutic modality for this disorder. Why? Because it is eminently gentle and addresses the problem's root cause: the malfunctioning of the cerebral cortex. The idea that the brain itself can learn to control its own seizures is an exciting one that offers a dazzling glimpse of human potential that is, as of yet, unrealized.

In chapter 2 we told the story of how Dr. M. Barry Sterman developed his antiseizure protocol. (Monomethylhydrazine, a rocket fuel, was giving astronauts seizures. Sterman's experiments with monkeys and rats showed that animals who produced a strong 12–15 Hz rhythm [SMR] over the sensory-motor strip were basically immune to seizures.)

By 1971, Sterman had begun SMR training with human subjects.[1] In 1972 he published a case history in EEG and Clinical Neurophysiology. His procedure soon was replicated by other researchers, a sign to the scientific community that the phenomenon under examination is robust.

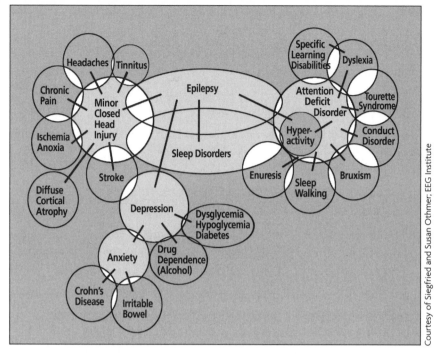

Courtesy of Siegfried and Susan Othmer; EEG Institute

Fig. 8.1. Chart showing interrelationship of symptoms associated with different conditions emerging from TBI and Seizure Disorder. (After a chart prepared by Siegfried and Susan Othmer, for use in training materials, ca. 1990–1995.)

Soon a four-person study was commenced, in which the subjects showed a 60–65 percent reduction in seizures. This study was published in the prestigious journal *Epilepsia* in 1974.[2]

Funding from the National Institutes of Health allowed Sterman to do larger studies using a rigorous A-B-A design—a design no longer sanctioned due to the fact that an intermediate "condition" of the experiment made the subjects worse. The protocol consisted of *suppressing theta and increasing SMR*. Again, the results were robust, and again Sterman published in *Epilepsia* (1978). Another grant from the NIH allowed him to undertake a study with twenty-four subjects over a three-year period.

With subsequent replications of Sterman's work in other laboratories, all told 174 subjects were treated, and 142 showed substantial clinical improvement. At this point, clinicians such as the psychologist

Robert Reynolds began to use the protocol to treat patients, with the same success that had been demonstrated by the experimental studies. A new, noninvasive treatment for epilepsy had been born.[3]

After this sturdy beginning, and the awarding of a 1982 NIH grant to do even larger studies, support for this research was suddenly withdrawn. "The proper place for Ph.D.s," Sterman was told, "is documenting the effects of drugs, which are the approved and mainstream cures used by doctors." His work was evidently not "mainstream" enough to warrant further support. (It may also have been perceived as threatening to the makers of anticonvulsant medications.) Sterman still fumes about these "political" slights, says Jim Robbins in his popular book on neurofeedback, *A Symphony in the Brain*.

Len Ochs's method is not as well known as Sterman's and has not yet generated enough significant experimental studies. But the clinical evidence is just as compelling as Sterman's. Here we might compare the protocols: Sterman's great discovery was that there was a rhythm, which, when learned and used, made the brain more or less *seizure resistant*.

With Ochs and his development of the LENS, the objective was to not allow the kindling of seizures through *entrainment*, or the amplification of existing slow waves. This thinking was, in fact, the reason for development of the *offset* procedure, and the *disentrainment* model as a whole. Brain waves *will try to follow, and entrain with, any rhythmical stimulus to which they are exposed*. By harnessing the stimulus to the existing brain waves, but at a higher (+5 +10 +15 or +20 Hz) frequency (negative offsets not producing such good results as the positive), Ochs felt he had designed in effect, an *antiseizure, anti-epileptic protocol*.

We do not know of any situation where the application of the LENS *with* an offset has ever occasioned a seizure. In fact the reverse seems to be true. Migraines are thought by some neurologists to be seizurelike in their action. Though we have never had the opportunity to intervene in an ongoing seizure with a patient, we have had lots of opportunities with incipient or even full-blown migraines. The results can be dramatic: often the headache is aborted on the spot or its severity is greatly reduced.

The case cited below is a vivid demonstration of how the LENS can intervene in a serious and chronic seizure disorder. Although it is only one example, the results are encouraging for many sufferers of epilepsy.

(Now all we can hope to do is to cure someone wealthy enough to fund some significant research!)

Michael: Transforming Seizures into Joy

Michael came to us with a heartbreaking story, but not so atypical among those who have suffered multiple head injuries. A father and husband in his forties, he came from a Catskills blue-collar, lumberjack family that encouraged a rough and tumble lifestyle, where a lot of time was spent in the local taverns. His father, Elijah, was a "good ole boy" with a severe drinking problem, an explosive temper, and a heavy hand. Even the police gave Elijah a wide berth.

Michael's older brother grew into the mold that had been established by their father. At age thirty (Michael was sixteen) the brother had been drinking heavily and was driving about ninety miles an hour when his car hurtled off the road and crashed. As so often happens, the drunk and floppy driver was virtually unhurt, while his younger brother's head smashed through the windshield. But Michael's feet were also trapped in the wreckage; he broke his left ankle and his legs and ribs were crushed. It took crowbars and sledgehammers (the "Jaws of Life" were not yet available in our area) to pull him from the wreckage. Michael's life as he had known it came to an abrupt halt.

Three years later, the seizures began. They were regular as clockwork and came on about once a month: *grand mal* seizures, lasting about three to five minutes. In their aftermath, Michael would be confused, incoherent, dyscoordinated, and moody, a state that might last for several hours or several days. Dilantin, Felbutol, Zyprexa, and SSRIs were all tried, and in various combinations, but without appreciable benefit. Rather, the patient experienced dumbing and numbing side effects from the medications.

Michael's condition was so severe that in 1998 his doctor recommended neurosurgery. Consequently, two-thirds of Michael's right temporal lobe, believed to be the foci for the seizures, was removed. But the seizures did not stop. Michael was on his way to New York City for a one-month postsurgery checkup when the car he was in got involved in an accident. Michael, in the passenger's seat, again broke the windshield with his head.

Now the seizures became far more serious. After this new trauma,

Michael was diagnosed with "post-ictal psychosis" in which it is recognized that, for a little while after the seizures, the person is "out of their minds" and literally uncontrollable. But in Michael's case, it was more like post-ictal *delirium*. Michael's wife, a strong woman, was unable to control her husband's more violent movements. He would try to climb out of windows, or rush into speeding traffic on a busy local highway. As the seizure began, their grown son who lived nearby would be summoned and he would race over to try and restrain his father and control his dangerous pilgrimages toward second-story windows, stairways, or highways.

Each month Michael could count on falling down a flight of stairs. He had broken most of his limbs, fingers, toes, and ribs, sometimes more than once, during the seizures and their aftermath. His head injuries began to multiply. It was a precarious and awful situation, compounded by the fact that the family lived on a second story—"the only apartment they could afford."

When we first saw Michael in January of 2000, his quality of life revolved around the seizures. It was awful to see him the day after one had occurred, as invariably he would have broken a rib, finger, or toe, and he would be in much pain. He had become sober a number of years before and converted to Christianity, which he felt had saved him in many ways. But he still needed marijuana in fairly large daily doses to keep the pain, anxiety, and depression away. And his temper, like that of his older brother and father, at times seemed uncontrollable, which adversely affected his marriage. Additionally, Michael told us that his dreaming seemed to have totally stopped some years before. He was on total SSI disability.

On the positive side, Michael had done a fair amount of work on himself. He had completed a two-year college degree, maintained his sobriety and, after a midlife conversion to Catholicism, he was participating in parish activities. But on the negative side, Hell was vying with Heaven in Michael's psyche. While his attitude seemed basically pretty good, his moods and his nervous system seemed uncontrollable.

Within the first few months of FNS treatment, Michael's sleep regularized and his mood improved. In psychotherapy and marriage-counseling sessions, I was able to help him interpret the rage attacks as subclinical seizures—such was their intensity. (He was totally unable to get out of them, sometimes for several days.) With my counseling, Michael's wife was able to understand that her husband's rages weren't really directed "at her" but were emotional events that Michael could barely control. These anger outbreaks began unmistakably, although slowly, to improve.

Around eight sessions into treatment, Michael came into our office, radiant. He had remembered his first dream in years!

After several months of treatment, the seizures were still present but were beginning to be erratic. Michael had a period of nearly fifty days without a seizure, and then two came a couple of weeks apart. He and his wife both noticed that the intensity of both the seizure activity itself, and the post-ictal psychosis, had lessened. A couple of times we saw him on the day of, or the day after, a seizure, and he looked and acted pretty good. He seemed less oppressed by them. His marijuana consumption began to decrease, effortlessly, as it were. He was remembering more dreams. His marriage was improving.

The antidepressant SSRIs were discontinued at the patient's request. The doctors changed his medication twice and finally agreed to take Michael off the Risperdal for the post-ictal psychosis, leaving only two medications—Dilantin 100mg and Moban 25mg—and "Trileptal" as needed. (Michael no longer needed meds to control other meds.)

July 30 of 2000 was Michael's last seizure, and it broke the mold. Heretofore all of his seizures had taken place when he was asleep in the wee hours of the morning. One afternoon he lay down for a nap. About 2:00 P.M. his wife saw his eyes fluttering, and thought he was having a seizure, which he was. It was mild, lasting a couple of minutes, and there was no post-ictal problem. About 5:00 P.M. Michael had a second seizure during which he was more confused than he had been during the first one, and although he bit the tip of his tongue, he was not aggressive, and he stayed on the couch. At 8:30 came the third and last seizure. He wanted to talk but couldn't. Dilantin, 500mg was administered, but it seemingly had no effect on him. That night, when he was sleeping, he sweated profusely, something that had often followed seizures. He had anxious "jamais-vous" experiences (he didn't feel "like himself").

These seizures were followed by a couple of days of restlessness and poor sleep, but then Michael began to feel better and his energy level improved. The doctor took him off Dilantin and put him on a new drug,

Keppra. Two weeks later, an enormously traumatic event happened when the teenage son of some close friends of his shot himself. The boy's family and the community were devastated, but Michael played a very supportive role. He organized a community benefit that raised fifteen hundred dollars for the grieving family. We continued treating Michael twice weekly with neurofeedback as well as the usual psychotherapy. Now the main topic in our talks was the recent tragedy.

Noticing that Michael was yawning after neurofeedback sessions (tiredness being a sign of overdose) we stopped using glasses with LEDs and used only the radio frequency stimulation. Immediately he seemed to respond with increased energy and clarity. Now he was getting up early and doing volunteer work for the church and for friends. All during the fall he remained seizure-free, and his mood and cognition radically improved.

In January of 2001 we were able to celebrate the fact that Michael had been seizure-free for six months (the longest time ever since the accident). I was able to record his own words about how he was feeling on this momentous occasion.

The FNS has given me a brand new positive attitude and the motivation to do something positive with my life. I can now step outside of my situation and make decisions based on what I see. Now I have more emotional distance from a situation. My interpersonal relationships have improved a lot. Before, I was depressed at the situation I was in, and I couldn't see past my troubles. I have a larger perspective. I'm more concerned with other people's feelings. I have improved my chess scores to the point of feeling almost "unbeatable;" maybe I'm winning 75% of the time. I can think and plan three or four moves ahead. (Michael played weekly chess sessions with the priest of his parish throughout treatment, and his success or failure became an interesting barometer of how he was doing in treatment. Recently he observed that the priest has a temper problem "and probably could use some biofeedback.") I carry around a positive attitude most of the time. You know, brother, it's much better to give love than try to demand it. It comes back anyway, always. My positive attitude has me jazzed; I feel like "Michael" again.

Michael continued neurofeedback treatment for about a year and a half, before slowly tapering off. He still asked for occasional psychotherapy sessions. He still remembers his dreams. When issues come up with his wife, he tries different strategies to resolve them. He acknowledges: "She's stubborn, but how else could she have put up with me for twenty-five years?"

With the blessings of his neurologist, and plenty of "referrals," Michael opened and led a community support group for people with seizure disorders, which was sponsored by our local hospital and head-trauma center.

Just as this book was nearing publication, I asked Michael if he would like to make a statement for it. This is what he wrote:

In 1975 I was a passenger in a car that struck a large maple tree going nearly one hundred miles per hour. I woke from a coma one week later with no memory of what had happened. I broke both feet, my left elbow, my left ankle, and I fractured three vertebrae in my back. I was sixteen at the time and seemed to recover quickly from the broken bones. But three years later the seizures began. I lived with epilepsy for twenty-three years. In 1998 I had a right temporal lobectomy that was supposed to stop the seizures. But after surgery the seizures continued, accompanied by a new condition called post-ictal psychosis. This was a very serious addition to my problem. I was offered more brain surgery to stop the seizures: a frontal lobectomy. I just couldn't face another surgery and turned to any alternative therapy available. After six months of psychotherapy and FNS treatments, everything started to change for the better. I had big memory improvements, more energy, and a better attitude about everything.

Henry: Exploding into Adulthood

One challenging case was a teenager we shall call Henry. Henry was fifteen at the time that he was seen at our center. We had received a tearful phone call from his mother; she was at her wit's end. At the age of nine, Henry had been hospitalized at Four Winds, a psychiatric hospital in Westchester, New York, for out-of-control rages. Now the rages were getting worse again, only Henry was bigger, so they were scarier. The family was considering shipping him out again.

Henry constantly felt irritable, and prone to explode at the drop of a hat. In the first treatment session he sat sullenly, not willing to talk much, just radiating the feeling that this treatment definitely *wasn't* going to help him. In the second week of treatment he was brought to our center with blood on his shirt and his pupils dilated. He was in a state of shock. On the way to the treatment session he had just put his fist through a storm door and gotten horribly cut. I told his mother that we couldn't treat him while he was in shock, and that she should take him posthaste to the emergency room, which she did. There he was given eight stitches and a tranquilizer. We rescheduled Henry for the following day and decided to treat him twice a week because of the precariousness of the situation.

Whence, the modern world seems to be asking, the terrible rage of the teenagers?

As we elicited the details of Henry's case history, we learned his mother and father had broken up when he was very young. After a little while his mother had remarried. From the beginning Henry resented his "new father." His new father also came with a son, six years older than Henry—who now became his new "half-brother." (It is with good reason that fairy tales present, again and again, the theme of the mean stepparent or stepsibling.)

The older boy, whom we shall call Tom, was easily able to master his little half-brother physically. Tom liked to tease Henry until he "blew," then he would knock him down and sit on his chest. However, at this point, one of those pivotal incidents that can change a life occurred. Henry was eight, Tom fourteen. On a wintry upstate New York day there was plenty of snow, and the boys wanted to go sledding.

They went to the top of a high hill that was great for scary rides— because you had to avoid the pavement at the bottom of the road. A "friend" of Tom's, an older boy with some problems, got angry at Tom but rather than take on an equal-sized guy, he decided to attack Henry. He stuck out his foot and diverted Henry and his sled down the scary side of the hill. When Henry hit the bottom of the hill, his sled stopped but—he didn't. He ploughed along the pavement with his face and banged his head numerous times. The frightened Tom grabbed his unconscious younger stepbrother in a fireman's carry and ran for home, leaving a trail of blood.

Henry was rushed to the hospital, and the boy who had caused the accident was arrested and arraigned in Juvenile Court for the misdeed. But that didn't help Henry, who now was scarred as well as traumatized. After this incident, Henry's "episodes" of rage increased exponentially.

Tom felt bad for a while, but the torture game didn't stop. It was too much fun to have his friends over, and then see what it would take to provoke little Henry until he flipped out and then throw him down and sit on him until he would almost self-destruct with impotent rage.

At some point Tom went into the Army, and it must have had a sobering effect on him, because he wrote Henry a long letter of apology; and when he returned home, he set about making amends for the years of torture. The military, as it sometimes promises, seems to have made a "man" out of Tom.

Henry complained of additional symptoms, which we decided to track: bad headaches, sleeplessness, constant irritability, mood swings, and depression. He had a pain in his chest, which got worse when an attack of rage was about to come on. His brain wave chart showed a mixed bag of moderately high delta, theta, and alpha, but then what I thought of as a "thundercloud" of high beta would roll through the chart, with amplitudes four times as high as any other brain wave. The delta and the theta would then shoot up as well when the "cloud" oscillated. These disturbances were so marked that when I saw the first one in the "offset" session, I checked to see if the electrode was falling off Henry's head. Henry's Power Spectrum graph on page 3 of the color insert shows his disturbed state (the high peaks) gradually calming and leveling out.

After about four sessions, Henry began to sleep better, and the headaches had vastly diminished. He always rated himself conservatively, but he said he felt one notch less "irritable"—the subjective measure that could register nervous instability and the likelihood of an explosion.

The following week Henry came to the session smiling. There was no sign of the hi-beta "storms" at all. There had been no explosions that week, and Henry felt much more "in control." In his psychotherapy sessions he was very verbal and cooperative and shared many things about his past that were useful. He discussed how particularly "abandoned" he had felt when he had been sent away to the hospital for two months when he was nine—and how desperately helpless he felt, at present, for being so "bad." We worked on insights about head injury and talked about how he would have liked to control himself if only he *could* have.

A positive transference with the therapist emerged, as did some positive additions to Henry's life, which included his friendship with Ed, an older, larger boy, who also had a rage problem. Ed, furious when the bike he had been riding got a flat tire, had thrown the bike into a swamp and then had to walk three miles home. Henry had accompanied Ed back to the swamp a few days later to fish out the bike, which was dripping with algae, and had frogs in its basket. As Henry told the story in the therapeutic context, we were able to laugh about the sometimes negative consequences of "losing it." Henry resolved to help his buddy more, even as he was really learning how to gain control of himself.

The next few weeks showed Henry doing just that. There were *no* rage attacks, nor even, he said, the urge to have one. Henry said his chest felt better. Reports began to come back from school that he was voluntarily staying afterward to work on English, his worst subject, and was seeking help from the teacher. He got fascinated by the story of *Oedipus*—and the idea of the "tragic flaw" in heroes. His mother reported that, at one point, anticipating her arrival home from an exhausting twelve-hour day at work, Henry had already put a dinner in the microwave for her—something he had never done before.

Henry wants to follow his brother into the military, because he said it "changed his brother for the better, and since 9/11 America needs really good soldiers." (But he thinks his best contribution would be in the realm of communication and intelligence.) Since he's not grounded any more, his favorite weekend pastime is to play "paintball" (a game where the players run around in the woods and ambush each other with guns that shoot paint-covered corkballs). "It's good at releasing all your frustrations," Henry said earnestly to me at our last meeting.

A Commentary on the LENS and Seizures

As the case of Michael showed, LENS is indeed an "antiseizure" procedure. By stimulating the patient at +5, 10, 15, or 20 Hz, we *disrupt* recruitment, or nip seizurelike beginnings in the bud. This is reflected in greater CNS stability overall, as sleep normalizes, and life apparently becomes less stressful. Often headaches decrease, as they did with Henry, and we remember that migraines are seizurelike in their action. With the decrease of physical pain, there is an improvement in energy because, as Len Ochs says, one recovers all the energy one previously spent defending against the pain.

Although it may not always be possible to find the causes of seizures, in some patients the seizure foci are rather obvious in that they are especially signaled by the standard deviation, or blue bar on top of the amplitude graph. In other patients, where we have seen no identifiable *nuclei* that are clear originators of seizure activity, the problems that initiate the seizures are diffuse. LENS provides repeated, gentle disruptions that ultimately strengthen the brain, increase its elasticity and flexibility, and ultimately help it develop *its own spontaneous ability to suppress seizures.*

This is not such a farfetched hypothesis. Something in most normal people resists seizures, or we would have them all the time—especially in response to traumatic events or sensory overloads—even a visit to a disco! We want the brain to find out how to do that suppression on its own, without pharmaceutical intervention, and that is the beauty of the neurofeedback approach. It is fully understood, by both proponents of medication and neurofeedback, that the real cure comes when the patient becomes higher-functioning, and his or her own behavioral and cognitive activity comes into the mix. In the same way as some studies show that a life of cognitive high-functioning seems to stave off or inhibit Alzheimer-like neural degeneration, it can also help the process of recovery of seizure or subclinical seizurelike instabilities.

That is why in the case of Michael, above, it was such a positive clinical sign when he began improving in *all* kinds of other cognitive and emotional areas. When you're not exploding all the time, it's just possible that your marriage might become a little better—at least you have a "fighting chance" to work on it. Likewise, if you're beating your priest at chess, your self-esteem goes up. If you're able to interact with younger, invariably irritating, siblings without exploding, read and concentrate for longer periods of time, or even to meditate or do yoga regularly, the stabilizing effects of those activities kick in, with the result being that you get calmer and become more centered.

However, one caveat here: if you try to do all kinds of things while your nervous system is destabilized and erratic, say in the wake of an injury, chemical insult, or emotional trauma, it is very hard to find inner stability or satisfaction. Those "little storms" that roll through our brains, as we saw in the EEG of Henry, are hard to resist.

In the Eastern traditions, even the ordinary mind is likened to a "drunken monkey," which can only be stilled by years of meditation. (The beginner can verify this for himself, by simply sitting down and asking his brain to have "no thoughts" for ten minutes.) Neurofeed-back can really help, especially in the early stages of that challenging, but ultimately very rewarding, attempt to calm the tempest in the brain.

Margaret Ayers may be one of the first people to have noticed that as people heal from epilepsy and TBI via neurofeedback, their emotional lives improve as well. Jim Robbins, in an interview with Ayers quoted her as saying:

> "These epileptic individuals were happier, smiling; they were talking about things," she says. "I thought to myself, you know, the sensory cortex is next to the motor cortex in the brain. We may be affecting emotions."[4]

It has been our consistent finding as well, in both conventional neurofeedback and with LENS, that there *is* an emotional improvement with our patients posttreatment. They seem kinder and more thoughtful. (We realize that these are very hard variables to quantify scientifically, but this is what people report clinically.) Henry thinks about his mother coming home tired and hungry and puts her supper on. Michael goes out of his way to stop in on an old lady parishioner who needs a chore done. A teenage girl with a closed head injury stops being "the sarcasm queen" and actually starts talking nicely to customers at the restaurant where she works. Little Damon (the "reactive attachment disorder" child) cuddles up more and says, "I love you." He pets the dog more and terrorizes it less.

Ali Turns His Life Around
Karen Schultheis, Ph.D., Neuropsychologist
(Presented at the Association for Applied Psychophysiology and Biofeedback, Las Vegas in March 2002).

Ali sustained a gunshot wound to the left side of his face in June of 1986. He was working as manager of a Pizza Hut when it was robbed. The robber took the money, then held his gun to the left side of Ali's face, and pulled the trigger. The bullet had shattered when it struck his facial bones. Ali was hospitalized, had several surgeries, and then was released to the care of his wife and family. Family members were never told about the implications of the brain injury or the possible effects it might have upon his behavior. But, as is so often seen, Ali's behavior changed radically. He became explosive and was referred to a psychiatrist.

At the time I saw him, Ali had been seeing this psychiatrist for about two years. The psychiatrist had diagnosed him with PTSD (post-traumatic stress disorder), and generalized anxiety. He was medicating Ali for the anxiety, and a Masters level therapist was doing psychotherapy, talk therapy, with him. I was asked by this therapist to do a neuropsychological evaluation on Ali.

My testing revealed that Ali had profound neuropsychological deficits. The most significant and disabling problems were his inability to effectively understand or use language (this is called *aphasia*). Talk therapy is the most inappropriate technique imaginable for someone with aphasia; a problem that was compounded by the fact that Ali's native language was Farsi. (Born and raised in Iran, he began speaking English only in high school, after his family had immigrated to the United States.)

Additionally, I suspected from Ali's description of his problems that he was having seizures. I recommended cognitive rehabilitation treatment and a referral to a neurologist for a seizure work-up.

Ali did receive about a year of inpatient rehabilitation treatment at an excellent facility renowned for their community reentry treatment program. He was also diagnosed with complex partial seizures and began taking anti-epileptic medications. But with this, the seizures were never very well controlled.

Medications were changed and combined but he continued to have breakthrough seizures, as well as other serious problems. He was unable to read or write effectively either in English or in Farsi. He had severe mood swings, going from nice and easy-going to extremely enraged and verbally abusive. The swings could be sudden and, after a blow-up, he could be very nice, seemingly oblivious to his previously angry behavior.

At times he would become physically abusive and throw things (although this was infrequent). At times he was extremely paranoid, suspecting his family members and any strangers he happened to see of all sorts of things. His memory was significantly impaired for both recent and remote memories, which exacerbated his paranoia. He couldn't remember doing and saying the things he did and said. He would often recall things incorrectly and then argue with his family about these things. His seizures were characterized by episodes where he had trouble breathing, his heart would race, and he felt like he was going to die.

At times Ali would hear voices that said, "Come with me. . . . You are dying!" This was an extremely frightening thing for him. He was so convinced that he was dying that he got to the point that he welcomed death as an alternative to having to live with his wretched symptoms.

I began seeing Ali again at the end of 1999. By that time he had separated from his wife and was living alone in an apartment. He was severely depressed, talking about just driving away and not telling anyone where he was going. His children would not speak to him and when they did, they would refuse to respectfully address him as "Father." This was especially traumatic for Ali because of his cultural traditions and the rules he had always enforced when they were living together. Allegedly, the separation had been precipitated by an incident wherein he had struck his oldest son (who was eighteen at the time). Ali could not remember the event but did not question the veracity of his wife's report.

Ali had difficulty finding his way to my office, an eighty-mile drive one way from where he was living. At every appointment he would rage about how badly he had been treated by the lawyer who settled his case, and about how incompetent and uncaring most physicians were. The monologue alternated with comments about his family and his sadness over losing them and was accompanied by tears and anger.

This went on for weeks. I could not do or say anything that would derail Ali's harangue. He would repeat the same thing each session as if he had an audiotape running continually in his head, and when he opened his mouth he verbalized the contents of that tape. I formed the inescapable conclusion that he could not stop or change that "tape."

I realized that I could not do anything to help him from a "talk therapy" perspective. I thought about FNS but was worried about the potential effects in that I was fearful that the treatment might destabilize his seizures (which were finally relatively stable after ten years of changing and adjusting his medications).

Finally, it seemed there was no other choice. Ali's depression was getting worse and he was talking nonstop about dying. He could not respond to anything I said to him. His medications were not effectively controlling his depression and his seizures still occurred occasionally.

Initially, the FNS treatment did not seem to be doing much. We were hampered by the fact that Ali lives alone and there was no one to report any possible changes. His level of self-awareness was almost nonexistent. Additionally, his memory was so impaired that he could not remember how he felt throughout the week between treatments. Finally, since he was unable to read or write very well, he could not keep notes on how he felt, or about any aspect of his behavior.

I could not have chosen a more difficult patient or one who was less likely to benefit from the treatment. Ali had undergone significant structural damage to his brain and bullet fragments remained embedded in his brain. His seizure disorder was *relatively* well controlled, but this meant that he still experienced breakthrough seizures, which could significantly interfere with his ability to function. The fragments reportedly migrated around the brain, periodically causing a change in symptoms. As there simply was nothing else to offer this man, I carefully began the subvisual EEG stimulation treatments.

Ali was extremely sensitive to this treatment, despite the huge doses of antidepressants and anti-epileptic medications he was taking. Because of his sensitivity, I treated him slowly: one site at a time, one second per site, one session per week or every other week. Sensitivity was indicated by his experience of being tired or sleepy after the treatment.

Slowly, he began to change.

Treatment continued for two years—weekly sessions for the most part—and is ongoing. The first symptoms to lift were his feelings of depression, of hopelessness, and helplessness. His insight improved and he began to examine the role his own behavioral problems had played in his marital separation. Although this was painful for him, he was able to face it.

There has been a great deal of improvement in Ali over these last two years. He has gone from being completely dependent on his wife to cook, keep track of his schedule, wash clothes, clean the house and take care of the myriad other responsibilities of running a household, to being completely independent. Ali's divorce is all but final. He was able to make the choice to end the marriage despite the fact that this was an extremely painful decision because it indicated his acceptance of the finality of his separation from his family. And while he continues to have episodes where he is sad about his situation, these episodes are short-lived and he is able to control this. Angry episodes also occur occasionally, but he is able to get these under control quickly as well. He remembers these angry episodes and attempts to keep them from occurring in response to the same situations again and again.

He is no longer socially isolated. He went from essentially being a hermit in his apartment and only going out for his doctors' appointments, to going out daily and spending time around other people. His social skills are impaired, but it is moving how earnestly he is trying to make contact with others. In addition to all this he has been able to cut his medications in half. Despite the decrease in medications his depression is gone and his seizures are under much better control.

This is a remarkable case. It is also atypical. It was a "Worker's Comp" case and as such, the insurance carrier was compelled to pay for the medical expenses associated with his injury. This allowed me to treat him for two years on a fairly consistent basis. He would not have been able to pay for the treatments from his disability income. We seldom get to treat patients this long so we are rarely able to see what the long-term treatment effects might be.

Ali represents a large population of patients who are significantly disabled and who have been bankrupted by their medical problems. Few of them have access to neurofeedback (actually to any type of treatment) despite the potential for significantly increasing functional abilities.

Travis: Living in the World of Tourette's

The syndrome called "Gilles de la Tourette's Syndrome" (after the French doctor who "discovered" it) is characterized by uncontrollable activities, tics, twitches, involuntary grunts or moans, even uncontrollable obscenities—in one of its more florid forms.

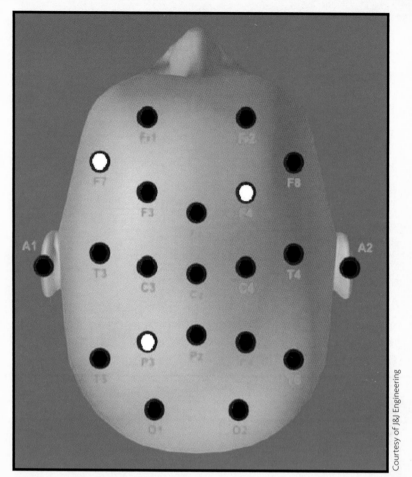

A Use3 screen that guides the practitioner to specific sites using the International 10–20 System.

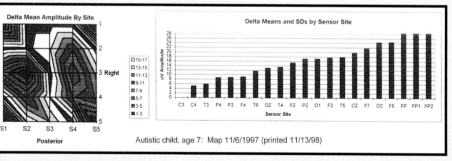

Autistic child, age 7: Map 11/6/1997 (printed 11/13/98)

...Map and site sort of seven-year-old autistic child. Delta mean amplitudes are so ...igh they go off the site sort chart at right; also none of the sites presents a standard ...eviation (which would have been indicated by blue caps on the bars).

Six minute baseline
allows clinician to
watch live brainwave

Four Minute Visual
Image of events
following each
offset with RMS line
for Alpha and Delta

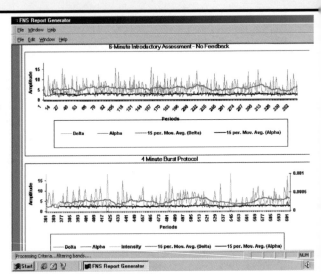

An Offset Protocol: Consists of a total of six
minutes of "baseline," and four one second *stim* periods
at +5,10,15 or 20. Usually recorded at FPZ (frontal) or CZ
(central) if frontal injuries.

Len Ochs's ingenious "Offset Protocol"

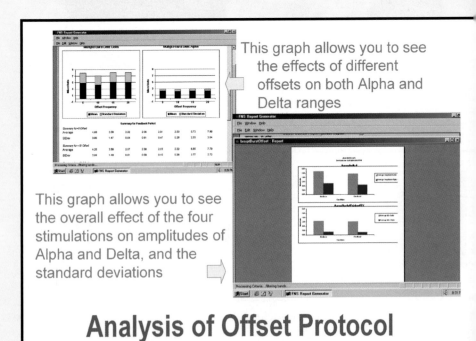

This graph allows you to see
the effects of different
offsets on both Alpha and
Delta ranges

This graph allows you to see
the overall effect of the four
stimulations on amplitudes of
Alpha and Delta, and the
standard deviations

Analysis of Offset Protocol

Analysis of Offset Protocol

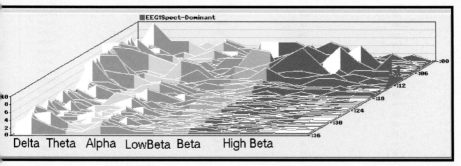

Henry's Power Spectrum graph reveals an underlying probably Bipolar constitution onstellated by a head injury. (See chapter 8, Henry: Exploding into Adulthood.)

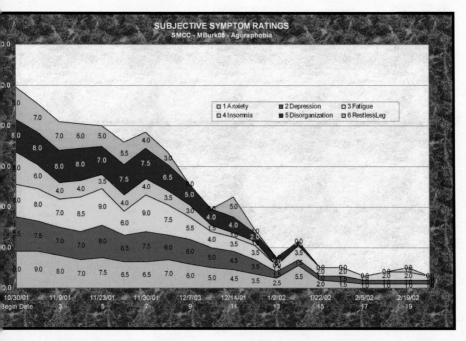

ubjective Symptom Ratings (Myrna). Already restricted by OCD, Myrna experienced n acute onset of agoraphobia after September 11, 2001. Here her symptoms were racked through the first twenty sessions of treatment. (See chapter 7, Myrna Breaks ree from Anxiety's Prison.)

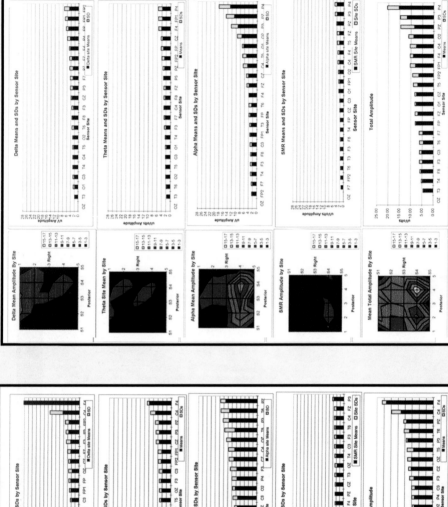

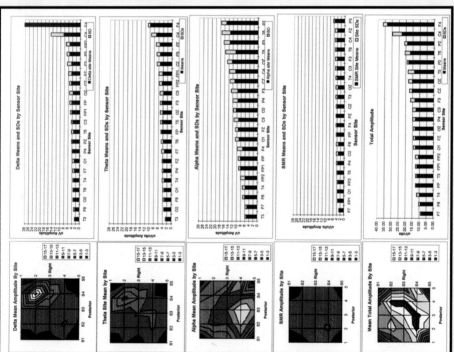

Two Map Comparison (Sharon): Multiple head-injured patient before (left) and after treatment (right); note decrease of brightly

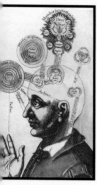

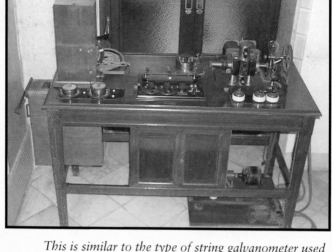

ow the Soul emerges
om the Brain, from
obert Fludd's Utrisque
osmi, 1617; the
ranger Collection,
ew York.

*This is similar to the type of string galvanometer used
by Hans Berger. We see his in the accompanying photo
of his lab. Courtesy of the Museu d'Historia de la
Medicina de Catalunya.*

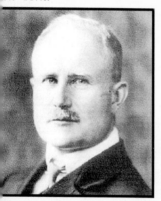

*Left: Hans Berger, M.D. (1873–1941), German
neuropsychiatrist who is best known as the developer
of electroencephalography. Below: Berger's Laboratory
where, from 1901 to 1938, he carried on his work
in secrecy, never admitting anyone to his laboratory
tucked away in a small building on the grounds of
the psychiatric clinic at the University of Jena in Jena,
Germany, where he was, for many years, director.
Photos courtesy of the Biomagnetic Center, Jena.*

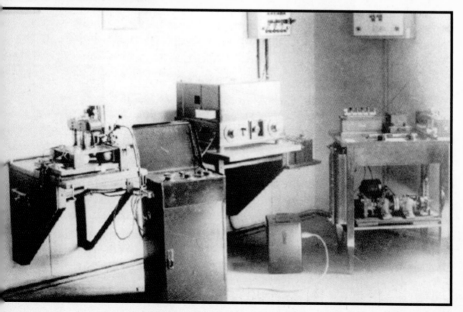

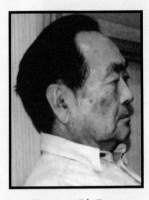

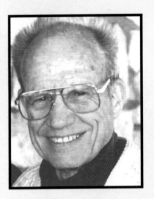

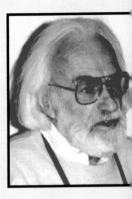

Joe Kamiya, Ph.D., in his early work showed the connection between brain waves and states of awareness.

Elmer Green, Ph.D., who with his wife Alyce, demonstrated that the body's autonomic functions could be voluntarily controlled and that states of consciousness corresponded to specific brain rhythms.

Karl Pribram, Ph.D., is the neuroscientist credited with the discovery of the holographic nature of memory storage.

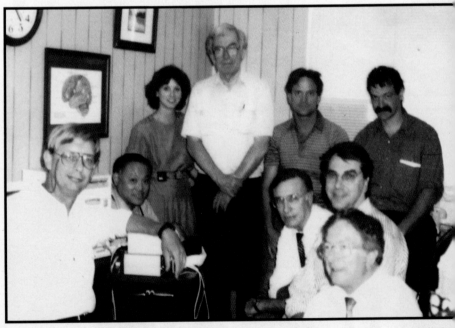

The "Nobel Prize Group" (as they were called) did early neurofeedback work with the head injured. Left to right: Bob Grove, Ken Tachiki, (unidentified), Harold Russell, Elm Wyler, (unidentified); seated in front with white shirts: Jim Smith, Len Ochs, and Herb Gross. Tachiki, Ochs, and Smith were influential in the founding of ISNR in 1993-199

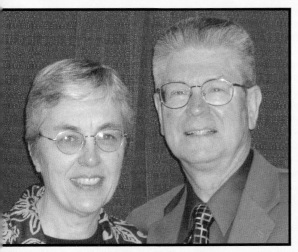

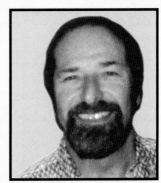

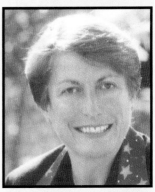

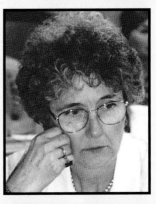

Clockwise fron top left: Susan Othmer, Ph.D., and Siefgried Othmer, Ph.D., are the founders of EEG Spectrum and have trained hundreds of clinicians.

Maurice "Barry" Sterman, Ph.D., developed the first anti-seizure neurofeedback protocols, using SMR (12–15Hz).

Margaret Ayers is recognized by the ISNR for her groundbreaking work, using neurofeedback, in the treatment of brain injuries.

Mary Lee Esty, Ph.D. worked with Len Ochs during the 1990s and conducted experiments in fibromyalgia.

Nancy White, Ph.D., is a clinical psychologist who has used alpha training in the healing of trauma and as a gateway to transpersonal and transformative experiences.

Thomas Budzynski, Ph.D., has done pioneering work on electromyography and "twilight learning."

Les Fehmi, Ph.D., is an early neurofeedback pioneer and the developer of the Open Focus method.

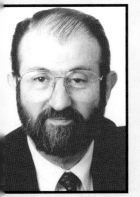

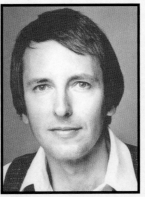

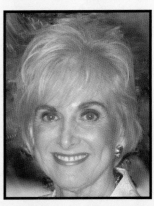

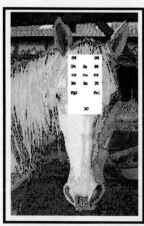

The LENS is used successfully on animals as well as people.

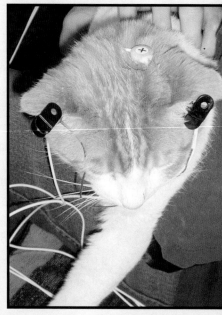

Silver demonstrates equine electrode placements, designated by Holliday and Williams; we have so far used only the nine central sites for treatment. (See Dr. Holliday's postings at www.neurovet.org for valuable information on animal EEG.)

Dizzy the cat undergoing treatment.

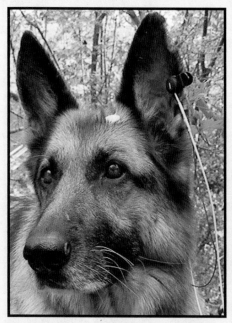

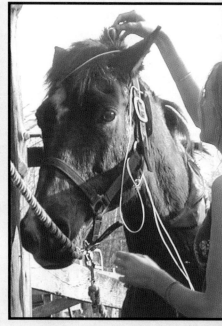

Della the dog undergoing treatment.

Claire Woolger administering electrodes to Dancer the horse.

When Travis, a frail, sensitive, highly intelligent young man was growing up, he began to develop involuntary grunts and twitches, and it didn't take long for a diagnosis of Tourette's syndrome to be given.

Travis's father was a psychiatrist and, naturally concerned about his son, began to treat him with the medicines that were at his disposal in the 1980s. Soon, Travis was on an unholy cocktail of psychotropics, which included the usual complement of medications to control other medications: stimulants, tranquilizers, anti-anxiety agents. SSRIs such as Prozac were rotated through, along with anticonvulsants such as Depakote. They probably made him worse, and they certainly didn't control the tics.

When Travis was first brought to us at the age of twenty-five, he talked and ticked incessantly with a rapid flow of disconnected ideas, which were flavored with apologies. His feet were beet red and quite fragrant from constant dyskinesia (writhing around) and his picking at them. (He was living alone on total disability, in a "bachelor pad" paid for by the Social Services Department.) He also chain-smoked. The whole staff experienced how hard it was to sit in the same room with Travis— given his constant movement, involuntary grunts and other sounds; it was like sitting in the presence of a small, odoriferous storm cloud.

Travis was in regular treatment at the Mental Hygiene Center and was stabilized on Methadone. But he was also on Luvox (a drug that combined Dexedrine and Ritalin), an SSRI (Depakote), and something to help him sleep at night—which was almost impossible given his agitation. He was in group therapy and also talked to his psychiatrist regularly. Despite all of the meds, however, and the therapy, Travis's Tourette's remained seemingly unaffected. His symptoms were incessant and almost explosive in intensity. He would stay up all night on his "speed," then fall asleep during the day in narcoleptic-like attacks, (which proved to be rather dangerous when driving).

Despite Travis's high IQ (which may have been over 140), he had failed out of school on numerous occasions. He appeared to have ADHD and was extremely disorganized and unable to keep track of anything.

As treatment progressed, however, Travis got a little better. The Tourette's did not go away entirely but was reduced by about 50 percent, with flare-ups that seemed to follow incidents that were emotionally upsetting or anxiety-provoking to him. He tried to attend school once again and made a valiant stab at it but then found himself dropping classes once more.

One of Travis's five symptoms that we were tracking was his "social isolation." After about twenty treatments, his social life started blossoming. We all were delighted when he told us he had "a girlfriend." The affair only lasted a few months, but Travis handled the breakup rather maturely, having realized that his girlfriend was "more emotionally needy" than he was.

Soon he was handling a lot more details and felt he was able to cope better. Traumas came along, ones like 9/11 and his father's remarriage. The remarriage was an event that Travis's father had insisted he attend. (His father had alternately bragged about Travis and berated him, an ambivalence-creating situation if ever there was one.)

Travis rose to the occasion and attended the wedding as best man, handling this meeting with his father and all of his estranged relatives (on his father's side) without coming apart. Subsequently, his psychiatrist, with whom he had a good relationship, left the clinic, and Travis was reassigned to a new doctor. Although he expressed sadness, he handled the transition very well. His relationship with his younger sister, a very delightful and grown-up young lady, was blossoming. Travis was now able to go out with his mother socially and to attend entertainment events without embarrassment. His mother and he started a "Tourette's support group" for other people with the same problem. It was a success and still continues to this day—with occasional referrals to our services.

As of this writing, Travis is off *all* medication, except for his maintenance dosage of methadone. Under normal circumstances, you might not know he has Tourette's, but it comes out if he's anxious or activated in some way. The swelling, irritation, and infection of his feet is a thing of the past, as hygiene apparently has become very important to him. (He has indicated that he is cleaning up and organizing his apartment.) He is more socially and politically active (he doesn't like war).

In retrospect, with 20–20 hindsight, it is hard to say whether what we cured was the illness—or its treatment!

A Summary on Seizure Disorders

EEG came on the neuropsychological map due, in part, to its ability to understand seizures as massive recruitment of neurons, measurable as very high amplitude, low frequency activity. Sometimes the prodromal of major seizure activity or partial complex seizures themselves can be seen as high-frequency spindles. The term "kindling" implies that the cortex is weak, and yet volatile. The strobe light in the disco that causes a pleasant state of intoxication in the ordinary brain can ignite wildfire in the seizure-prone brain.

When I asked Len Ochs about seizures, he said, "Remember I told you I was puzzled, as I was refining this method, why some of the lower amplitude sites were harder to treat than I expected, and some of the high amplitude sites were easier. I began to think that the 'blue bar' (a feature of the brain map that measures standard deviation) was the key to that. If the blue bar is really high, compared to the overall amplitude, you've got what I call 'an Instigator.' It's basically like a 'seizure focus', where kindling starts. But the blue bar is also the 'life' in a site, so if there is too much it's no good, and too little, it's also no good—probably worse, because there's nothing, no energy to work with."

In general, seizure disorders, Tics and Tourette's tell us about things that happen in the brain and CNS that are unresponsive to conscious control. As such, they fill us with a fear about the "uncontrollable" things in life—of which there are, alas, far too many. Given half a chance, the brain can learn to inhibit seizures, whether through anti-convulsant medications, SMR training, or the LENS. More importantly for our understanding of general human psychology, we now know that certain compulsive behaviors, rituals and repetitive behaviors, tics, emotional outbursts, and even *grand mal* seizures, all have their basis in the neurology of the brain. In the LENS we have found a valuable, often effective and drug-free approach to calming the nervous systems in its hurricane and tsunami moods.

LIFE HURTS

Post-Traumatic Stress Disorder, Pain, and Bereavement

Stephen Larsen, Ph.D.

He tries to read, but the sentences don't hold together. He opens letters that have been left lying on his desk for weeks, and then tears them to shreds before completing them. He chain smokes. The light of the sun or a bulb burns his eyes. He doesn't wash, he doesn't fraternize. He doesn't clean his room, but he never leaves it either. He can't stop trembling. . . .

J. D. SALINGER'S PORTRAIT BASED ON HIS WWII EXPERIENCES,
QUOTED IN *WAR AND THE SOUL* BY DR. EDWARD TICK

It is an amazing thing to think that, after thousands of years of engaging in war, people have just recently begun to identify something called "Post-Traumatic Stress Disorder" (PTSD). The DSM IV-r defines PTSD as: (either oneself or one's significant other/s) having been threatened with death or mutilation, or having been raped—one of the worst human indignities imaginable. PTSD is also defined as follows: Incidents where one witnesses large numbers of people experiencing such horrors as subway fires or gassings, nightclub conflagrations, or bombings. Far-reaching, traumatic events such as the World Trade Center tragedy also qualify, not to mention outright war in which even the *victors* are traumatized (as clinical experience has shown).

Survivors of the above-mentioned experiences are likely to be hypervigilant, insomniac, anxious, phobic, depressed, alcoholic and/ or addicted, mood-unstable and, at worst, delusional, suicidal, and/or homicidal. People with PTSD typically experience nightmares, which are the rule rather than the exception; these nightmares often remain monotonously fixed upon the traumatic event, as do (waking) "flashbacks," in which the event is experienced over and over again.

In *The Iliad,* the horrors of the Trojan war brought on the madness of Ajax, seasoned and formidable warrior though he was. (Podalirius, son of the healing god Asclepius, was called upon to cure Ajax, and thus Podalirius became the first psychiatrist; his brother Machaon became the first battlefield surgeon.) In the three millennia since then, it was the Vietnam War, allegedly one of the most unpopular in history, that revealed and gave name, currency, and clinical actuality to wartime PTSD.

Some have called PTSD "soft trauma," in that, instead of an actual physical blow to the head, there is the psychic and emotional "blow" of witnessing the unspeakable, knowing the unknowable. Neuropsychologists have likened PTSD to physical or chemical traumas, and though the neurological damage cannot be shown to be *structurally* identical to the massive damage done to neurons and glia from a physical blow (visible in X rays, CAT scans, or MRIs), the *functional* effect is the same. Parts of the overwhelmed brain can shut down, or spin into hyperdrive—or both at the same time—depending upon which region of the brain we are looking at.

When this latter event happens, sometimes the EEG clinician sees hi-beta waves: fierce, energetic little squiggles clustered up and down the looming waves of delta. The image is telling: there is a futile, frantic reactivity (including muscle "artifact"—neuronal discharges from tense muscles) to something overwhelming, implacable, and monolithic—the trauma. Another way to envision this is to picture a car that's stuck in the mud. The anxiety-driven higher frequency waves are the wheels spinning, while the car sinks further and further down into the mud (some drivers think if they just "step on the gas" they're bound to get out).

Memories seem to be stored in different places in the brain depending upon their emotional intensity. How this happens is largely controlled by a limbic horseshoe called the *hippocampus,* which also has bundles of neuronal connections to the *amygdala, thalamus,* and *hypothalamus,* along with nuclei in the brain stem. Frontal, more ordinary cognitive storage of memories, for example, seems to be more or less available to consciousness, and amenable to change. This frontal storage of memories can, in fact, be "elaborated" by consciousness, so that, for instance, different people can have differently "colored" memories of the same event—the *Roshomon* effect. These memories can also be "worked with" by consciousness, as in psychotherapy or hypnotherapy: the skilled therapist helps the client "reframe" or recontext the memory.

But traumatic memories of the kind we are concerned with, indelibly stamped by the hippocampus with an *eidetic* form—like images in a wax museum, frozen in time—seem to be largely inaccessible to such verbal or cognitive interventions. Think of them rather as neurologically "locked away," like the forbidden room in Bluebeard's castle "that must never be opened." It is obvious that, in certain kinds of extreme trauma, the brain will try to isolate a toxic memory, so that the rest of the brain may function in a more or less normal way. On the cortical level, these toxic memories tend to be stored in a more central, temporal, or parietal position in the brain.

As with Dr. Freud's repressed traumatic or conflicted memories in the "unconscious," it is thought by clinicians that a brain with an abundance of such buried "psychic landmines" can be perilous—and *explosive* indeed. Dreams can exquisitely reproduce such a perilous landscape of the mind, as when you walk on a cracked and broken sidewalk, fall into a quagmire, or enter a shell-cratered, battle-torn region with undetonated bombs lying around.

Traditionally, theta training is the "gateway to the unconscious." As we have mentioned earlier in this book, Elmer and Alyce Green of the Menninger Foundation showed in the 1970s that theta training was associated with the recovery of memories laden with deep emotion. These could include traumas, but also quintessential childhood experiences, religious or creative insights. Biofeedback clinician and researcher Ken Tachiki has talked about specific theta (4–7 Hz) frequencies where traumas of different levels can be accessed, and worked with in ways that psychotherapy sometimes seems to grope for but seldom reaches.

Lower level theta, 4–5 Hz, is close to delta, in other words, it is close to the "deep unconscious." The upper levels, toward 7 Hz, connive with alpha, which begins, by convention, at 8 Hz; the prudence of alpha-theta training in clinical protocols is that alpha is supposed to "soothe" the rawness of the memories—oil poured on turbulent water— retrieved through theta. We have discussed how Eugene Peniston's work with Vietnam vets, and Matthew Kelly, who repatriates alcoholic and drug-addicted Pueblo

Indians of Arizona and New Mexico to the shamanic landscape of their original culture, their ancestral spirits, and animal totems, has shown that the alpha-theta "crossover" facilitates the recovery and integration of the traumatic memories that cause self-destructiveness and alcoholism.

Anna Wise is a California clinician and author who was trained by British researcher Maxwell Cade. She has hypothesized that an abundance of lower frequency delta and theta waves indicates an instinctual attempt by the human mind to "drop down" to the fundamentals of existence, to fathom, as it were, the "mind of God," the deep place where we all contact ultimate existence. It's an intriguing idea. In her book: *The High Performance Mind,* she argues that all of the brainwaves contribute to human psychological health.[1]

Although clinicians since Arthur Janov have imagined that if their patient's scream was truly "primal" enough, the trauma would slink away and disappear, perhaps there are other approaches, which involve less emotional melodrama. And that are as efficacious as weeks of such cathartic discharges.[2] Biofeedback clinician and researcher Michael Tansey claims that there is a higher frequency, 14 Hz (perhaps a harmonic of 7 Hz), that provides a window where traumatic memories may be retrieved and released without the individual being retraumatized in the process. In this range, a curious emotional detachment seems to accompany the recall and reprocessing of the traumatic memories, and the overall effect is therapeutic—without the *sturm und drang.*[3]

These studies raise the intriguing question as to whether or not, as some psychodynamically oriented therapists have postulated, "recall with affect" is really necessary for these emotionally loaded experiences to be integrated and healed.

Wounded and Walking

At Stone Mountain Center we have had no lack of traumatized patients, and those presented in this book are just a sampling of literally hundreds of patients who have come to our rural New York center for some relief from the debilitating aftereffects of trauma. The explanation for such a large number of referrals is that once some people have found relief, and have returned to some level of normalcy, they are grateful enough to want to help others.

Vietnam vets went to war for a government that not only drafted them against their will but then exposed them to the horrors of war and, on return, gave them, at best, perfunctory treatments and no viable assistance integrating back into ordinary civilian life. Many of these men were, in fact, vilified upon their return. The self-destructiveness of this population (which has become legendary) is due, in large part, to these contributing factors, as well as possible damage done to the men from exposure to Agent Orange, a known neurotoxin, and other hazardous substances.

Gulf war vets likewise were put firmly in harm's way when they participated in that theater of war and in so doing were exposed to radioactive materials such as depleted uranium, unknown infectious diseases, and the mysterious combination of agents that contributed to Gulf War Syndrome, characterized by fatigue and disorientation. (The predicament of the war veteran may be glimpsed in the movie *Born on the Fourth of July*, with Tom Cruise.) Often all these men have is each other; and their intrinsic compassion and humanity is an amazing testament to the resilience of the human spirit.

In the 1980s I became good friends with Dr. Ed Tick, a psychologist who specializes in working with veterans. I had read his moving book, *The Sacred Mountain: Taming the Vietnam Beast.* At one point, Tick visited our small private school with a number of vets he had worked with and, through the caring and compassion of this very skilled therapist, I saw that very wounded people could be helped. We began to refer patients to each other.

My first application of neurofeedback to this population was in 1978. A returning Special Forces vet had now become a New York State Trooper. When I came into the evening Psychology of Consciousness class I taught at the community college, I found the uniformed trooper standing by the lectern. I read his badge, "Trooper Moore."

"Dr. Larsen," he said, "may I have a word with you?" (I thought he might arrest me on the spot for some malfeasance I did not yet know I had committed, so to avoid public humiliation, I invited him into the biofeedback lab.) But the man just wanted to tell me his story and as he recounted it, I listened, fascinated as, out front, the classroom filled up with students waiting for class to commence.

When Moore was a Green Beret, he found that he had an uncanny ability to anticipate when "something" was going to happen. He had, in fact, saved the lives of many of his friends, and undoubtedly his own, with this skill. But he remained troubled by mood swings and his marriage was on the rocks.

I invited him to sit in on the class, in which we were discussing brain waves and states of consciousness. Later, I was able to offer him some EEG training in the lab. He took to this training like a duck to water and spent hours each week in the lab, working with EMG, GSR (lie detector), and Temperature Training, in which the person learns to raise the temperature of body parts that are vascularly constricted—cold, or "blue." His mood swings subsided, and he began to sleep better. His life was (slightly) less chaotic.

However, it was the EEG that seemed to give him what he was looking for: an enhancement of his already well-developed intuitive capabilities. In fact, Trooper Moore now began showing up, in the most uncanny way, *before* a robbery would occur, which made him able to confound the perpetrator on the spot. Eventually Moore was hired as a staff trainer for the troopers and taught some of his techniques to other troopers. He would eventually go on to train FBI agents.

In 1996, I began trying the LENS approach (then called EDS or EEG disentrainment) with Vietnam vets and the Gulf War population. We already knew that disentrainment could energize and balance the nervous system, helping with anxiety, depression, and sleep disturbances, but at first, we were uncertain as to whether there would be enough therapeutic effect to heal the deep psychological and emotional problems represented in PTSD.

Since the procedure does not specifically aim at *abreaction* or *catharsis*, we wondered if it could possibly have a therapeutic effect on deep inaccessible nervous-system trauma? Both Peniston and Kelly reported psychological *content* emerging through their biofeedback procedures, and traditional psychodynamic approaches have postulated that it is the release, understanding, and integration of such content that constitutes the therapeutic process.

Joe Rock: Ears Still Ringing

The following case is a relatively recent one and shows a dramatic example of how PTSD, along with fibromyalgia, may be helped by neurofeedback. I will give enough details of this case and its treatment to impart to the reader how LENS works in actual clinical practice.

Joe was not tall, but stocky and strong, with a blond crewcut. But his eyes were haunted, and his face carried a gentle, intense sorrow, as if he had seen many more things than ever he wished to see. Joe had not enlisted in the Vietnam War but was drafted. However, he made the best of his time of service, earning five Bronze Stars and a Purple Heart. Joe killed people, rescued people, watched friends dismembered before his eyes, saw unconscionable and stupid wartime errors, cried and laughed at the barbarous enormity of it all, and like so many Vietnam vets, returned to a country that seemed suddenly to have lost interest in what he had gone through.

The Vietnam War had been over for thirty years when Joe first came to our center. The return itself was precipitated by the event that had caused his ears to ring deafeningly for every one of those thirty years: A "rocket-grenade" had hit the tank he was in and disabled it. All the other men were killed. Joe was picked up half-alive, and taken to a field hospital. When the extent of his injuries was fully assessed, he was sent Stateside to a Veteran's hospital.

For most of the thirty intervening years, despite endless group therapy sessions and much medication, Joe was permanently insomniac, anxious, disoriented, confused, and explosive. Each night he experienced *myoclonia*, or little seizures. Each night the undead of those Mekong valleys swirled and swam reproachfully before his eyes, and bombs and shells went off as he jerked and cried out. When he slept at all, he always woke in a sweat, night after night, *every* night.

Once, during the war, after an intense period of engagement with Vietcong raiding parties, there seemed to be a lull in the hostilities. Needing a release, Joe and a friend found a bottle of rum and split it between them. They were very drunk and having a good time when the next mortar attack came and blew a nearby tree to smithereens. Suddenly, mortar shells were going off all around them, and they were surrounded by Vietcong. Joe and his buddy were "shit-faced" as he said; his fellow soldiers were dying all around him.

After that, unlike so many of his buddies, Joe had stayed away from drugs and alcohol. At the point that he came to our center, he was married to a professional woman, the family breadwinner; the marriage was an unhappy one. They had two young children and, as Joe was disabled and unemployed, he took care of the children, more or less full time.

Like many people with physical as well as neurological damage, Joe had developed profound pain throughout his body. He could not move without suffering, and he was perpetually exhausted. The diagnosis "fibromyalgia" had, in fact, been offered, but no one seemed to know what to do about the debilitating condition. "All those doctors say is 'more meds,'" he told us. "No thank you. The only one I'm on is Remiron, because without it I can't sleep at all." Joe felt cognitively impaired: "I can't think like I used to. I can't really read, I'm too distractable."

We decided to use both LENS and photonic stimulation on Joe because of his muscular soreness and weakness. Joe turned out to be in the top 10 percent in terms of sensitivity; even during *no-stim* mapping, he felt twinges running up and down his arms and legs. Joe had been shot or blown up at least four different times. He could feel tingles and "electric shocks running up and down my arms and legs." Sometimes he perspired. The offset made him very tired, so we knew he would only take a couple of seconds of treatment.

The photonic treatments (which use a "diffuse" laser of infrared lights to stimulate the muscles and nerves), revealed an even greater sensitivity. After the low level stimulation Joe was stiff and aching— with even more pain. (This is a result we have seen with fibromyalgics, advanced neurological Lyme disease, and a few other disorders. On the other hand, people with anxiety, depression, even TBI—without fibro- myalgia—can take fairly intense stimulation and feel eased, energized, and more flexible as a result.)

I decided to administer Joe's biofeedback treatments myself, rather than have one of our clinicians do it, because after the actual LENS treatments began, proceeding through the site sort, two or three sites at a time, one second each, the "fireworks" really began. (My colleague Sebern Fisher has communicated personally how she feels it may be very important to have the biofeedback clinician and psychotherapist be the same person, to help people emotionally "detox" in really subtle and discerning ways.) Make no mistake, catharctic release is sometimes therapeutically helpful; I have found that by itself, it is often insufficient to resolve deep and painful wounds, but paired to neurofeedback, the healing process can be awesome!

The following is a step-by-step description of a typical LENS treatment with Joe:

The patient is sitting in a comfortable chair, eyes closed. When I have ascertained that my connection is good, I inspect the raw EEG to make sure that it looks clean and "real" (with little or no artifact caused by blinking or muscle tension). I begin the treatment cycle, which is usually about thirty seconds long. One of those seconds, the programming menu I have previously set, will deliver the stim, wordlessly and soundlessly. It is certainly "single-blind" and often "double-blind," as I am often preoccupied with observing the power spectrum and writing notes.

As that second of stim "pops on" I glimpse it out of the corner of my eye on the screen. The EEG spikes, Joe writhes in the chair, his face distorts in fear, and he breaks into a sudden sweat. Some twenty seconds later the computer "beeps" to signal the end of that trial. "What is it Joe?" I ask gently.

"Mortar attack!" he says through clenched teeth.

"What's happening right now?" I ask.

He looks sick. "I just got a little shrapnel myself, it wasn't bad, but I'm, I'm wiping my buddy off of me!" Tears well up in his eyes, and I fall silent as I realize the implications of what he is saying.

After a little while I ask, "Tell me about him," and Joe tells how just a few minutes before the attack they had been talking, and his friend was smoking a cigarette, just as normal as can be, and now he is gone—forever—except for his gory residue, which is all over Joe. I ask Joe if the scene is still vivid, and although it is painful, I ask him to hold it in his mind as we do the next site. (Remember that the LENS is a "disentrainment" procedure, and I want to break up the traumatic memory at its source.) This stim produces a little myoclonia—a muscular jerk—at the moment of stim, but no content.)

As we do the last site (we are only doing three this time) Joe heaves a sigh. I ask him to open his eyes, we do a little EMDR, and I ask him to please visualize the trauma spatially "behind him," an NLP (neuro-linguistic programming) technique.

After a short break, we do a little more talk therapy and work on some life-related strategies to address a situation he is working on at home. The difference between the relatively normal insight-oriented psychotherapy and the starkness of the war memories emerging intact seems dramatic to me. (It's why "talking about" never seems to get to the *core* of the overwhelming emotion that Joe experiences in our therapy sessions.)

The next week the procedure is repeated, and again he flinches at the moment of stimulation. This time, "It's a guy in black pajamas that jumps up right next to the tank. I have no time for reflection, I'm trained, and I shoot him right between the eyes. But what I can't forget is the expression of surprise on his face as I shoot him. We're looking right into each other's eyes." During the ensuing psychotherapy session, Joe is able to dig in to what it means to be trained as a soldier, and to have those kind of lethal reflexes. It is a useful session.

As the weeks unfold, event after event rises to the surface, some of them so horrible that Joe talks in a hushed whisper as he recounts what is happening. To both of us it seems remarkable how exhaustive his memory by memory sequence is.

As the course of treatment progresses, Joe reports that he is feeling a little better physically, he has more energy and is a little less depressed. At one point Joe says: "Three months here and I've made more progress than I did in thirty years back and forth to the VA hospitals!" He looks more cheerful when he arrives in the waiting room. His sense of humor is returning, and he is joking and flirting with the many attractive women on my staff. One day he enters our office beaming. He says that, not only was he able to play golf again, but "I didn't do as badly as I thought I would!" (given what was his apparently long absence from the game). He is having fewer "wall to wall nightmares," sort of "flashbacks" from the war; his dreams now are much more ordinary in nature.

Joe is on the mend.

Our not-for-profit Center for Symbolic Studies offers Native American programs—including sweat lodges and vision quests—and Joe attended one such sweat lodge. The Native Americans, a wiser, older civilization, developed many ceremonies of departure and return and reintegration. Many of our patients who are vets have been helped by these timeless traditional rituals. The shamanic work, in particular, provides immeasurable help to this population of vets.

Bereavement

I had the sad experience of having, as a patient, a man who had tragically lost a child. It is a truism that nature prepares us for the death of grandparents and parents, but not of children; and both common wisdom and professional literature agree that this is the most painful form of bereavement imaginable. Mingled in the equation are guilt at not protecting the child—irrational though such guilt might be, the lacerating anguish of love that now has no object, and the loss of all that was imagined for the future.

Randall and Bereavement

Randall had had a painful separation in his marriage before tragedy arrived. He and his wife Sheila had adopted two children, a girl and then a younger boy, both Korean. The beautiful little girl, Clarissa, unfortunately had damaged hearing, which developed due to an untreated ear infection that had festered as she lay in a Korean orphanage awaiting adoption.

As the children grew into teenagers, tensions developed in the family. Randall and Sheila were not getting along. Neither were Sheila and Clarissa—the latter had a very strong will and was very popular socially. After the couple split, the fights between Sheila and Clarissa grew. Now fifteen, Clarissa's mother was jealous of the time that Clarissa spent with her friends and her dad. She accused Clarissa of acting out sexually, whereas Randall, more tolerant, said, "No, she's just enormously popular. The other kids just love being with her." Naturally Clarissa started spending more time with her dad.

One afternoon Clarissa was downtown with a group of friends, talking and laughing by the highway while waiting for a ride. Clarissa, still hard of hearing, didn't hear the car rapidly approaching as she stepped backward directly into its path. Randall was summoned from his business immediately and drove in a frenzy to the Westchester ospital where Clarissa had been flown by helicopter. Clarissa was dead on arrival.

Randall went numb. It seemed the blackness of his despair was overwhelming. He laughed grimly at the depth of his own despair and the injustice of life. At some time in the past, Randall had realized that alcohol could be a serious problem for him and he had entered a Twelve-

Step program. The AA community was there for him in enormously helpful ways. Randall was already in psychotherapy with me, dealing with the breakup of the family, when the tragedy of his daughter's death occurred.

This was a man who had overcome an emotionally abusive childhood with alcoholic parents, been rejected by older siblings, gotten out of a difficult marriage, and now this? Could his gentle, intelligent spirit bear it?

Over a year and a half of bereavement psychotherapy, Randall was able to look at the tragedy from every side, deal with his ex-wife's blame and anger, and pretty much banish his own guilt—there was absolutely nothing that he could have done to prevent the accident. But still the black, crippling depression persisted. There was also a cognitive cloud that made previously easy tasks seem overwhelming to him. Keeping his successful business together and operating normally took everything he had.

I must say that I was so focused on my "psychotherapist's hat" that I didn't even think of putting on my "neurotherapist's cap" until that time. I was thinking, rather lamely, that bereavement was primarily a psychological problem, if you will. I hadn't yet peered into the neurological face of tragedy, and come to understand that it functions just as a TBI does.

Randall's 21-site cortical map told the tale. There was the depression: huge delta waves spread through his frontal area, whereas there were other areas of the brain that looked normal, flexible, and intact. It took the better part of a year before those frontal delta *tsunami* began to relent, but slowly they did, coming down gradually from 20µv (20 microvolts), to 15, and finally to 10. As the treatment really began to "take"—at about fifteen months—the delta dropped to about 5–7µv.

Randall's cognitive abilities rose to where they had been before the tragedy, perhaps even higher. He enrolled in self-improvement courses at Omega Institute, our local spiritual growth center. He began to go to meditation retreats with the Theravada Buddhist teacher Thich Nhat Hahn, in whose teachings he found inspiration. He was able to join with like-minded seekers and begin a regimen of Zen that turned into a routine of daily meditation.

It is a strange thing, but today, Randall, who had no formal training in psychotherapy at all, is sought out by all kinds of people—relatives, friends, acquaintances—simply to talk. People find something comforting in his gentle presence.

When interviewed by me recently about the bereavement, he said: "Nothing will ever bring Clarissa back, that I know. But I don't live in the Black Hole of Calcutta any more either. I get depressed every now and then, but now it's often an hour or two at a time instead of weeks!" Wonderfully enough, Randall's relationship with his estranged son, who had favored his mother, began to improve, and at this point they are roommates, eating meals and working out together, and generally enjoying each others' presence.

Summary

The theory that emerges from our work with wartime trauma victims as well as those who have suffered bereavement is that the CNS effects of "soft-trauma" are no less real than those of "hard-trauma." To be sure, neurons are not destroyed, as in the latter type. Some of the most complicated cases, such as that of Joe Rock, combine both kinds—and this is what we must learn to anticipate in the survivors of wartime, or the victims of terrorist attacks. It's not rare in these violent environments, to sustain both kinds of trauma at once: a knockout blow to your tank, thence to your head or your ears (physical trauma) that also kills all of your buddies (emotional trauma).

We realize through this work that the neurological environment is intimately tied to the psychological. The causality operates in both directions. A traumatized brain hurts the psyche, and the traumatized psyche affects the brain. This is the level at which the "functional" impairments of the CNS dominate. The sequelae are subjectively overwhelming for the victim. It is amazing how many people are sensitively attuned enough to realize that "something is wrong" despite not knowing "how wrong the something itself (the neurological effect of the trauma) is."

Just as in the history of neurology, we didn't really begin to get a very detailed picture of how intimately the psyche and the brain were connected until we studied the effects of various localized injuries that caused various cognitive impairments: the dyslexias, agnosias, and various aphasias. We need a far more modern sensitive psyche/brain synthesis. Whereas X rays, CAT scans, and MRIs show us clear evidence of *structural problems*, EEG—along with neuropsychological testing—are the main objective indicators that can show us *functional problems*. However, never to be dismissed are the subjective indicators. After all *this is where the patient lives.*

With this subjective analysis, we turn the awesome introspective capabilities of the brain on itself. Though there are no sensory receptors in the brain that tell us whether it is lacerated or stunned, sensitively attuned human beings assess their own behaviors through the prototype of biofeedback: self-assessment, or introspection. People say, "I'm not doing well. This isn't like me." Or, on the other hand, "I can feel I'm getting better. I'm sleeping better, I'm thinking better." These subtle, but irrefutable, markers tell us that the soul dwelling in this body is in dis-ease, or at-ease.

It is doubtful, as Karl Pribram showed, that a single state or symptom can be made to correspond with a specific cortical location. The processing of complex problems and situations by human beings involves rolling waves of coherence—frequency and amplitude both—sweeping through the brain and inviting the many kinds of intercortical communication. This intercortical communication allows us to reconcile feelings and thought, instincts and impulses, and allows us to respond to human social situations, the natural world, gender issues, art. The brain also corresponds to the subcortical environment, with projections of the reticular, hypothalamic, and thalamic nuclei.

In regard to this complexity, the only sufficient analogue to the shades and textures of human experience is the multisite, multilevel way of stimulating and evaluating the brain. In this regard we believe the LENS is a method of treatment that is unique—because it charts and relates the topography of the brain to the nuances, day by day and week by week, of human experience.

Sometimes "touching" a particular site on the 10–20 system, either with or without stimulation, produces a very specific response. In the most sensitive patients, this can correspond to a whole cognitive/affective domain of experience. In keeping with the theory developed and first clinically tested by Len Ochs, "less is more." That is, touch and stir the pot, if you will, and wait respectfully and attentively to what comes forth. If the procedure produces discomfort, or "overdose," lower the stimulation by half next time, and see how the site responds.

The majority of sites will respond obligingly to the clinician's contact and request for lowering the amplitudes (through the *disentrainment* effect, as explained), but some will surge and raise the amplitudes, as the request asks the site to do something it is not used to doing. Another explanation, suggested by Ochs and borne out by the theory of EEG coherence, is that though the site itself is responsive, or compliant, nearby sites press the treated site to go back to what they all are used to, their own *status quo*.

In any case, we are asking the brain, the most complex structure in the known universe, (a whole, a *holistic* organ in fact), to respond to a very slightly disruptive stimulus and come back to a new, more harmonious way of being. If this procedure, this *opus contra naturam*, the "work against nature" is to succeed, it must *permit*, not *force*, nature to change in a healthful direction. In this way alone can we avoid joining the darker forces in this shaded world by reevoking the trauma, or making the situation worse.

BRAIN ATTACK

Aneurysm, Stroke, Alzheimer's Disease,
Parkinson's Disease, and Headache

*Stephen Larsen, Ph.D., Joan Piper Mader, M.A.,
and Beth Hanna, R.N.*

When you consider all the billions of cells within the human brain, with each one affected by an unknown number of transmitters, peptides, and other "messenger" substances; the amount of information quickly escalates to a figure approaching the number of particles in existence. . . . To this extent, no matter how much we learn about the brain, we can never learn it all. There will always be something to astound us, to amaze us, to keep us humble, while at the same time stimulating us to greater efforts toward understanding the brain. The human brain is simply the most marvelous organ in the known universe.

MILES HERKEMHAM, NEUROSCIENTIST

We begin this chapter with one of the most extraordinary narratives in the history of the LENS treatment, by Joan Piper Mader. Joan was a biofeedback/neurofeedback practitioner who suffered a brain aneurysm and became hemiplegic, about which her physicians told her: "Get used to it. Neuronal damage, once incurred, is permanent." But, fortunately, that did not stop Joan from believing that she could be helped by what she knew, and even what she didn't yet know: a nascent form of neurofeedback, which in those days, (the early 1990s), was called "EDF." It was an early precursor of the LENS.

In our practice of the LENS, "seconds" of stimulation treatment has been the rule. However, in Joan's case, her stimulation sessions would last as long as 24 *minutes*, and transpire every day or every other day for weeks on end. (In the early days, following other biofeedback protocols, that is just "how it was done.") As Joan herself says, "sometimes it was very challenging." Her story now serves as an exquisite chronicle of human life inside the pressure-cooker of such intense therapy, living within the alchemical *alembic* of transformation. The detail and texture of her self-observation make it extremely worthwhile to include here: Joan's story is a moving, instructive, and compelling narrative.

CNS Specific Biofeedback: Neuronal Regulation from the Patient's Perspective

JOAN PIPER MADER, M.A.

In 1986, at the age of thirty-nine, I suffered a cerebral aneurysm of my right middle internal carotid artery and a cerebral vascular accident. The injury resulted in left hemiplegia and hemiparesthesia, as well as cognitive and perceptual deficits consistent with right temporal and parietal lobe damage. I underwent surgical repair of the defect, and at that time, I was told that whatever level of recovery I had achieved by one year post-surgery would probably be my maximum recovery. Whenever I ventured to express a more optimistic outlook, I was emphatically admonished, "brain tissue, once damaged, can never be repaired or replaced."

After two months of rehabilitation in a residential facility, I engaged in eighteen months of physical and occupational therapy as an outpatient. Dr. Harold Russell and I began working with EEG biofeedback nine months after the rupture of my aneurysm. Over the last seven years, Dr. Russell and I have employed EEG biofeedback, AVS (audio-visual stimulation), and the EDF technique, as this knowledge and technology became available.

All of the neuronal regulation techniques have had favorable effects on my physical and cognitive functioning. However, our most recent efforts with EDF have resulted in the most dramatic and rapid changes. During the past twelve months, EDF treatments were conducted at the average rate of one 24-minute session every 2.1 days. These have produced three major shifts in my brain reactivity.

First, the average amplitude of my brain wave activity has been reduced across all frequency ranges, with the greatest decrease evident in frequencies 19 Hz and higher (beta and hi-beta). Second, changes have occurred in all frequency ranges in regard to the total percentage, with each frequency range contributing to overall brain activity. The most noteworthy alterations include a 50 percent decrease in the percentage of hi-beta, and a 60 percent increase in the percentage of alpha.

Last, pronounced changes have occurred in overall stability of my brain activity. The most marked stability has been seen, once again, in the 19 Hz or faster frequencies. In my case, the preliminary data suggest that neuronal stimulation initiates the process whereby brain wave activity undergoes a shift from poorly organized activity to less variable patterns. In addition, for me it appears that an optimum relationship exists among the various frequency ranges. In my personal experience with CNS biofeedback, the shifts in my brain's electrical activity reflected in the graphs were accompanied by equally dramatic physical, emotional, social, psychological, cognitive, and spiritual alterations.

I do not believe my experiences have been unique in any way. . . . Every patient who undergoes it may experience a kaleidoscope of reactions to the experience, ranging from joyful excitement to profound bewilderment and even distress. Changes in all these areas do not occur independently or sequentially; dramatic shifts occurred in several areas simultaneously. Undergoing EDF required that I make very rapid adaptations to an ever-changing brain environment—an often confusing and fatiguing task.

What I am talking about is a treatment that can alter a person's full experience of reality. Determining the optimum training schedule was important to avoid undue cerebral fatigue. Initially, I underwent twice daily EDF sessions, then once daily, and currently thrice weekly. I learned that signs such as tinnitus, persistent vague nausea, extreme mental and physical fatigue, exaggerated startle reflex, photophobia, and increase mental confusion were my body's signal to suspend EDF for a few days. The "no pain, no gain" maxim does not apply in this situation.

The brain is continuously in a state of flux, reordering itself every second of the day and night. Therefore, the brain you wake up with in the morning is literally not the same brain you went to bed with the night before. Alterations in cerebral functioning set in motion during a CNS training session do not cease at the end of the session. The patient's brain will shift, stretch, and wiggle every minute of the day and night until you train again. Thus does the brain seem to have a native intelligence regarding the rate and progression of its reordering. Since we have limited understanding of the process, we have limited understanding of how it *should* progress. It is best to *let the organ set the pace for this intricate sculpting of neurons and juices.*

Consequently, during the time between appointments, the patient may need to discuss a change that has occurred. Therapists need to be aware, and to offer reasonable telephone accessibility to these patients between office visits. As practitioners must be alert to the signs of cerebral fatigue and tailor treatment schedules accordingly, key words for any therapist venturing into CNS work are "caution" and "compassion."

The earliest effect of my EEG and AVS work was a diminution of my left-sided spasticity, along with a proclivity for spontaneous movement in my left arm and leg during treatment. This movement was initially of a jerking nature. A diagnostic EEG ruled out seizure activity as the cause of the movement. Over the ensuing months, the nature of the movement changed from random jerking of arm or leg, to a slow controlled stretching of more comprehensive muscle groups.

An additional dramatic reduction in my muscle tone occurred almost immediately with the EDF. I found this rapid reduction of tone to be exhilarating. However, this event was both good news and bad news. I discovered that, although I could move my limbs more freely, walking was actually more difficult. Unknowingly, I had been relying on my spasticity to hold myself erect, to hold my joints rigid. Without this prop, I found my affected muscles to be far weaker than I imagined; my limbs flopped about because I lacked the strength and coordination to stabilize or control movement. In short, I found myself prone to falls as well as extreme muscle fatigue.*

My reduction in muscle tone was rapidly followed by enhanced abilities to isolate muscle movements, recruit additional muscle groups, and integrate muscle activity into more coordinated and efficient movement.

---

*Patients need to be aware of these possible changes at the start so that they do not become alarmed by what may feel like regression in their progress or recurrence of their CNS injury. The families of more fragile individuals should be alerted to safety issues and an increased risk for injury. Patients should be advised to exercise caution and to perform daily strengthening exercises as advised by whomever directs their ongoing physical rehabilitation.

Prior to this, I had recovered many muscle movements but had a poor understanding of how to put them all together in a meaningful way. For instance, if I was standing up, to reach out to touch an object on the table, I tried to do it all by simply straightening out my elbow. I had no conception what adjustments—in the position of my neck, shoulders, spine, hips, ankles—were needed to perform this simple movement. In some manner, the neurofeedback allowed me to reach this integrated understanding.

While the necessary communicative pathways were being established within my brain, I also learned how better to integrate movement through a dual process of memory retrieval and mental rehearsal. I regained memories of the "feel" of certain movements. During treatment sessions I had mental images of certain movements being performed, in an "imaged" rehearsal.

The process is sometimes complicated by the sudden acquisition of another component of gait or movement. Sometimes these additions occur so quickly that I have difficulty making the necessary adjustments, and may be thrown off balance, or walk with an exaggerated awkwardness for a day or two.

My fine motor performance has also progressed markedly in the past six months. I can now write with my affected hand. (I am strongly right-handed.) The writing is not very legible, but at least it is possible. I have also been able to resume some of the handicraft hobbies I once enjoyed, such as crocheting. On a more subtle level, I now have the sense of being a two-handed person once again. I find myself automatically using both hands, without having to make a conscious effort to include the use of my left hand.

Changes in my sensory awareness have also occurred. Postinjury, I was left with total anesthesia of the left side of my body. The first return of sensory awareness occurred during EEG biofeedback. This presented as a vague awareness of the existence of my left hand, which was accompanied by visual imaging of the hand's appearance. The return of my tactile perception has also been greatly accelerated with EDF treatment.

Initially, my experience was once of transient episodes of extreme burning or coldness in my left hand or foot. These sensations occurred in the absence of any changes in skin temperature. The experience was unsettling and sometimes uncomfortable. Usually after two or three days of these temperature aberrations, I would begin to experience increased awareness of light touch and pressure on my left arm and leg. While my perception of skin sensation still is prone to error, and some isolated areas of anesthesia remain, I continue to see gradual improvement.

My awareness of muscle and joint sensations has also improved. This is another one of those good news/bad news things. I am more aware of muscle spasms and painful joints on my left side. At times I feel as if my muscles are crawling on my bones. Another strange sensation is a deep itching, as if my very bones were itching. However, the improved voluntary control I now have over muscles, joints, and appendages as a result of this improved sensory awareness has been well worth the discomfort.

I have also enjoyed enhanced auditory acuity and peripheral visual acuity. Unfortunately, all of this increased sensory input to my brain often has created sensory overload. I find I am distracted, confused, and slightly disoriented at times when my sensory awareness is most keen. At these times, I also experience a deterioration of my other cognitive processes. I experience a mild reoccurrence of old right temporal lobe cognitive deficits such as a left side neglect, and scanning and sequencing difficulties. (CNS patients may need reassurance about these things.)

Improvements in my proprioception, and sense of position, have been marked. Although I generally know the whereabouts of all of my parts, sometimes my "mainframe" short circuits with humorous results. Recently I experienced several hours of feeling as if I was tilting to my right side; the sensation subsided by the next morning. However, every night for the next three nights, I fell out of bed, something I haven't done since I was a child. Eventually, things righted themselves in my brain, and these incidents did not recur.

My overall cognitive functioning has also improved since we began the CNS therapy (the neurofeedback). Some of the changes include: increased fluidity of thought, enhanced flexibility, increased attention span, and reduced distractibility. Functionally, this means I can now process several different tasks, move back and forth between them quickly, and do so with less fatigue and frustration. Prior to this I could handle the tasks, if they were presented to me one at a time in a controlled environment. If I was interrupted, I might have to start all over again when I resumed the task.

Next, I'd like to relate some of the psychological and emotional responses that I've had to the CNS work. I find that these areas are difficult to describe, partially because I have trouble putting the experience into words, but also because these experiences are unfamiliar to me. The initial, occasional, and recurring emotional response I've had to the AVS and EDF has been related to a sense of "being out of control," or rather, of "being controlled" by something external to my self. This has created feelings of anxiety, apprehension, and fear. At times I've felt trapped and had to resist running from the room. Over time, thanks to my therapist's support and reassurance, I have come to trust my brain's aversion to taking me anywhere I'm not prepared to go.

It is simply not possible to remain emotionally neutral during the sessions. EDF is an especially persuasive cathartic for any sort of emotional blockage. During the sessions, I often experience a collage of emotional responses that, on the surface, seems to erupt from nowhere and seems unrelated to anything I am thinking or experiencing at the time. This occurrence does not happen every session, only at those times when I sense that I am emotionally constipated. At those times, I have felt intense sorrow, sheer terror, rage, and gleeful giddiness—all within 20 minutes time. The emotions are usually fleeting, vanishing at the conclusion of the session. It is a little like aerobic exercises for the emotions. Generally, I come out of the session feeling tranquil and refreshed.

However, there have been times when an emotional response seems to linger on for hours or even days. These instances seem to occur when the emotional response is related either to a memory I have retrieved during the session or to some unattended grief work that has surfaced.

The implications of this emotional roller coaster are obvious. First and foremost, a patient should never be left unattended. The patient should be given the option to take a break in the session should he or she become too uncomfortable. And, of course, the patient must be allowed the opportunity to process their experience with the therapist.

Although I had been emotionally labile during the sessions, I have experienced fewer mood shifts and more appropriate control over my emotions outside of treatment. My sleep pattern has improved markedly, with frequent dreams of an instructive nature. An occasional period of two or three nights of restless sleep generally precedes a major shift in my brain's electrical activity.

Another era of my experience that I have found fascinating is that of memory, both long-term and short-term. In some manner, the EDF finely tunes the process of long-term memory retrieval. This is yet another one of those good news/bad news things. I have remembered events I didn't even know I'd forgotten. However, each memory was of a part of my past that I needed to remember, and it surfaced at precisely the best time for me to remember it. Of course, not all of my recollections have been pleasant ones. Those that prove painful are revealed in stages during and between sessions; a glimmer here, a glimmer there, perhaps a related drama or two, and then, when I'm ready, the full-fledged memory emerges in a form I call *experientially enhanced memory.*

For me, experientially enhanced memories are not simply past events "remembered"; they are past events "relived." These memories always come replete with many of the properties—emotional responses, physical sensations, sights, and sounds—that accompanied the original event. If the emotional response to the memory is particularly intense and unsettling, I can walk around with it for several hours or even days. This lingering emotional climate seems to serve several purposes: it keeps me preoccupied with the memory, it forces me to process it, resolve it, and eventually move away from it feeling more comfortable about the experience that I have recalled.

This process had been repeated many times for me, unearthing events from as early as when I was nine months of age.

My short-term memory has also been affected by the neurofeedback work. Overall, I have noticed improvement in my short-term memory. This improvement seems to wax and wane depending on my level of fatigue and distraction. (This inconsistency may be an important factor in evaluating patients who seek CNS treatments for short-term memory disorders.)

Another area I wish to mention is that of "spiritual" experiences. Many of my experiences are similar to those reported by persons engaging in various forms of deep meditation. These are the "twilight zone" happenings, which are most difficult to elaborate in words. Although I have had some of these experiences since the beginning of my CNS work, they have become more frequent, and more accentuated with my more recent EDF exposure. I include in this category episodes of precognition, prolonged episodes of deja vu, communication with my deceased father, and out-of-body experiences.

I know I take a risk in relating these experiences. But I feel it would be negligent of me not to alert other practitioners to a possible occurrence that may provoke a major spiritual crisis in one's CNS-therapy patient. While I have been amused and comforted by these experiences, others might find them profoundly disturbing. Our current society does not seem well prepared to deal with spiritual happenings or to talk about them. The therapist utilizing CNS therapies should be open and accepting toward the mystical, and establish a patient/therapist relationship that conveys a sense of safety to the patient.

All of which brings me to my final area, the social implications of CNS therapy. As a patient, I sometimes feel an extreme sense of social isolation as a result of this work. While every area of myself is in a state of flux, I have difficulty communicating these experiences to others. There is simply little basis of shared experiences to others. This has evoked periods of my feeling disconnected from the mainstream of life and more than just a little off-center.

Even my dearest friends look uncomfortable, and more than just a little concerned, when I relate that *I can actually feel my brain working.* When I explain that I have learned how to move alpha activity around to various places in my brain, my friends start looking for that white coat with buckles. Although I can laugh about this much of the time, there are times when feeling like the "odd man out" is painful and depressing. It's hard to have something this fantastic happening in my life and no one—apart from my therapist who, fortunately in my case, also happens to be a friend—to share and validate the experience with.

The therapist who provides CNS services should also be prepared to encounter a little isolation of a professional sort. The drawbacks of CNS specific practice are: few colleagues to share ideas with; limited acceptance of these novel modalities by the medical community; the frustration of working with unknown variables; the lack of studies documenting guidelines for applications, efficacy, and outcomes; etc. All of these factors may contribute to a sense of approach/avoidance when considering the use of the CNS-specific feedback modalities.

Commentary on Joan Mader's Account

The above is an edited version of Joan's journey, which she wrote and gave to Len Ochs in the early 1990s, the very dawn of this kind of treatment. Her treatments were lengthy and are seldom, if ever, of this length anymore. However, despite the atypical nature of her treatments, her document provides not only a journal of how it felt to have an overdose (all your familiar symptoms get worse, and you get "mighty cranky" or exhausted), but also how the simple remedy of stopping all treatments for a while, during which time everything "righted itself," felt as well.

Her account is extremely important for the would-be client who is leery of "overdose" or the biofeedback therapist who has heard alarming stories of such, and steers away from the LENS because of them. In our contemporary clinical protocols—as taught by Len Ochs and myself—Joan Mader had several thousand times the usual and customary dose. The situation is analogous to how the toxicity of most pharmaceuticals are tested (since most drugs given to people are toxic or lethal above certain doses). Higher and higher doses are given to animals until the animal is dead, and then an autopsy, and extensive analysis of tissues, etc., is performed. In Joan's case, given the length of stimulation, she probably got grouchy and couldn't function very well for a few days, but there was no other damage or impairment—since nothing alien or toxic was put into her body.

As a biofeedback provider and trained health professional herself, Joan Mader looked at her own emotional—and even spiritual—response in very textured, nuanced terms. These are very useful insights for the clinician or prospective patient. We are indebted to her perspicacity and transparency in toughing out what was, no doubt, an extremely difficult personal ordeal, and growing from it, thereby enriching *our* knowledge in the bargain.

Alan Returns to the Black Diamonds

Alan Carey is a member of a prominent family of artists and filmmakers who live in Woodstock, New York. Alan was the photographer of the family and, over many years, his photos appeared in all of the Hudson Valley area's newspapers and journals, as well as in numerous exhibitions. However, when the cold weather came, his passion was the ski slopes. In his fifties, a fit, vigorous man, he still loved the "black diamonds," the hardest slopes on the mountain.

One snowy day, while enjoying himself skiing in central Vermont, he suddenly fell over, unconscious. The ski patrol brought him down at some speed to the base lodge, and when it was determined that Alan's condition was serious, perhaps even life-threatening, a Medivac helicopter was summoned.

By this time quite a snowstorm had developed, and the helicopter pilot did not think he could safely make it to Albany Medical Center, the most comprehensive facility in the area. Consequently, Alan was driven by ambulance to Hanover, New Hampshire, to the Dartmouth-Hitchcock Medical Center, where a serious brain-bleed, an aneurysm in the subarachnoid area, was diagnosed.

His frightened wife was told that an operation had to be performed on the spot and that her husband would be a "goner" if the operation was not done. However, the operation itself was risky: the doctors gave the injured skier a 50 percent chance of survival, and *if* he survived the operation, there was a 50 percent chance that he would become an epileptic. In addition, if surgery was performed, there were many other potential complications that were considered unavoidable. In one of the most agonizing moments of her life, Alan's wife gave the doctors permission to operate on her husband.

Alan's skull was cut around the entire head, and the bony "cap" lifted off so that the brain itself could be lifted out, enough to get to the ruptured artery (in the space beneath the brain) and clamp it. The brain, the piece of skull, and the scalp (in the correct order!) were then delicately reattached.

Alan made it against all the odds that had been offered. (And before we discuss our part in assisting with his healing, I want to say that the success is largely due to his excellent health, both mental and physical, before the event—not to mention the support of a loving family.) He did have some seizurelike events that began after seven months of recuperation, but these did not develop into anything like the threatened *grand mal*. Fortunately, he was referred to Dr. Richard Brown, who skillfully prescribed both pharmaceuticals and nutraceuticals to help Alan's damaged brain balance and rebuild itself.

When Dr. Brown referred Alan to us, he still suffered from headaches, extreme fatigue, difficulty sleeping, cognitive and speech problems. But Alan's brain map offered us hope. The high functioning, flexible, disciplined organ that his brain had been before the trauma was still there. It just needed a little renovation, and a tune-up. While Dr. Brown managed the Aricept, CDP choline (for brain restoration), and Rhodiola, we performed regular neurofeedback on Alan.

After the first treatment, Alan was able to drive himself the twenty-five miles or so each way to our center. We moved slowly and delicately through the site sort, going even slower when we hit a troubled area, near the fracture, or the "shunt" that had been put in to release fluid pressures. Alan did well at HeartMath, and soon was scoring in high percentages of "entrainment"—80–90 percent, meaning that he was able to get his heartrate variability balanced and regularized, which helps with emotional life, cognitive clarity, and even correlates with physical health. (See www.HeartMath.com and www.HeartMath.org for more details—the latter for experimental research.) He said it made him feel calm and comfortable inside.

This combination of treatment, along with some psychotherapy, was to work wonders. Alan became increasingly functional and noticed that he was less fatigued, and his speech improved. He was not working, however, and this was a source of great distress to him.

In the fall of this past year (2004), Alan seemed to go through a quantum leap. His energy was better, and his sleep was markedly improved. He decided to try photography again, but all his old Nikon equipment had become more or less obsolete, given the digital revolution. He needed to get up-to-date with the new equipment—so he did, with a state-of-the-art digital Nikon—with *beaucoup megapixels!* Suddenly Alan was publishing his photos again, in an entire issue of *The Woodstock Times*—Alan was back! The spreads were beautiful; his eye had lost none of its visual taste.

Sometime in the early winter we had started Alan on the Interactive Metronome, a device that measures the brain's timing and processing speed. (See www.interactivemetronome.com.) An initial test showed that his were way off because of the injury, particularly on his right side (left hemisphere damage), and coordinating across the corpus callosum (right to left and vice-versa). At first the exercises were extremely fatiguing and we found that we had to keep the repetitions low or he would be sweating and exhausted.

On Alan's next visit to Dr. Brown, he told him about the work on the IM. "I bet it will help your skiing!" Dr. Brown said. In January, Alan and his wife proudly observed their son doing well in the national stunt skiing competition in New Hampshire. (Yes, the ones where these young athletes do amazing full-twisting double gainers, and somehow manage to land skiing in the same direction they had started).

At his most recent metronome session Alan did much better and wasn't tired, even though we upped the repetitions. "Been skiing?" I asked.

"Oh yeah!" He grinned from ear to ear. "On just about every black diamond at Windham." (Windham is one of our local ski areas.)

I allowed myself a moment of awe. "Was Dr. Brown right?"

He mused: "I skied most of the day and wasn't tired, and come to think of it, my turns were linked and easy. Wow!"

"Well," I said, "I think the inverse is true too—your skiing might have helped you on the IM. You did very well this week, averaging thirty milliseconds of error when before you had eighty."

"Most important of all," he said, "I'm working again!"

"Amen!"

Evan: A Grumpy Santa Claus

Evan could be called a grumpy Santa Claus. Not tall, but weighing over two hundred and fifty pounds, with a bushy white beard, he would come sailing into our center on his *Moto Guzzi*, an extremely snazzy Italian motorcycle known only to the *cognoscenti*. Invariably, Evan would be wearing a sweatshirt with rolled-up sleeves, and *Grateful Dead* suspenders with little skulls all along them. During the 1960s he had been politically active in the war protest movement and worked on and marched with a ten-foot model of a yellow submarine. But he loved nothing more than to put away can after can of Pabst and some smoke (along the lines of the *Fabulous Furry Freak Brothers*).

But after many catastrophes, including a broken marriage and failures in business, Evan had come to terms with his alcoholism and become sober. He had worked at many jobs: electrician, business owner, teacher. However, at this point in his life, Evan began leading twelve-step groups and doing a lot of philanthropic volunteer work. He was certainly an imposing figure, and when he was smiling everyone wanted to hug him (or sit on his lap). But when he was grumpy—watch out! (All the dwarfs would scatter and hide behind the reindeer!)

About ten years ago Evan had a stroke that took the wind out of his sails. He lost memory, speech, movement, and coordination and was a shadow of his former self. Worst of all, his benign and beatific persona seemed lost in his new persona: that of a rage-oholic. He was angry at the world's stupidity and his own, and *everything* seemed to make him angry. At times he seemed like a large, wrathful storm cloud moving across the horizon. His wife said he kicked her in bed every night. She loved her big fuzzy bear, but she was thinking of sleeping without him.

Evan blew up at co-workers, people in groups, merchants, and doctors. Most of all, he hated corrupt political figures or other questionable authorities. (Sometimes we were afraid he would do something unwise vis-à-vis this group.) Evan was also quite forgetful. All in all, he was practically on the verge of a nervous breakdown. His doctor had put him on medication, and Evan reported that, while initially this seemed to help him, he now was angrier than ever.

Through his work as an electrician, he and his mild-mannered assistant, with whom he formed a kind of Laurel and Hardy team, one day were at work installing a pair of backup generators at our center. When a frustration was encountered, the calm voice of the assistant could be heard wafting through an open window: "Gosh darn it to heck!" while Evan's own offerings: "*#@&" could wither houseplants and terrify small animals!

We really wanted the LENS treatment to work for Evan—otherwise he would be pretty unbearable. We approached the stroke area in his brain very slowly through the site sort, and when we got there, there were some minor flare-ups—in the form of explosions, of course.

We won't say Evan's course of LENS treatments had no ups and downs, and it certainly went on for a while, perhaps for as many as thirty sessions, during which time we wondered if *anything* was actually happening. But what became increasingly evident was that Evan's "other side" was becoming visible. Clearly a heart of gold beat within his shaggy exterior. He initiated warmer, more genial, exchanges with me and/or with the staff; he seemed to be coming back into his own.

Recently Evan and his assistant were fixing a rather complex electrical problem. I heard what sounded like a massive, highly profane explosion from Evan and, as I approached the two of them to determine what was wrong, I saw that both Evan and his assistant had big smiles on their faces. *Evan had been lampooning himself in a rage*, which was irresistibly funny.

A recent questionnaire showed that he was not kicking his wife in (or out of) the bed any more. "So," I said, to Evan, with a little smirk on my face as we sat in the therapy room, "you've stopped kicking your wife?"

"Only," he growled back at me, "when she deserves it."

Tom: Alzheimer's with Parkinson's and Cancer

Tom was brought to our center by his wife Alice, a social worker, who was his main caretaker. Alice had been helped out of insomnia and an anxious depression by the LENS, so she knew that it could help with cognitive problems. Tom was in his late sixties, with a nonaggressive, but malignant, cancer that had stabilized. But he also had been diagnosed with Alzheimer's and Parkinson's disease at the same time—a "triple whammy."

Tom was a large man, over six-foot-three-inches tall, and his wife was tiny, more than a foot shorter than her husband. To get him to go "in the right direction," Alice had to kind of "herd" him, like a sheepdog, nipping at his heels or trying to head him off from a single-minded lurch in this or that direction. Tom was also very forgetful, awakening her several times each night to ask for help with the "remote" for the TV, which he never seemed to be able to find or figure out.

In bed at midnight and up by 5:30 A.M., Alice did not appreciate being awakened so frequently in this fashion. As a result of these nocturnal disturbances, Alice became hypervigilant, and her migraines got worse. But Tom was not only forgetful and cloudy, he was childlike, unable to dress or care for himself and needing constant reassurance. His walk was accompanied by a shuffle—characteristic Parkinson's Disease—and a substantial tremor.

We began treatment with an offset protocol (one second of stimulation at four different offsets). The offset alone produced one of those miraculous recoveries, according to his wife's report of the following week. On the seventy-mile drive home from the treatment, Tom, socially inept since his decline, delighted his wife and one of her co-workers with the aptness of his comments, and his suddenly regained, dry sense of humor. He seemed far more clear, asking sensible questions, responding well to the answers, and, not only able to produce, but to respond to humor (the latter is truly a sign of CNS health!).

The following day, Tom was able to dress himself and tie his shoes; this improvement continued throughout the week. Alice was sleeping better too, and the following night she got her first whole-night's sleep in years due to the fact that Tom didn't wake her up. She noticed he was walking more normally—without the shuffle.

Overly enthused with these results, I decided to introduce one second of stimulation per site into his map, instead of no stimulation. Wary of overdosing him, though, I did only half the map—which would amount to a total of 11 seconds of stimulation at 11 different sites. He left the session ebullient and energized, but when he arrived home, all hell broke loose. Again Alice would awaken with befuddled Tom standing in his pajamas, the "remote" dangling in one hand, asking for help. He shuffled and was once again asking inappropriate questions.

Alice was so upset, she wondered if she should take the seventy-mile trip to bring him in. I said, "Ouch, sorry, yes bring him in." That week I did not even resume the mapping but gave Tom a single second of stimulation on his forehead site of FPZ ("fp" meaning prefrontal, "z" meaning "center line"), where we had done the successful offset.

Almost immediately, the report came back that he was better. He was dressing himself again and tying his shoes well. I mopped my brow: "Another disaster averted, and another object lesson in what Len Ochs calls 'The Wonderful World of Overdose.'" Too much of a good thing, it seems, is not a very good thing at all. In the long run though, even these disruptions can be helpful, as the organism rights itself whenever the resources return.

Tom passed away just a month before this writing. He will be missed; but our memories of him are enriched by the times that he was at his best during those last years.

Coping with Advanced Parkinson's Disease

The following is a condensation of a letter of support for a Parkinson's research project proposed by doctors Stephen Larsen and Richard Brown, to the Michael J. Fox Foundation. Ultimately, the grant would be denied. However, the letter is included here because it describes the remarkable improvements that the LENS made in the life of a long-term Parkinson's sufferer, Richard Henson, a distinguished retired professor of philosophy who had taught at the University of Utah, Cornell, and Rutgers during his long and distinguished career.

The letter was written by his wife Amie Brockway-Henson, the talented director of The Open Eye Theater, originally founded in New York by Joseph Campbell and his dancer-wife Jean Erdman, and now located in the Catskill Mountains in Margaretville, New York, where Dick and Amie reside.

Dear Grants Panelists:

I am writing in support of Dr. Stephen Larsen and Dr. Richard Brown's application for funding for their collaborative work on Parkinson's Disease. My Husband, Richard Henson, is a patient of Dr.'s Brown and Larsen. His ability to function with Parkinson's Disease has changed remarkably for the better under their care and guidance.

Dick was diagnosed with Parkinson's Disease ten years ago, in the fall of 1993, when he was 68 years old. He had been suffering from a wide variety of ailments that eluded one specialist after another for several years: laryngitis, difficulty running, tremor under stress, stiffness, depression, an inability to complete tasks, etc.

He improved for a while on the medicines prescribed by our first neurologist, but before long, he was experiencing severe hallucinations, cognitive cloudiness, forgetfulness, increased depression, increased nightmare activity, and decreased participation in our family life. It was difficult, if not impossible, for him to write a letter or to follow complex thoughts. He slept a lot, and listened to the radio some, but did little else.

At Beth Israel, Dr. John Rogers, a neurologist, determined that Dick was undermedicated (he hadn't been taking his medications on his own). Monitoring his medications saw some improvements, but we also saw that the medications were causing serious side effects. So Dr. Rogers recommended that we see Dr. Richard P. Brown, a psychopharmacologist based at Columbia University, who specializes in alternative treatments, especially nutriceuticals. (He also happens to live and have an office upstate, about an hour from our home in the Catskill Mountains.)

Dr. Brown introduced us to the nutraceutical SAM-e, which he had found to be helpful to Parkinson's patients, before it was readily available in stores in the U.S. We imported it from Italy, and started with a low dose, gradually increasing to the maximum of 4000mg/day. Other nutriceuticals, Rhodiola Rosea from Siberia, and Maca from Peru, were introduced to Dick one at a time, so that we could see their effect. They were kept in the regimen or discarded according to their ability to increase cognitive clarity and physical stamina.

Within a short time, Dick was free of hallucinations and was functioning at a much higher level than before. However, he still had problems with cloudiness and depression—some difficult problems that created awkward and dangerous situations. Dr. Brown recommended that we look into Dr. Stephen Larsen's neurofeedback treatments. These are the LENS treatments developed by Dr. Len Ochs of California, using radio waves to feed back brain waves.

Dick had some initial problems after the offset, and seemed worse. But after the map he was better. After only a few sessions more, we could see a marked change for the better. Dick began to write again, and sing. He participated in discussions and family life. He was *present*. Dr. Larsen also used a device called a Photonic Stimulator [discussed in chapter 12], which considerably eased the muscle spasms and the pain in Dick's shoulders, neck, elbows, knees; he got stronger and more flexible. Most recently he introduced Dick to "HeartMath," which slows the heartbeat and promotes harmony between the heart and the brain, helping to produce unified positive feelings, and soothing discordant emotions.

During the past year, as a direct result of our work with Dr. Brown and Dr. Larsen, Dick (now 78) has been able to do some travelling. We crossed the country by train to visit his children, and took an ocean cruise together. Dick has pulled together a collection of poems he has written through the years, and submitted three of them for publication. They were accepted and appear in an anthology of Catskill Mountain writing.

He has at times appeared socially, without obvious symptoms of Parkinson's, done public readings, and resumed singing lessons. I believe Dr. Brown and Dr. Larsen are at the forefront of Parkinson's research and treatment. Dick and I have reaped tremendous benefits from their collaboration. Without the benefit of the extraordinary research and collaboration between Dr. Brown and Dr. Larsen, Dick would not be functioning as well as he is—much better today than four or five years ago! We have been far more fortunate than most.

Please give the strongest consideration to Dr. Larsen and Dr. Brown for a Michael J. Fox Foundation Community Fast Track Grant, so their work can continue full speed, and their discoveries can make effective treatments available to the thousands of other patients with Parkinson's Disease who could benefit from them.

Sincerely,

Amie Brockway-Henson

On Richard Henson's eightieth birthday, a party was given for him and, at that party, Mr. Henson made the following speech to seventy assembled guests:

Some may see this birthday as an achievement; but I regard it more as the result of good fortune. I've managed to avoid being eaten by a cougar or stepping in front of a bus, and I learned at an early age that "inflammable" isn't the opposite of "flammable."

Of course Parkinson's disease is no slice of birthday cake. There are days when bitching is my only honest response to the unwary neighbor who asks how I feel. But that is the exception—much more often, I feel blessed in the loving care of my wife and many friends, notably my devoted team of doctors, therapists, and caregivers.

We are all familiar with what is said to be an ancient Chinese curse: "May you live in interesting times." Parkinson's is certainly interesting, and sometimes without early fatality. I can only feel lucky that in my case, at least, it has been so. I feel especially blessed to have so many good friends here today.

Richard Henson,
Margaretville, New York, August 13, 2005

One More Headache

People routinely use "headache" as one of the most painful metaphors that can be evoked. Accounting ordeals, ungrateful spouses, unyielding tasks all may be called "headaches" (and may indeed play a part in evoking the actual pain itself). Headaches are of three general varieties: tension, cluster, migraine. Epidemiological studies show us interesting things, such as the fact that tension headaches are seven times more prevalent than migraines, and cluster headaches far less common than either.

Women are more than twice as likely as men to get migraines, and there does seem to be a perimenopausal dimension to them. Tension headaches may be episodic or chronic, while cluster headaches are known to be periodic, vicious attacks of a half-hour to three hours in duration. Migraines may last much longer, may be chronic, and are sometimes accompanied by auras, light and sound sensitivity, strange visual phenomena with images appearing and disappearing, nausea, and often almost total incapacitation for days at a time.

According to some psychological studies, those people who have an external focus of attention, and believe that most of life's events are beyond their control, seem to be more susceptible to headaches than those who believe that life circumstances are often in our control through inward changes or the modification of one's own actions. This interesting feature brings up the biofeedback treatment of headaches, because clearly biofeedback is biased toward acquiring control of one's inner states. Biofeedback is more natural for the second group, and not so natural for the first group—the "external controllers"—who are far more likely to look for a cure in something from the outside, like a pill they can take, "to make it all go away."[1]

Headache medicines are, in fact, rated in strength from normal to "extra-strength" depending upon the ferocity of the headache. For ordinary occasional tension headaches, over-the-counter remedies may work fine: aspirin (buffered or otherwise), Ibuprofen, and Tylenol (acetaminophen). More serious migraine sufferers find these remedies inadequate and head for the Imitrex, Feurinol, Darvoset, which have much more profound action; or even the infamous opiatelike Oxycontin (which certain conservative radio personalities use to quell their inner contradictions). The only problem is that the stronger the drug, the stronger the side-effects, and the more profound the backlash when the drug is discontinued.[2]

During the 1970s, Elmer and Alyce Green (then associated with the Menninger Foundation) were pursuing the vascular aspect of migraines and thought they had found a cure—certainly an amelioration. In many migraine conditions, blood rushes to the head—overloading the capillaries—and drains away from the extremities, often causing a comorbid condition called Raynaud's Syndrome, which is typified by chronically cold hands and feet. The Greens found that if they could teach people to warm their hands, and later, their feet, through autogenic imagery and temperature biofeedback, they could redistribute the blood flow, take the pressure off the head, and largely abate the severity of the migraine.[3]

I tried this approach clinically with many patients and with student sufferers of migraines in my biofeedback classes and found it to be fairly effective. It was more effective when combined with EMG or muscle-relaxation training, however, especially if the headaches had something of a *tension* headache flavor, with or without migraine. The downside was that the procedure took quite a bit of work—on the part of the patient—and the therapist and was far from completely successful.

Coming from this background, I will have to admit that I was skeptical that any EEG procedure, like the LENS, could do much for headaches, especially migraines, given their pronounced vascular aspect. After all, it was the engorged blood vessels, not the brain itself that was the problem—or was it? At that point, I had a few opportunities to treat clients who were courageous enough to come in to the office with their migraines in full bloom. Applying the LENS stimulation, I could see the tension leave the faces of these patients following what had been just a few seconds of treatment. Depending on the severity and the length of time the person had been suffering from migraine headaches, they might come back again for treatment sooner or later. But we found ourselves with some dramatic successes.

One such patient was Martha, an intellectual, urbane New Yorker who was initially quite skeptical when her doctor referred her to us for intractable migraines of some twenty year's duration. (I had quite a challenging first interview with her but persuaded her to give the LENS a try.) To our mutual surprise, Martha's migraines began to abate almost immediately, both in severity and duration. Then Martha incurred some serious professional stresses that involved a bullying boss, which caused her to leave one job and begin a new one. (Talk about "headaches"!) We both expected her familiar "basket case" reaction to this stressful situation, but she did better than ever before, and the migraines continued to abate after the stressful period was over.

"Wouldn't it be wonderful," I said to her one time, "if your headaches came knocking, and you just weren't there?" (And then you could stop coming every week and doing this weird procedure!) We both laughed. But a few months later, that day did come—Martha had been headache-free for weeks. The mutual decision to stop Martha's therapy was a joyful one.

I did more research on headaches and found the world of physiology had changed a little since my early biofeedback work. In those days, the vascular theory seemed center stage. It was the scalp that hurt, not the brain; the brain lacked the sensory neurons to experience severe pain.

In time, however, a fuller physiological understanding has shown that there is indeed a cortical (brain) component to migraines, along with the vascular component—not to mention the influence of the extra-cortical trigeminal nerve, which indirectly seems to instigate a cortical kindling not so very different from seizure activity. I found that many clinical studies cited psychiatric or medical "comorbidities" (other problems) that frequently accompany chronic severe headaches. Often sleep disorders, depression, anxiety, mood instability or explosiveness, and/or cognitive or concentration problems are found as well. These are all symptoms of an irritated or destabilized brain.

When the photonic stimulator was added to our practice (see chapter 12), we found an additional tool to relax muscles of the shoulders and the neck and help reduce neuromuscular pain signals. This combination seemed very soothing and balancing to people with active headaches. Acute chronic headache, the tiger of personal pain, was, with skilled practice, in danger of becoming a domestic cat.

The following case account was obtained by Beth Hanna, R.N., a recent trainee in the LENS work. She also had years of clinical nursing practice, so no one was more astonished than she was at the efficacy of her new magic tools.

Darryl: Making Headway with Migraines
Beth Hanna, R.N.

One day I received a call from a man named Darryl, a forty-four-year-old engineer who had suffered from migraines for most of his life, as well as from ADD (recently diagnosed). He had heard about the LENS and thought he would give it a try since he had tried many, many treatment modalities over the course of his life.

Darryl's migraines had started around the age of five, at which point his parents took him to many doctors to rule out life-threatening causes. He was treated with histamine shots and learned traditional biofeedback; both brought temporary relief. He tried many, many other medications as well as supplements, always with only temporary relief. He said his best relief came from two Excedrin tablets and a can of Pepsi. As a teenager Darryl learned to mask his migraines to participate in normal teenage life. He was considered shy and quiet by most people he met. In truth, he was either dealing with a migraine or trying to avoid one.

About ten years ago Darryl started treatment in Ann Arbor at the Michigan Head and Neck Pain Institute—a major, internationally renowned center for the treatment of migraines. His intake forms included a standard list of medications; he was asked to check off any that he had tried. The sheet was 8½ x 11 and filled with at least three columns of medications. Darryl checked "yes" to having taken approximately 90 percent of the medications. He was, at that time, taking Concerta for his ADD, and Methergine (Methylergonovine), Corgard (Nadolol), and Exedrin for his migraines. He was undergoing biannual CT scans for his doctor to continue to prescribe Methergine because the Methergine can crystallize in the kidneys.

Darryl was also asked to check off any items that would trigger a migraine. This list included food, light, noise, smells, sensations, and many other items. Darryl again checked off approximately 90 percent of these items. (Chronic pain was obviously a way of life for him.) As with most chronic pain sufferers, depression also became a way of life for Darryl, and he had been taking antidepressants for three years, with little success. All of his energy was spent in a coping mode, instead of enjoying himself.

Darryl stated that he had had six head injuries throughout his life, dating back to when he was five years old. Three of the injuries were from car accidents and one was from a motorcycle accident. After filling out the CNS Questionnaire, it was noted that Darryl also had sensory problems (light bothered him—8 out of 10) and he had problems with his sense of smell (8 out of 10). He showed clarity problems such as feeling "foggy" (10 out of 10), problems with following conversations (10 out of 10), confusion (8 out of 10), problems following and understanding what he had just read (10 out of 10), concentration (9 out of 10), and attention problems (8 out of 10). He also had daydreaming problems (10 out of 10), organizational problems (8 out of 10), and problems with stamina (8 out of 10). He had some memory issues and stated that his head pain was steady and throbbing (both 9 out of 10). His wife commented on his emotional issues: irritability (9 out of 10), mood changes (7 out of 10), depression related to his pain (6 out of 10), and minor problems with explosiveness (2 out of 10).

Darryl was treated, on the average, twice per week with the LENS and the photonic stimulator (this was done on the front and back of his fingers and toes for one second per site). We started with a no-stim map because we assumed that Darryl was very sensitive. We did not do an offset and started with one or two sites for the first month (his offset was set at 20).

After the first few sessions, Darryl stated that he felt "cautiously optimistic." By the end of the second month, we gradually increased the number of sites to seven sites per session. Darryl was titrating his migraine medication down slowly. By the middle of the third month we remapped him and performed an offset (which came out to be 15).

Darryl filled out the CNS Questionnaire again wherein he rated his head pain a zero. His problems with light and smell had improved (both 3 out of 10), as had his irritability (also 3 out of 10). His clarity had gotten better, specifically his fogginess. Problems following conversations, and his confusion levels, had dropped to 3 out of 10. He stated that his reading comprehension problems had improved (5 out of 10) and that his issues of concentration and attention had improved (both 4 out of 10).

Darryl's problems with sequencing, prioritizing and not finishing what he had started got worse (2 out of 10). His daydreaming problem improved (3 out of 10). He rated his energy problems between 2 and 1, with problems related to his inability to fall asleep weighing in at zero. Darryl rated his memory problems on a par with what they had rated pretreatment, but he rated his procrastination and ability to learn from experience a 3 out of 10 instead of a 5–6 out of 10.

After three months of neurofeedback, I received a call from Darryl's brother thanking me for giving him his brother back. Over the three months, Darryl would comment to me that he felt calm, his energy level was much improved, and he felt rested. His migraines were not as intense as they had been and he felt that his fogginess had lifted.

Darryl had a few major emotional strains about three months into his LENS treatment. He claimed, however, that he would not have been able to handle these upheavals very well prior to his LENS treatments. He has been able to reduce his migraine and ADD meds to half, while maintaining improved mental clarity as well as a 50 percent reduction in migraines. The sense of control that he gained by minimizing both his migraines and his medications has given him an emotional strength that he did not possess before undergoing the LENS.

An interesting footnote to Darryl's migraine occurrences is that they are, at this point, more easily treatable and much less severe. As a matter of fact, he feels good enough to start challenging his depression meds. I feel that this is significant because his travel and work schedule are as busy, if not busier, than they have ever been. His hobbies are extremely technical in nature, yet he keeps at them, something he would not have done in the past few years.

Another thing worth noting here is that Darryl likes us to stimulate two brain sites when he has a headache, even if he has had a session the day before. He swears this reduces his headache pain and sometimes even completely *ends* the pain. If he has a migraine prior to his scheduled session, it is gone after his treatment.

Summary on Headaches

It would not be fair to conclude this section without saying we have also experienced failures. Careful probing usually reveals these are often the patients who have rebound headaches caused by years of medication overuse.

Dr. Steve Baskin, a biofeedback practitioner who is very versed in the research and the clinical treatment of headache, as well as being a President of the Association for Applied Psychophysiology and Biofeedback, says that, as chronic migraine is frequently caused by medication overuse, the first stage for these refractory patients is a detoxification procedure and withdrawal from all medication—in other words, an enforced period of privation from quick relief coupled with a willingness to try the way of inner awareness and self-management.

ALTERNATIVE APPROACHES TO EVALUATION AND TREATMENT USING THE LENS PERSPECTIVE

Stephen Larsen, Ph.D., Len Ochs, Ph.D., Karen Schultheis, Ph.D.,
and Mary Lee Esty, L.C.S.W., Ph.D.

We need to be quite humble about the enormous range of human possibility that can come in and confound our efforts.

LEN OCHS, PH.D.

I get chills when I think about the possibility that I might have treated this child (with the LENS) and his parents could later have found out that he had seizures caused by a brain tumor. Would they have wondered whether the LENS treatment caused the problems? Would they have thought that the treatment had made him worse than he would have been without it? I'm glad I did not have to find out.

KAREN SCHULTHEIS, PH.D., NEUROPSYCHOLOGIST

A Different Understanding of Diagnosis

In this chapter, but also present throughout this book, you will find a new type of evaluation or diagnosis, boldly proposed. More and more, in our clinical practice, we rely on what people tell us they want and need help with and attempt to address that need, rather than try to pin a clinical diagnosis of their condition to some nomenclature developed to help doctors talk to one another or to justify treatment to third-party reimbursers.

These diagnostic categories *come from the patient's own sensations and expressions of discomfort* ("I don't sleep so well. . . . I don't have the energy that I need. . . . I'm upset far too often. . . . My thinking is cloudy. . . . I don't organize well, etc.). For the clinician, the *reason for diagnosis* is to identify one disease or problem entity to guide the *decision tree* leading to a cure, or to a therapeutic procedure that addresses the problem. The language of diagnosis also facilitates conversation between professionals about a particular case, as they seek to apply the general rule to the individual instance.

For the patient, a diagnosis may provide reassurance that their problem is identifiable and can be matched with a treatment or cure. On the other hand, however, it also provides a label that ignores one's unique personhood. ("Doctor, the *borderline patient* is here to see you," not "Anita Schwartz is here to see you.") While it helps the clinician to know that a person is *obsessive-compulsive,* for example, and thus may in some ways resemble others in that category, most people *would rather be known as individuals, than by some collective attribute!*

For third party reimbursers, of course, diagnosis must be linked with procedure. Just as the actors in Gilbert and Sullivan's *Mikado* prance about and sing, "Let the punishment fit the crime!" so also for managed care. If the punishment fails to fit the crime—"*This* procedure code does not match *that* diagnostic code!"—reimbursement will not be forthcoming.

Diagnosis is dependent upon human judgment, of course, and human judgment is not hard science. It is governed by the paradigm in which it is taking place. In the "medical model," certain problems are "diseases" and need to be treated with "medicines." In the social-behavioral model, such problems are seen as the result of "reinforcement history," or socio-economic problems. In the cognitive model, the cause is habitually inept or catastrophic thinking. In the humanistic approach, it is a bad set of relations between the individual and society, coupled with limiting beliefs about human potential. From the religious or transpersonal perspective, the same problems may be seen as fundamentally spiritual. In each of these cases, there is a guiding set of causal assumptions, a language, a set of therapeutic procedures or remedies for the problem, and a way of adjudging the outcome.

Bridging the gaps between these different perspectives and approaches is typically very difficult. For example, it took a virtual paradigm war in legislative bodies for psychologists and psychiatrists to arrive at a common and reliable professional vocabulary. In the mid-twentieth century, psychiatry, eager to display its clear and effortless dominance of the field, initially tried to control the entire process of diagnosis through the creation of the definitive *Diagnostic and Statistical Manual of Mental Disorders* (DSM IV). Standing upon its affiliation with medicine and biochemistry, it drew its paradigm from the work of pioneer psychiatrists such as Richard von Krafft-Ebbing, Emil Kraeplin, Sigmund Freud, and their successors.

The resulting diagnostic language used archaic and antiquated Greek and Latin terms based on *physiology and psychosexual attachment*. Despite this attempt to standardize diagnoses, certain experiments conducted during the 1960s and 1970s revealed that seasoned psychiatrists demonstrated an extremely low (25 percent) agreement with each other, a miserable performance according to the statistical *reliability* criterion.[1, 2]

In the newly unfolding realm of LENS neurofeedback, diagnosis is something quite different from all of the above, if it can even be called "diagnosis" at all. A wide variety of diagnoses—traumatic brain injury, Autism, stroke, early stage Alzheimer's, Parkinson's, and multiple sclerosis, Cerebral Palsy, ADD, ADHD, depression, anxiety and panic attacks, and fibromyalgia, for instance—are all helped by this one LENS approach. As a result, assigning some conventional and particular "name" to the patient's problem—so important in conventional diagnosis—is virtually irrelevant.

The most important factor in determining whether LENS is suitable for a patient is whether or not they have a CNS dysregulation. The many different types of problems treatable with LENS often have in common something neurologists call "EEG slowing": high amplitude, low frequency brain wave activity. This kind of activity can have a wide range of origins. It does become necessary to make certain whether this kind of EEG slowing exists (or potentially exists when such activity may be suppressed by stimulant medications).

Further, it can be critical for the LENS practitioner to determine whether or not such activity originates in a cause that would be better treated by medication, surgery, or other medical approaches. However, just as the LENS approach is no substitute for competent medical treatment (when appropriate), medical (or psychological) treatment is no substitute for competent use of the LENS.

LENS practitioners employ a variety of measures to identify the existence of impaired central nervous system functioning and EEG slowing, actual or potential. They consist of a Central Nervous System Questionnaire (CNSQ), a Reactivity-Vitality-Suppression Questionnaire (RVS), an Offset, and a Map Evaluation. These measures provide a reasonable assurance that the LENS is the right approach for a potential client.

Tools for Determining Impaired CNS Functioning

The Central Nervous System Questionnaire, which was developed by Ochs, broadly indicates whether there is a global functioning problem, and whether it occurs at work, at home, or while driving. It further tells us what kind of problem or problems the client sees in him- or herself: in the area of clarity and cognitive functioning, in mood, in energy, or in the domain of pain. The questionnaire—our primary screening instrument—is also an extremely useful prognostic tool. It's amazing how many people ask, after completing it: "How did you know?!" ("How did you know about all of my exquisitely individual symptoms?")

The questionnaire reflects Ochs's ability to be aware of an entire *gestalt*, a "pattern, or configuration, *which is more than the sum of its parts.*" Often he has confounded patients who have told him just a little about their symptoms by suddenly "filling out the picture" for them, that is, knowing—without being told—a lot of what else they are experiencing.

The Reactivity-Vitality-Suppression Questionnaire (under revision, hence not included here), tells us how reactive and sensitive to stimulation the client judges him or herself to be, the degree of vitality or strength the client feels, and the odds that we may encounter the releasing of suppressed activity such as seizures, tics, or even violence, during a course of treatment. It also gives us another way to look at any hypersensitivity, which bears on how to choose the dose of feedback that is useful for the client.

THE CENTRAL NERVOUS SYSTEM QUESTIONNAIRE

CNS Functioning Assessment

Name _____ Date of Birth _____ Age _____

Today's Date _____ Time _____ Diagnosis _____

Are you able to drive a motor vehicle? ____Yes ____Partially ____No

Are you able to work or study? ____Yes ____Partially ____No

Are you able to sustain a close relationship with someone? ____Yes ____Partially ____No

How frequently, *in the past 24 hours,* have you had problems in the following areas? Please pick a number from 0-to-10. "0" means *Not at all,* and "10" means *All the time.*

If one or more of your parents had this, or a similar problem, place a *P* in the column headed by "Parents."

If the problem came on suddenly, put an *S* in the column head by "Suddenly?"

Sensory	Frequency (0–10)	Parents?	Suddenly?
Light, in general, or lights, bother you	_____	_____	_____
Problems with the sense of smell	_____	_____	_____
Problems with vision	_____	_____	_____
Problems with hearing	_____	_____	_____
Problems with the sense of touch	_____	_____	_____

Emotions			
Problems of sudden, unexplained changes in mood	_____	_____	_____
Problems of sudden, unexplained fearfulness	_____	_____	_____
Problems of unexplained spells of depression	_____	_____	_____
Problems of unexplained spells of elation	_____	_____	_____
Problems with explosiveness	_____	_____	_____
Problems with irritability	_____	_____	_____
Problems with suicidal thoughts or actions	_____	_____	_____

Clarity			
Feel "foggy" and have problems with clarity	_____	_____	_____
Problems following conversations (with good hearing)	_____	_____	_____
Problems with confusion	_____	_____	_____
Problems following what you are reading	_____	_____	_____
Realize you have no idea what you have been reading	_____	_____	_____
Problems with concentration	_____	_____	_____
Problems with attention	_____	_____	_____
Problems with sequencing	_____	_____	_____

Clarity	Frequency (0–10)	Parents?	Suddenly?
Problems with prioritizing	_____	_____	_____
Problems not finishing what you start	_____	_____	_____
Problems organizing your room, office, paperwork	_____	_____	_____
Problems with getting lost in daydreaming	_____	_____	_____
You cover up that you don't know what was said or asked of you	_____	_____	_____

Energy			
Problems with stamina	_____	_____	_____
Fatigue during the day	_____	_____	_____
Trouble sleeping at night	_____	_____	_____
Problems awakening at night	_____	_____	_____
Problems falling asleep again	_____	_____	_____

Memory			
Forget what you have just heard	_____	_____	_____
Forget what you are doing, what you need to do	_____	_____	_____
Problems with procrastination and lack of initiative	_____	_____	_____
Problems not learning from experience	_____	_____	_____

Movement			
Problems with paralysis of one or more limbs	_____	_____	_____
Problems focusing or converging the eyes	_____	_____	_____

Pain			
Head pain that is steady	_____	_____	_____
Head pain that is throbbing	_____	_____	_____
Shoulder and neck pain	_____	_____	_____
Wrist pain	_____	_____	_____
Knee pain	_____	_____	_____
All-over pain	_____	_____	_____
Joint pain	_____	_____	_____
Other pain _____(specify)	_____	_____	_____

Other Problems			
Problems with nausea	_____	_____	_____
Skin problems	_____	_____	_____
Problems with speech or articulation	_____	_____	_____
Dizziness	_____	_____	_____
Noise in ears (Tinnitus)	_____	_____	_____

We also look closely at the five to seven factors that have been selected for the subjective rating scale reports. Thus, a "headache" patient may also be anxious, insomniac, irritable, and have "tinnitus," or ringing in the ears, along with being smell-sensitive or *osmophobic*, an unusual symptom. The clinician will also want to know if any relatives have these same problems or anything similar, or perhaps anxiety, mood, or metabolic disorders.

Finally we use something that few other modalities employ: a topographic EEG map, *which includes all of the standard International 10–20 sites*. It shows us both the amplitudes for the different frequency ranges all over the head, and the predominant frequency activity at any spot in the head. Most important, the LENS topographic map tells the clinician exactly where to place the electrodes during treatment. LENS treatment follows the topographic map and its accompanying site sort, moving from where the brain is the strongest (most regulated) to the least. In the realm of brain wave neurofeedback, the astute clinician is looking at many things, including the relationship between the topographic brain map and the offset and what the patient has said in the clinical intake interview, as well as other neurological information, such as psychometrics or tests such as CAT scans, MRIs, X rays, or PET scans that may have been done.

LENS practitioners have benefited from the example of Len Ochs's exquisitely honed clinical skills that—as he describes it—draw on his training as a psychologist, as well as his finding:

> that medical factors play a part, along with physiology (the brain, the way the cortex is able to respond to stimuli), and the environment. I look at the etiology, which may, for example, include depression, problems with sequencing, problems with retaining information, and short-term memory and organization problems. These symptoms can be generated nine different ways: from traumas, to a virus, to a protruding lump or disc on the spinal cord, to diabetic neuropathy, to peripheral problems such as Lyme Disease. So diagnosis may be almost a completely separate problem than treatment.
>
> A diagnosis is often a set of symptoms with a statement about causation, and a lot of emphasis on what caused the problem, which

we don't necessarily need. In the LENS, we don't have to have an exquisitely refined diagnosis, because we're just asking the cortex to quiet down a little. I only treat according to the EEG, what I see in the map, and what I know about the person's sensitivity, and not according to any diagnosis. I also carefully note the reactions to the treatment. *The reactions to the treatment guide future treatment, rather than the diagnosis.*[3]

However, conventional diagnosis may guide the speed with which we move through the sequence and how we estimate the length of treatment that may be required. For example, endogenous familial depression will take far longer to ameliorate than a reactive depression due to a sudden adverse circumstance. Conventional diagnoses also may guide how the treatment is understood and the results evaluated. Some people have relatively simple depressions, while others have anxiety-driven depressions, with quite different brain wave configurations, which will probably require longer treatment times.

While diagnosis is not integral to the LENS treatment, LENS practitioners do recognize the importance of diagnosis in ruling out problems that require medical treatment. That is why all of our intakes at Stone Mountain Center are commented on by a physician, our supervising psychiatrist. We also do "case conferences" to see if a person's problems might really be best addressed by a skilled psychotherapist, marriage counselor, physician, social worker, or even a dietician or physical or occupational therapist.

A Dialogue with Self-Regulating Systems

It is important to note once again that LENS clinicians do not assay a diagnosis to *tell the brain what to do:* procedures are not used to clear up slow-wave problems (depression, fatigue) through training higher brain waves, nor to relieve fast-wave irritability by training up the lower frequencies. All of these changes occur automatically through the disentrainment effect, *as the patient's own brain figures out what to do.*

Ultimately, of course, the goal *is* to see the slow waves reduce their amplitude and prominence in the chart or to see the freaky hi-beta spindles—that can betoken either muscle spasms, hyperactivity, or subclinical seizures and tics, explosive disorder, and so on—shrink and regularize. One sure sign of improvement could be described, in Paul Simon's words, as a "Bridge over Troubled Water," such as when a person suddenly experiences a reduction in depression, fatigue, and frantic "wheel-spinning," and, concurrently, their EEG shows that their dominant brain wave frequency moves freely up and down through the middle ranges. It's a wonderful outcome, but we don't even *presume* to tell the brain how to do it; *after all, it may be smarter than we are.*

The "Taoist" part of this whole procedure is that rather than *doing something*, we are instead setting up *the preconditions for the brain to heal itself.* That truth cannot be overemphasized. The clinician is the *manager* of a self-healing feedback loop, in which the brain is "fed-back" its own waves in the most elementary form: at a slow frequency, with an offset, tacked on to a weak (but much faster) radio frequency (Hertz information on a carrier wave of Megahertz). Our work proves the "self-healing" capacity of the human being: no real substance or measurable energy is put into the system; it is just "tweaked," or very gently stimulated.

The clinician's task is to monitor the specifics of this awesome process—Nature healing nature; the brain healing itself—while making sure that the treatment itself doesn't get in the way or freeze things up. This is clearly what *overdose* does, so a very important part of the initial diagnosis, as well as ongoing session-by-session evaluations, is devoted to determining how sensitive or reactive the patient is. The experienced LENS clinician is *ready for exponential increases (and decreases) in the levels of sensitivity during treatment,* and ready to respond with smaller and smaller doses.

Our culture's Cartesian-Newtonian emphasis says, "If the force introduced into the system is not enough to budge the object, increase the force!" This paradigm is often unconsciously embedded in modern medicine—"Let's try a stronger dose," and even in biofeedback—"Let's double the amount of time"—or double the sessions to enhance improvement, or to get the desired result more quickly. But in this subtle domain, where energy meets frequency, physiology, and chemistry, the intensity of the stimulation is *lowered* until it works, with the recognition that we are working with a dynamic, resonant, adaptive system. Thus LENS involves post-Einsteinian *relativity*, or *dialogue*: working with the client as an intelligent self-observant center, who is capable of *both conscious and unconscious forms of self-regulation*, if the necessary energetic or informational conditions are met.

We not only support dialogue between client and therapist but also with third-party payers, helping them increasingly to realize that, in the long run, holistic and preventative measures may be far cheaper to underwrite than escalating surgeries and more catastrophic measures. We also support dialogue between paradigms, working to create a collegial attitude of cooperation to help deflate the professional posturing and condescension that too-often characterize the practice of allopathic medicine. We work to substitute the recognition of each person's exquisite biochemical, bio-electrical, and genetic individuality for an approach that continues to blame patients for *failing to conform to the norm of a given diagnosis*.

The importance of teamwork and dialogue is continually reinforced by the experiences we have as practitioners, such as those related here by two of the finest diagnosticians in the LENS field: Dr. Karen Schultheis, Neuropsychologist, and Dr. Mary Lee Esty.

A Case of Diagnosis Using a LENS Map
KAREN SCHULTHEIS, PH.D.

Ryan came to me as a twelve-year-old student who was in the seventh grade at a local public school. His mother (who was one of my patients undergoing treatment for fibromyalgia) had been talking about him, stating that he had ADD, and wondering whether the LENS would help him. We discussed the fact that attentional problems could have many different causes, and that while LENS might help Ryan, there were certainly no guarantees. His mother described his difficulties—his teachers were complaining that he was inattentive in school and not doing well as a result—but also reported that, overall, he appeared to be a bright boy. Ryan's mother could not understand why her son was having so much trouble.

When Ryan came in and I reviewed his brain map, it showed three areas that concerned me: elevated delta, very high occipital alpha, and significant elevations of theta. His total amplitude map indicated extremely high amplitudes in the back of the head and throughout the right hemisphere. I did not want to alarm his mother but I had only seen maps like his in seizure patients, so I reluctantly asked if he had any symptoms that might indicate the presence of a seizure disorder.

To my surprise, she said, "Yes, he has staring spells and sometimes when I call him, I have to call several times before he responds by saying, 'Huh?'"

I asked if his teachers had ever said anything to her about the possibility of his having seizures. She said, "No," but she would ask them at a meeting she had scheduled for the following week. I instructed her to also make an appointment with a neurologist and gave her the name of one I trusted to diagnose and treat seizures.

The next week Ryan's mother came in and reported on the meeting with Ryan's teachers. When she had asked them if they had seen anything indicative of seizure-related behavior in Ryan, they had all agreed that his behavior *was* consistent with seizures. (I have no idea why they had not mentioned this to her before!) The mapping I did was in February, so Ryan had been in school long enough for them to get a good look at his behavior, and to let his mom know if there were concerns. Even this meeting had only taken place because she had called for it, and it is doubtful if anyone would have brought up the possibility of seizures if she hadn't.

When Ryan went to the neurologist the next week the doctor did an MRI and found a brain tumor. The tumor was pressing on the aqueduct in the ventricular system and had restricted the flow of cerebrospinal fluid. The neurologist was actually enraged that none of this child's physicians had ever considered his symptoms significant enough to warrant further testing. Nor could he understand why the teachers had said nothing.

The moral of this story for LENS practitioners is threefold:

1. Get help from the appropriate medical experts if you suspect underlying problems that need to be dealt with.
2. Don't trust teachers or the school system to identify problems to the parents. (In Texas a big issue is that if the teachers identify a problem in a child then the school system becomes responsible for helping the child cope with the problem from an educational perspective. The rule seems to be that if the parents don't bring it up, the teacher is not to say anything.)

3. The maps not only direct treatment but can also be valuable indicators of serious problems that need immediate medical attention. It is better to make a referral to a physician that results in a clean bill of health than to attempt to treat a problem, the underlying cause of which may be something as serious as a brain tumor!

I get chills when I think about the possibility that I might have treated this child (with the LENS) and his parents could later have found out that he had seizures caused by a brain tumor. Would they have wondered whether the LENS treatment caused the problems? Would they have thought that the treatment had made him worse than he would have been without it? I'm glad I did not have to find out.

Dr. Esty's Insights

I've often been dazzled by Dr. Mary Lee Esty's capacity to pinpoint the presence of pharmaceuticals or other foreign influences in a patient by examining brain waves. In her discussion, Dr. Esty shares some of her insights and guiding principles in a wonderful story that exemplifies the dialogue, interaction, and synergy between the disciplines that we try to model in our practice of LENS.[4]

Treatment Complexities
Mary Lee Esty, L.C.S.W., Ph.D.

Medications may be chemicals, but they make their presence felt in the brain waves. Generally medications cause a reduction of amplitudes, although stimulants register in the higher frequencies. We can't tell for sure, though, until we see what the brain looks like when it is not on medications.

The amplitudes of the waves and the standard deviations in the charts of people on heavy painkillers or on SSRIs such as Prozac just seem to be flattened; sometimes I think they provide a metaphor for what they are experiencing when they say: "I don't feel anything. Yeah, I am not depressed now, but so what!" In the study I conducted on the effect of FNS on fibromyalgia, we didn't allow anybody who was on Prozac or the benzodiazepines to participate because of their dampening effect on the brain waves, which makes treatment with FNS very hard.

We have been able to help people get off of a variety of psychotropic drugs, but to do so requires that the person really wants to get off and that they have a doctor who is willing to help them plan to get off. Recognizing that they are the ones who must work with their doctor, I make it clear to people that that is *their* choice, not ours. Prozac takes such a long time to get off—it has a "half-life" of a month—which makes it harder to discontinue. In general, the longer people have been on a psychotropic drug, the longer it takes to get them off, because of the impact of what is called "down regulation": the brain actually degrades some of its own neurons in response to the overstimulation of the medication. So the brain has got to have time to recover. Still, we have been able to get people completely off of huge amounts of medication, down to none. They are still doing well.

We have also been able to help patients get off antipsychotic and antiseizure medications as well, as in the case of the daughter of one of my early patients. He had cancer and was dying and asked me to treat her. She was in her thirties, a college graduate, but had been diagnosed variously with bipolar, schizophrenia, multiple personality, PTSD, depression, and manic-depressive disorder. She was on total disability, having been hospitalized at different points for being suicidal and homicidal.

Although I didn't have much hope, under the circumstances I couldn't say no. She was on lots of medication, Risperdal and things like that: it was quite a list. Being on disability, she had been transferred from psychiatrist to psychiatrist. Thus there was no stable physician relationship of any kind, and certainly no one who was very interested in helping her change, her social worker being the only constant. This was far beyond anything I had ever done, so I had no expectations. I saw her twice a week, and she would pay me a dollar. (I think people should pay something for their treatment, even when they are unable to pay the regular fee.)

We started before her father died. Her therapist had expected that when he died, she would probably have to be hospitalized again, but was pleasantly surprised when she didn't have to be. And I was also encouraged: maybe we *were* going to have a positive impact.

Not long afterward, she had to face another big challenge. The mayor of Washington had appointed a crony to be the head of the housing department, who proceeded to embezzle $600,000 worth of funds. As a result, people with subsidized housing were not getting their rent paid. My patient's rent had not been paid in six months. When her landlord kicked her out, she had no recourse but to move in with her mother, who was very critical of her. The various members of her therapeutic team all felt that it was going to be a difficult test of her recovery process.

Amazingly, the patient kept it together. She even tried taking some classes again. She started with a couple of easy things and did very well, so she started taking harder courses and getting straight As. Still, we were floored when she announced: "I've started volunteering on the suicide hotline at night." (She used to be a customer, so she certainly knew the ropes.) She did great at that, and last I heard she was in graduate school getting her master's degree. She was functioning so well that everyone was amazed.

Another patient was on an antiseizure drug, as psychiatrists are gravitating toward using antiseizure medications such as Neurontin, Tegretol, and Dilantin to correct the instabilities of bipolar and schizoaffective disorders. She was on Dilantin, which gives a clear signal of overdose: a very specific kind of rash. As she started taking in the benefits of the neurofeedback treatment, the same amount of the Dilantin was causing her to get the rash. So she went to her doctor and he reduced her meds. The rash went away; we continued our treatment; the rash came back; he reduced the Dilantin. This continued in a kind of step-down procedure. If every drug had some neat little flag like that, it would make the process of helping patients reduce their medications much easier.

Conclusion: A New Model for Diagnosis

In treating the brain—even with the extremely gentle and safe LENS treatment—we are exploring uncharted territory. That is why LENS practitioners foster the possibilities for different disciplines to work together in a synergistic, democratic way, rather than supporting the kind of misguided aristocracy of treatments in which, for example, a doctor's opinion cannot even be compared to that of a person's Feldenkrais worker or nutritionally-versed friend, *because he can charge more for doing something really powerful (and often toxic) to his patients.*

Why shouldn't physicians make more use of QEEGs to see if their meds are working or are perhaps overdoing it? And why shouldn't biofeedback and neurofeedback clinicians be extremely sensitive to other factors, such as when Mary Lee Esty "sees" Prozac or Ritalin in a patient's brain waves, or Karen Schultheis sees really high occipital alpha and, realizing that something may be very wrong, consults a neurologist.

Certified LENS clinicians are trained to interact with clients, diagnose CNS dysfunction, and apply their treatment in the most discerning and sensitive ways. They also are encouraged to see, holistically, the most hopeful picture possible of the person who is paying their fee. Because of this training and orientation, they are less likely to do harm by counteracting or negating the treatments of other doctors or therapists. This promotes positive outcomes in situations where therapists use more than one kind of treatment. We examine this topic in the next chapter, as we consider a new kind of therapeutic alchemy: the creative mixing and matching of the LENS with other treatments, enhancing the effectiveness of both.

The LENS and Other Modalities

Psychotherapy, Conventional Biofeedback/Neurofeedback,
HeartMath, Photonic Stimulation, Interactive Metronome,
Deep Vascular Relaxation, Nutritional Support,
Sudarshan Kriya Yoga, Qi Gong, and Open Focus

*Stephen Larsen, Ph.D., Wendy Behary, L.C.S.W.,
and Len Ochs, Ph.D.*

When Len Ochs began to see the extensive potentialities for the treatment method that was evolving under his guidance, he was astonished. The method is so effective for so many people that it would have been easy for him to believe he had discovered a type of *panacea*, an "all heal." But he was an astute enough biofeedback clinician and clinical psychologist to recognize that *the LENS couldn't do everything*. He understood that other modalities could and should be brought in at crucial points, to do things the LENS couldn't do.

When Ochs and other clinicians began doing just that, an even more amazing property of the LENS came to light: *It could facilitate the other treatments*. Its action was like a catalyst that seemed to jump-start other kinds of healing and self-regulation therapies. Thus, recognizing its limitations actually opened even broader new horizons.

Those of us who offer professional LENS training try to make therapeutic discernment about the best option for any given patient *the core of our approach*. We have found a piece of street wisdom to be a very helpful guide for our decision-making about which modality or combination of modalities might be best: "Different strokes for different folks."

All treatments should be tailor-made to the patient's constitution, robustness or fragility, and availability of inner resources. After just a few LENS treatments, some might do best by going to regular biofeedback; perhaps EMG (muscle relaxation) for spasticity or chronic tension, or classical hand-warming for migraines. Good results have been achieved in all the specific EEG ranges: alpha-theta for trauma, SMR for seizure disorder, beta for ADD. Here, treatment is geared to specific psychomental goals—"I want to think faster," or conversely, "I want to learn to daydream or fantasize at very deep levels." Some people may start with the LENS and then go on to achieve advanced levels with HeartMath, the Interactive Metronome, or Open Focus. Many patients benefit from nutritional support, yoga and qi gong, during or after their LENS training.

In this chapter we share some of our own favorite complementary modalities and offer some examples of how they have been combined, for specific patients, in an integrative holistic approach.

LENS and Psychotherapy

Many LENS practitioners are psychotherapists, trained in various schools—Freudian, Jungian, Transactional Analysis, gestalt, object-relations, as well as cognitive-behavioral, rational-emotive, family systems, and so on—enabling us to observe firsthand that a combination of psychotherapy and neurofeedback can lead to life-changing transformations of a truly positive nature.

Years ago I read a study by Johns Hopkins psychologist Jerome Frank, which showed that no one method of psychotherapy was measurably or experimentally superior to another. What *did* translate to therapeutic success was the bond between the therapist and client, and the successful emotional atmosphere of their first few encounters. The study also seemed to indicate that psychotherapy is less effective as time goes on. Therapist and client alike may experience therapeutic "doldrums," where nothing seems to be happening. When the client's resources are inaccessible or seem to have run out, the therapist's may also do that shortly thereafter—thus the therapeutic "slough of despond."

It is often said that we typically use only 5 percent of our brain. When our brains are locked in the hysteria of anxiety or the torpor of depression, this expression seems doubly true! A client who is a classical pianist once told me, "The anxiety makes me feel like I'm playing Bach with mittens on!" CNS distortions, depression, and anxiety ruin our precision and our nimbleness. When our neurological sea is choppy or full of evil-looking *tsunami*, we cannot hope to get our bearings and steer a course. The inflexible brain leads to an unquiet, locked-up mind.

A key phrase on our CNS Questionnaire is: "Failure to learn from experience." A surprising number of our clients check this off with a high score. When a person's nervous system lacks flexibility, he or she makes the same silly mistakes over and over again. An elderly Viennese man—who had been in psychoanalysis for most of his adult life and knew he was still terribly neurotic—put it this way: "You know vat a neurosis is? It's ven you discover that something don't verk and you just keep doing it!"

"Talk therapy," in whatever form, has limitations, particularly where underlying neurological conditions persist. It's probably why most psychoanalysts who are also medical doctors shrug their shoulders at a certain point and head for the prescription pad.

Many problems, whose *field of effect* is psychological, stem from *neuronal dysregulation*, rather than classic psychoanalytic dilemmas. These include variants on the classical list: anxiety, depression, panics, obsessions, insomnias. In response, psychiatry provides psychotropic drugs whose action is chemical/pharmaceutical, but whose *field of effect* is the psychological symptom.

Biofeedback and neurofeedback represent a third approach, relying on the energy dynamics of the brain or body, and the power of *feedback itself* to intervene. The LENS has proven to be very useful in treating the neurological underpinnings of problems not amenable to psychotherapy. Time and time again, we have seen neurofeedback breathe fresh life into therapy. The CNS is activated, the neurological "pot is stirred" and the lumps (as it were) come boiling to the surface.

We know now, from over ten years of experience, with hundreds of therapists and thousands of clients, that *the LENS stimulates dreaming*. (For those who use dreaming therapeutically, this is a bonanza!) However, long-dormant feelings and traumas may also arise as a result of LENS treatments. Interpersonal spaces between people, or in families, can become recharged. Symptoms can be brought to the surface, or "layers" of defense mechanisms reveal themselves. More awareness *does not always lead to more tranquility*—especially with codependent neurotic habits or psychopathologies.

Ochs has warned his clinicians—as well as patients—that things that have been tidily "under wraps," such as buried memories of childhood neglect or abuse, may constellate suddenly and dramatically, and require expert psychotherapeutic attention. Good psychotherapeutic or counseling training is an unmistakable asset to the practitioner, who can then, with skill and compassion, help the patient resolve or integrate such constellations. The results can be remarkable healings of long-neglected, intransigent complexes, decades-enduring knots of obsession or emotion.

As we have noted earlier, Freud said that psychoanalysis "speeds up the process of maturation," a very desirable thing in a society as immature as ours. (A Westerner once asked Gandhi what he "thought of Western Civilization." "I think it would be a very good idea," said Gandhi.) The combination of LENS and psychotherapy *palpably* "speeds up" the process of maturation. People seem more capable of taking responsibility for themselves. They reason more clearly and blame, or overdramatize, less. They find themselves more sensitive and discerning, but less reactive, than they were before.

The LENS also can lead to Jungian *individuation*, that is "becoming more and more oneself," one's evolving self—in a good way. By its neurological disentrainment action, it breaks up stagnation. The recursive neurological process, found in the LENS, as well as in generic biofeedback, meditation, and psychotherapy, is like heating up the contents of an *alembic* (a vessel originally used in alchemy). With the heat, the contents of the vessel begin to mingle and bond chemically. New compounds may be formed. Jung believed that the therapeutic process itself was such an alchemical alembic; my practice of the LENS for ten years and psychotherapy for thirty-five years, leads me to the belief that neurofeedback seems to act as a catalyst in the therapeutic process. Nothing new, really, is added, yet the *cooking* is more intense.

This is observable in children, where the sandplay environment, or any kind of expressive arts therapy, shows the *gestalt* of the process taking place as a result of adding the LENS to their treatments: more central control, more metacognition, more ability to recognize another's perspective, more emotional intelligence emerge in their little symbolic worlds. The same thing goes on in adults. They become better able to see things about their own narcissism, self-preoccupation, social inhibition or fear, or other self-limiting behaviors *but without the awful bite of existential angst.* In effect they see themselves more fearlessly and objectively, in a way that leads to subtle change.

These are changes that are preached from pulpits, exhorted in classrooms, and dinned in private therapy offices, but when people *really* change, from the inside, by themselves, a type of magic has taken place, and everybody who is around them knows it! They are more flexible, alert, and not infrequently kinder, because they are more empathic. They seem better equipped to accept things as they are.

Along with these changes, there is an added grace with perennial appeal: the sense of humor. Ochs taught his clinicians early, by example. The ability to accept and see the absurdity of life is healthy, and the ability to laugh (joyously, and intermittently, not continuously and sardonically) at it, a definite sign of personal evolution. Meetings of LENS clinicians (especially those who practice the method on themselves) often abound in laughter and warm camaraderie.

LENS and Psychotherapy: A Conversation with Wendy Behary

The following is a conversation that took place in January of 2005, between Stephen Larsen and Wendy Behary, an experienced psychotherapist, who had treated a patient we shall call Connie, for over five years before we began LENS neurofeedback with her early in 2004.

Connie, a dark-haired, pretty, athletic young woman, had alternately been diagnosed with depression, mood instability, panic attacks, dissociative identity disorder, including depersonalization. She wasn't exactly suicidal but felt certain she *would soon die an untimely death.* Connie had little self-esteem. She had shown herself highly sensitive and reactive to medications that had been tried along with the psychotherapy. She was referred to our practice by Dr. Sharon Sageman—an innovative psychiatrist on staff at Columbia Presbyterian Hospital—who felt she had run out of medical treatment options. At the time of this interview with Wendy Behary, Connie had been doing neurofeedback for almost a year.

Interviews with Connie had brought forth her personal history of early trauma and abuse, along with the expected dysfunctional family configuration. Due to Connie's overwhelming neurological anxiety, Behary reported very limited therapeutic success with her; nonetheless their contact was one of the only lifelines for this exceedingly fragile patient.

Stephen: I wanted to interview you because of some things you mentioned when we had our first "case conference" about Connie, whom we've both treated. I think it has been almost a year since she started with us, though she's worked much longer with you.

Wendy: I think that's about right. I have an intimate knowledge of her history over the years, which included hospitalizations and various in-patient and out-patient therapeutic settings, medication trials, and even mindfulness training. But Connie seemed to have an inability to make much use of these things. She was still in terror. There were memories we couldn't get near, because she would dissociate.

Stephen: And you didn't know much about neurofeedback, right?

Wendy: Not really. My primary approach to treatment is Schema Therapy (Jeffrey Young, Ph.D.). I also draw upon concepts from Interpersonal Neurobiology (Daniel Siegel, M.D.). I am a firm believer that the nervous system plays a pivotal role in people's mental and emotional well-being. It was not long after Connie told me she had come to see you and been mapped on your system that I noticed something: it was like an easing or a relaxation response, even a sense of hope and relief. Then I saw her making more use of the psychotherapy, which was frankly astonishing. That was not long before we first talked.

Stephen: Yes, thank you so much for being collegial in that way. I appreciate all the hard work you did with Connie before we even met her, and it seemed that the LENS treatments helped her start to be able to make more use of it.

Wendy: After the map she didn't have so much of her awful self-negation: *the feeling that she should cease to exist.* I think her self-esteem went up because there was a scientific, neurological, explanation for why she was feeling so lousy and so desperate. There was an explanation to mitigate the shame and self-blame.

Stephen: There was certainly enough in her map to warrant that she'd been having a tough time. Sadly, we have often seen that people naively blame themselves for what their nervous system does; they even think they're defective because they can't fix it!

Wendy: Yes, Connie felt she was "broken," irreparably damaged. Simultaneously she was incredibly tightly wound and overwhelmed. She would be so socially uncomfortable around people that she couldn't talk and would often detach. After a couple of LENS sessions I noticed she was smiling more, and she became more genuinely vulnerable in therapy. There was an amazing feeling of her beginning to connect with her emotions for the first time. Over that first month I noticed her being increasingly able to approach the emotions related to the traumas. Before that, she would go rigid or dissociate if she got close to them.

Stephen: That's so very interesting. Would you say that it was like an "edge" of really fierce anxiety was softened?

Wendy: It was almost as if there were interior passageways opening up. My recent training in Interpersonal Neurobiology made it possible for me to appreciate how potentially remarkable some of these changes really were. People have their stories, their narratives. In a really pathological case, the person tells their story over and over, but there is no real feeling attached to it. And there's a rigidity about the way the person relates to their own narrative. Then, for the first time, Connie was able to tell her story with more fluidity and flexibility. When she approached overwhelming emotions, she wouldn't just flit away or dissociate. I think she also began to really feel and be able to make use of the safety of the therapeutic situation, as if for the first time.

Stephen: This is very helpful information. We couldn't track the subtlety of what the neurofeedback was making available to her without your reflections, with a corresponding degree of therapeutic subtlety and sensitivity.

Wendy: She was able therapeutically to approach her childhood memories—explicit and implicit, both real and imagined, and all the faulty thinking tied up with them—instead of just being ruled by them. Before, her dread had been so huge that it ruled everything about her, making it very difficult to do therapy. Now she's able to engage and progress is emerging. When I sit with her she has the capacity to breathe more evenly.

Stephen: Speaking of breathing, has she mentioned that she has been doing HeartMath training? HeartMath is a biofeedback technique that teaches inner self-management by regulating the breathing and visualizing positive scenes and emotions. In the beginning Connie could only do it for a very brief period, indicating that anxiety was in the driver's seat, making her a restless soul that couldn't let herself be. But slowly she has been able to use it for longer and longer periods of time, and benefit from it.

Wendy: I think that's great. She expresses that she feels really good about the whole encounter with your center; it has empowered her. She's definitely more motivated in therapy. And I can tell if she's skipped her neurofeedback for a couple of weeks.

Stephen: What do you notice in those instances?

Wendy: The flow of communication is more stifled again; her posture is different, more rigid; she can't quite get her thoughts together and communicate them to me, or be receptive and open to me.

Stephen: I have seen the same thing myself, with other patients. I don't think Len Ochs ever intended his neurofeedback to be a "stand-alone" procedure, but he saw enough of that improvement in flexibility you mention to realize his method could help other areas of functioning. Thank you so much for this enlightening conversation.

LENS and Conventional Biofeedback/Neurofeedback

Using Jung's phrase, we have described the principle behind both biofeedback and neurofeedback as "the self-liberating power of the introverted mind." As therapists, our real skills lie in knowing how to help any person acquire the tools for inner balance and self-regulation that characterize a healthy human being.

Sensory stimulus, motor activity, and social interaction all exercise our brain and thus increase its flexibility and resilience. Sensory isolation and social isolation both breed underdeveloped nervous systems and bodies, as illustrated by "failure to thrive" syndrome, where institutionalized children are smaller, lighter, less active, and less developed than their normally raised counterparts. The extreme of this is *reactive attachment disorder* (such as was seen in the case of Damon, presented earlier); future sociopaths and serial killers are bred by absent, neglectful, or abusive parents, or in sterile institutional wards, full of abandoned children, making this a very good syndrome to "head off at the pass!" In this regard, it is important to remember our discussion of chapter 3 regarding the rats raised in three environments of varying stimulation, wherein the most stimulating environment produced the heaviest brains, better dendritic growth, and a pervasiveness of neurotransmitters and AChE channels.

Neurofeedback is one of the most gentle and yet powerful methods of *exercising* the brain; a person who learns to produce more alpha *or* more beta *or* more SMR has greased up his or her mental/emotional gearshift and is better able to shift easily and comfortably to any level of arousal. As the brain has its own internal feedback loops, *they* are probably being trained as well: not only the layers of the cerebral cortex itself, but also the subcortical pacemakers in the limbic system and brainstem. Mere speculation? Many people who respond well to treatment seem less "driven." As Ochs says, "The question is not: "Do you have issues?"— everyone does—but "How much *grip* do your issues have on you?"

The LENS focuses its regulatory activity on the brain. But we also suspect the training may reach further down the neural tree, as the autonomic nervous system becomes involved. The vascular (heart and circulatory) and muscular systems are also touched. For example, the LENS seems to be a vasodilator: a very few seconds of stimulation can cause palpable warming in the hands or feet. Rather dramatic increases in the temperature of the extremities, of as much as five or ten degrees, have been recorded within a few minutes. Thus the treatment helps with Raynaud's syndrome, in which the hands and feet are usually cold. We have even seen people with quite active migraines or vascular headaches walk out of the office, after twenty-five minutes, headache-free. Likewise, muscle spasms, especially of the scalp and neck, can also be relieved by the disentrainment stimulus.

People also notice increased gastrointestinal activity after the stimulus, or a slight worsening, and then amelioration, of stomach or abdominal cramps. Sometimes patients produce a nice audible sigh, as their breathing and whole physiologies relax just a notch or two. Parkinson's or TBI patients often have muscle cramping, which may be CNS based, because no amount of massage or treatment of the muscles themselves seems to help. However, a single centrally administered stimulus helps the sensory-motor strip in the brain relax, and they find relief.

What is being trained then is the entire *soma* (a lovely Greek word for the entirety of physiology) as innervated by the CNS. In the context of asking not just the brain, but the entire body/mind system, to change itself, as we are doing, it is small wonder that sensitivity becomes an issue. Sensitive or reactive people already have mechanisms in place to guard against trauma. After all, that is what their lives have taught them. They already know about hard shoves—behaviorally, energetically, or medically—and they make them brace and resist. But with neurofeedback, a small, sneaky stimulus just walks past the guards. The core of the dysregulation producing the brain waves is "tweaked" and has to reconfigure itself. As these little disruptions accumulate, the invigorated system balances itself and finds a slightly new way of being that it can tolerate. It is often "a gradual enlightenment."

The variety of conditions treatable by generic neurofeedback are pretty much the same as those treated by LENS: depression, anxiety, ADHD, chronic fatigue, and so on. Siegfried and Susan Othmer have proposed that really only two major conditions are being treated: *underarousal* or *overarousal*. Beta training is done for those patients who are underaroused, and alpha or even theta for the hyperaroused. Conventional neurofeedback is believed to produce its considerable therapeutic effects by training the brain to increase its frequencies in certain areas or, in other cases, to slow its rhythms, as in the Peniston protocols for alcoholism and PTSD. And in general, these models seem to do a satisfactory job of explaining the data.

But there is a hidden variable, which we have become aware of by practicing both kinds of biofeedback. When, for example, an underaroused cortex in an inattentive child is sped up by beta training (at C3), it is not desirable for the child to stay "sped-up" or hyperaroused all the time. If this happens, the protocol then needs to be switched to an alternate training, such as SMR (at C4), because this is known to give more composure and stillness. We have found that, in general, earlier training with the LENS protocol allows a client to slip in and out of these states more easily and not get stuck.

Conversely, clients can often experience an impasse when conventional biofeedback treatment is given: session after session may unfold with the client "trying as hard as he can," and failing to achieve what the protocol asks for. We remember that the LENS tills the soil of the brain, so that it is ready for new learning, new possibilities. Once flexibility has broken the unyielding soil of neural rigidity, and life "rains on our parade," gardens grow all around!

A corollary to the question: "What method?" is always: "What dose?" *People must be able to make use* of the stimulation or feedback they are given. Many people are resistant to ordinary reward-based or "operant" biofeedback because they are in a secret war with themselves. Their organic selves resist all conscious agendas or programs coming from the intentional mind. That is why most biofeedback practitioners suggest that results most readily occur when *the patient stops trying* so hard. Nature takes over and the Tao prevails. The best strategy most conventional biofeedback practitioners have come up with is just *watching*, not *trying* to do anything. In this regard the LENS starts out one existential step ahead of other kinds of neurofeedback involving reward and inhibit protocols, for with it, there is truly *nothing to be done*. People are very astonished and pleased when they get better for just showing up, and, as we have said before, *sitting and doing nothing*.

The important "Yerkes-Dodson Law" from psychophysiology says that the *arousal level of any activity* should roughly correspond to the activity itself. A cup of coffee might help you to take that final exam, but five cups might make your thoughts race and your hands shake so that you miss the subtleties in the questions. Rage might help you in a fight, but not while making love. Daydreaming is wonderful for creative schemes, but not when you're paying for an education, and sitting in class—and so on!

The LENS might get faster results than other forms of neurofeedback because it lets the brain (the most intelligent and complex thing in the known universe) find its *own level* of activation, rather than trying to "micromanage" it. Thus, nature itself is enlisted as an ally, rather than antagonized. This is probably why LENS works so well with complementary self-help efforts, including meditation, bodywork, yoga, qi gong, and so on. It subtly invigorates whatever else a person does.

The LENS and HeartMath

In his autobiography, *Memories, Dreams, Reflections*, Carl Jung describes a profound encounter with Ochwiay Biano (Mountain Lake, a Taos Pueblo shaman):

> "The Whites always want something; they are always uneasy and restless. We do not know what they want. We do not understand them, we think that they are mad."
>
> Jung: "Why do you think whites are mad?"
>
> Ochwiay Biano: "They say they think with their heads!"
>
> Jung: "Why of course. What do you think with?"
>
> Ochwiay Biano: "We think here." (He said, indicating the heart.)[1]

Jung wrote in his biography that the encounter with Mountain Lake revealed to him a face of his own predatory, acquisitive race that was inescapable. He pondered what it meant to "think" to dwell, to immerse, in the world of the heart.

The heart itself has its own built-in brain (of some forty thousand neurons plus glial cells). The heart resides just above the solar plexus—the mesenteric complex of three hundred million neurons—and is exquisitely interconnected with it. Nearby is the diaphragm, the organ of our involuntary respiration. The heart talks to (and is talked to by) both the diaphragm and the solar plexus. It also talks to the "roof-brain" at the top of the head, in two ways: through ascending afferent nerve pathways, and through an electromagnetic field thousands of times more powerful than the one produced by the brain.

According to research done by the HeartMath Institute, it is the simple, rhythmic power of the heart that makes it the body's central pacemaker. It is like the big bass drum in a marching band, whose profound, inescapable throb regulates all the other instruments. Cardiac health, it seems, is also visceral health, including endocrine regulation, and it is intimately related to brain, or "mental," health.

Forty years ago, most doctors thought that a "rock-steady" heart-beat was a measure of cardiac health. We now know that just the reverse is true. In fact, an unvarying heartbeat can be used to diagnose the likelihood of a serious cardiac event of some kind. The heart *should* be able to leap at the sight of something beautiful: an attractive person, a spectacular waterfall, or a crackling lightning storm. It *should* accelerate easily and rapidly in response to momentary exertions, and calm quickly when the exertion is done. Even while a person is asleep, there should be heart rate variability from beat to beat.[2]

HeartMath, developed by Doc Lew Childre, is a system of heart rate variability (HRV) training and technique, one of the best-researched and documented areas in all of biofeedback. Doc had been through many harrowing situations, especially while in the military and had developed an inner method based on the heart to keep himself emotionally balanced. Although he had no advanced degrees, he was called "Doc" after his dad, the man who founded the Grand Ole Opry. Doc Senior had such a kindly and healing way about him that everyone called him "Doc." Over time, the name stuck to his son, too. Soon talented people began to congregate around him, eager to learn his method and share it with others.

Eventually Doc and his associates founded the Institute of HeartMath in Boulder, California, in the mountains among the great redwoods and tumbling, mossy-banked streams. Doc and his associate Howard Martin co-authored *The HeartMath Solution,* a book that has sold over one hundred thousand copies. In this book they have simplified their carefully developed method of cardiac regulation and psycho-emotional balancing into some simple steps that can be done as a biofeedback technique, or simply an experiential, stand-alone process.

HeartMath methodology uses exercises that shift emotional states by breathing, along with acknowledging an appreciation of positive experiences. More can be learned from reading any of the books on Heart-Math, going to the Web sites www.heartmath.com and www.heartmath.org, or training as a professional provider in HeartMath.

Unlike the LENS, which is based on *disentrainment,* in HRV (Heart Rate Variability) training, *entrainment* (between the heart and the brain, or the sympathetic and the parasympathetic, branches of the autonomic nervous system) is what is desired. When the heart and brain are rhythmically entrained, the autonomic nervous system is balanced, the person is alert and relaxed, and thinking clears out, because there is less "static" from the afferent pathways through limbic arousal organs such as the amygdala, to the cortex. It is a very powerful process, which can be documented. One way to do this is with the Freeze-Framer sensor and computer program available from HeartMath, which provides real-time biofeedback. When the person's brain is well entrained with their heart, a beautiful undulating sine wave appears on the computer, a green button lights up, and a bar graph rises. The robust and well-documented research indicates the efficacy of this process for almost anyone.

The group of talented people who gathered around Doc to learn his method included therapists and research scientists who recognized the power of HeartMath and set out to document its areas of effectiveness. The placebo-controlled studies published in peer-reviewed journals that have been slowly accumulated by the Institute of HeartMath form one of the most impressive collections in all of biofeedback literature. Within just a few years, HeartMath clinicians were helping children with ADHD and other problems, calming students with test anxiety, and helping adults or children with panic. They were assisting with emotional self-management, including rage and anger; decreasing dangerous cardiac markers, like essential hypertension or cardiac arrhythmias; and helping athletes achieve peak performance.

There were also medically/biologically significant outcomes: Heart-Math, practiced consistently, was shown to increase the amount of salivary IgA (Immunoglobulin A), a measure of disease resistance. In other studies monitoring body chemistry, HeartMath was shown to decrease the amount of the stress hormone cortisol, which contributes to aging, brain-cell death, and other physiological problems, and to increase the amount of DHEA (di-hydro-epi-andosterone), which is associated with anti-aging effects, general vitality, and well-being, as well as with improved sexual vitality.

HeartMath scientific research also shows that the practice enables a person to have beneficial effects *on other people*, through the magnetic energy field of the human body. The *torus,* the energy field from the heartbeat, can be up to fifteen feet in diameter, as measured by magnetometers. Some research shows the entrainment effect on other human beings, and even on pets, such as dogs, with whom the subject practicing the HeartMath is associated.

HeartMath supplements the LENS neurofeedback in a marvelous way. While the LENS is basically a passive procedure, HeartMath is volitional. It is *something to practice.* Like any other biofeedback exercise, it rides on an autonomous physiological process—in this case the heartbeat and its variability. This can be measured and quantified with the Freeze-Framer to give an objective indication of how well the person is doing. The real goal, though, is to carry the practice of HeartMath into everyday life. *After all, our heart is always with us.* The biofeedback device is built into our own physiological responses and, after a while, is relatively easy to lock into.

In chapter 1, I mentioned that Ginny—the young Montessori teacher who had been shot in the head by a sociopathic killer—had been helped by HeartMath when she had come to a sort of plateau in her neurofeedback treatment. Even after her explosiveness (probably involving partial complex seizures) had abated, she often still found herself irritable and impatient around the children in her classes, and sometimes around other teachers. She was also still having bouts of insomnia, and occasional headaches.

Ginny took to the HeartMath process like a real natural, that is, in her first couple of sessions she was able to hit a fairly high entrainment level of 70 percent. This early success indicated that she would do very well as she became a more advanced practitioner. As she worked her way through the first half-dozen sessions, however, she soon saw that her heart rate varied enormously, depending on the amount of stress in her day. Sometimes it was rather smooth and easy to reach higher entrainment, and sometimes harder, as you can see on the charts on pages 314–15.

If there was a lot of disentrainment visible on the screen, we would pause the session and process the events of the day in a conversation. For example, one day an assistant teacher had treated Ginny disrespectfully and then walked off in a huff, failing to apologize. Ginny had come home upset, and then she and her mother had fought.

In our appointment, seeing the HeartMath disentrainment, we moved to the psychotherapeutic mode. We talked about Ginny's relationship to this person—and others like her—who have appeared in her life. Ginny made the observation that the teacher is kind of immature and does such things to everyone: she didn't need to take it personally. We replayed the

TWO MODALITIES OF BIOFEEDBACK (THE LENS AND HEARTMATH) WORK TOGETHER

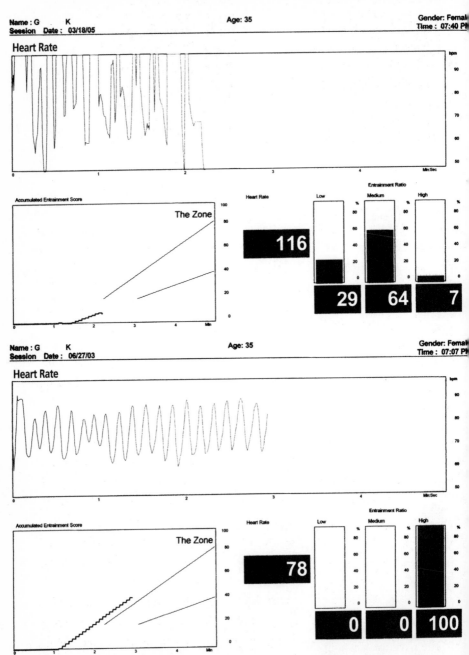

Fig. 12.1a. Two examples of HeartMath screens. Top: Ginny struggles with tachycardia (rapid heartbeat). Bottom: Ginny's heartbeat settles down. Compare the shape of the waves representing her heart rate variability in the two figures.

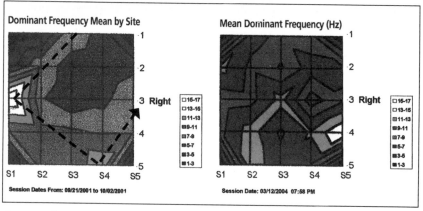

Fig. 12.1b. Two map LENS comparison, dominant frequency Ginny.
Left: Beginning of treatment, October 2001, amplitudes suppressed by
medication. Right: March 2004, Ginny is now off medication. Ginny's maps
show with uncanny precision the probable path of the bullet. This is evidenced
by the "hotspot" in the map on the left. While the map on the right looks
quieter, the clear "hotspot" in the lower right portion of the map indicates the
probable location of the bullet. See chapter 1 for a discussion of Ginny's case.

contretemps with her mother, and Ginny was able to laugh and state,
"There's no doubt about her love, but she gets me so mad!" Then we
resumed the HeartMath.

The results of the psychotherapeutic work were immediately visible
on the computer screen. Ginny had chosen one of the "games" instead
of straight biofeedback, in which the task is to fly a balloon over houses,
trees, and large stone walls. She did it magnificently, grinning softly, till
the balloon cleared everything, sailed past airplanes and fluffy clouds,
and began its scheduled descent among some cows in a pasture. I checked
the ratio of entrainment: 100 percent! This gave Ginny tangible proof
about how stress affects our bodies and our minds. Most important, she
had *learned a skill* that she can use as her stress levels rise.

By about the seventh HeartMath session (done right after the LENS),
Ginny gave a really good report: she was less irritable and was sleeping
better (if she found herself lying awake, she would practice HeartMath
and soon be asleep—something I have heard from other clients).

Ginny had the following to say about her experience with
HeartMath:

It has a definite calming effect. My emotions are more modulated, especially after I come in for my appointment on Friday night, tense from the week. After we do the LENS session, and then HeartMath, I feel so much better. When I'm in that state I find I can handle whatever happens much better. Of course, *it does still happen!* But I have realized that part of the stress is how I react to the stress itself. The HeartMath training helps me not to react, or to react much less. Of course sometimes I still do anyway, it depends on "how stressful the stress is."

At the point when I started therapy, when someone upset me I would have a huge fight with them. Now I react more rationally, rather than being emotional right away. The one area where I still have trouble is my mother. She comes at me charged with emotion. I find it difficult not to come back with the same intensity. But it's better than it was.

I was injured in 1998. I guess in the beginning I thought I would recover and be "back to normal" in a few months. At first it was very frustrating that I wasn't. Now, after seven years, I find it is emerging that I am *still recovering.* I don't have to be totally happy with myself the way I am *now,* or say "OK, this is how or who I am." I've come from *back then*—when I was banging into walls and yelling at everyone—to *now.* And I'm doing kind of OK. I have a full time job, and am a contributing member of society.

I think that at any time in making up our reality, we weigh possibilities: "I'd like this to be over, I'd like to be back to normal, thank you." Maybe that was kind of impatient of me. Nowadays I make little strides, and say, "That's OK, Ginny, you're doing fine."

We introduced another client to HeartMath after the LENS: Joe Rock, the Vietnam veteran whose case is cited earlier in this book. As Joe got better, with the help of the LENS neurofeedback and photonic stimulation, he found himself wanting to stretch his lifestyle more, especially with regard to sports and music. After training with HeartMath (as mentioned earlier) he was soon back to playing golf, a game he had been good at in the past. It was at that point that he was invited to join some musicians for a set and found he could readily keep up with them. He did the HeartMath not only daily, but each time before he played—golf or music. Soon his golf scores were dropping to where they had been before his tour of duty in Vietnam, and even lower. Coupled with this, he began playing music quite a bit.

Many other LENS clients also swear by the HeartMath practice. Our heart is always with us; the skill, once learned, uses the exquisite capabilities involved in the dance between the brain and the heart. The practice also fosters other qualities, which are metaphorically associated with the heart: emotional intelligence, perhaps chief among them, but also warmth, empathy, and compassion. I think of Ochwiay Biano talking to Dr. Jung. There is a *wisdom of the heart*: a different thinking organ in the body is involved in the processing of the world. It complements and supports our (poor, Faustian, frightened) brain.

LENS and the Photonic Stimulator

The photonic stimulator is a piece of equipment that provides modulated infrared light to stimulate nerves and muscles—as Len Ochs says, "It's just an infrared flashlight." The original instrument that intrigued Ochs was engineered by inventor Maurice Bales to energize and heal peripheral nerves and blood vessels. The effects were immediately visible on the CTI or Computer Thermal Imager, a much more complex piece of equipment that in a noninvasive way measures the temperature gradient of the entire body to thousandths of a degree. It can be used to spot neuropathies, ischemias, and when used on human breasts, early signs of breast cancer.

The dramatic effects the stimulator produces are visible to the camera: as blood vessels relax and expand, warmth in the part of the body treated goes up. Subsequent studies of the stimulation, generally active in the 8–900 nanometer range, show that it reaches down even to the mitochondrial level of cells.

Len Ochs encourages practitioners to use photonic stimulator as a useful adjunct to the LENS, especially for people with neuropathies, chronic pain, and fibromyalgia. He felt strongly enough about this that in 2004 he designed his own, more portable and less expensive machine, and saw it through to production. His rationale for using it for peripheral pain syndromes is that *a brain being bombarded by continual afferent pain* cannot focus or process information very well. The experience is sort of like a siren or a buzzer that won't turn off! The infrared stimulation is able to soothe chronic muscle spasticity that may have started with alarm signals from the brain; the brain is then reassured that it doesn't have to be so vigilant, enabling it to relax.

In the Bales machine, a wand attached to a console is moved over the body with an (invisible) infrared light coming out of its lens. A computer in the console allows you to set intensity of the stimulus and time. In Len Ochs own, far more portable version, a small, self-contained unit with its own lens and LED (light emitting diode) is passed over the injured areas (the clinician is responsible for keeping track of the time of the application and the intensity—the further away the unit is held from the body the weaker the stimulation. In relatively strong, robust people with an acute injury, many minutes of treatment may be used and are remarkably effective. On fibromyalgia, chronic fatigue, or Lyme patients, a few seconds might do just fine; with the wand just swept lightly over an aching limb, or even scalp, in the case of headache. (The treatment must be *always* modulated to the sensitivity of the client.)

Len Ochs on the Photonic Stimulator[3]

Psychology, as we learned in *Psych 101*, is concerned with human behavior/learning/adaptation. Humans adapt on many levels, from the microphysiological on upward. One view of pathology is that it's the process and state in which things are no longer adaptive. As psychologists become more sophisticated, we intervene with these maladaptive processes on more and more levels. We've gone from verbal interaction to EMDR (Francine Shapiro's Eye Movement Desensitization and Reprocessing) to desensitization (behavior modification), to visual and auditory stimulation, to biofeedback or neurofeedback reinforcement protocols, to Interactive Light Technology or photonic stimulation.

When we use infrared light, the stimulation is interactive with the person at the conscious level. The person reports reactions to the light stimulation: warming, pulsing, reductions in tension levels, reduction in pain levels. In using the photonic stimulator, we seek to match the exposure duration with the sensitivity of the individual. It is interactive in the sense that it is used to progressively desensitize the individual's hyper-reactivity to stimulation. It is at all times to be used within the behavioral context with humans (and in the reactive context with animals), rather than as a procedure in which the client is not conscious. Fundamentally, the way we use it is to retone various response systems of the body, so that the body learns to ameliorate its reactions to stimulation, allowing functioning to become flexible once again.

There is an art to the use of the photonic stimulator, which requires a clear assessment of the sensitivity of the individual, and a good understanding about the reactivity of the autonomic, neurovascular, and muscular reaction systems and how they respond to this kind of stimulation. Not only will each person's reactions be different, but a person's reactions will also change from one time to another. The clinician must be aware of differences in reactivity and be able to switch approaches, locations for applying stimulation, and exposure durations.

As pain abates, the clinician will need to be familiar and comfortable not only with changes in physical status and function but also with changes in consciousness (both cognitive and emotive), such as increasing ease, increasing clarity, brightness and sharpness of visual and (perhaps even imaginal) field, as well as decreasing mental fog. In addition to needing to be aware that dream processes and sensory acuity can reestablish themselves, the clinician needs to be familiar with energy in all its contexts. When the amount of energy exceeds the person's ability to use it, it can appear as anxiety, rumination, worry, hyperactivity, restlessness, gastrointestinal problems, or even as the tendency to make up for lost time, and increasing one's activities in an excessive fashion, as a result.

Thus, it seems much more reasonable for photonic stimulation to be provided by a psychologist or another behaviorally-trained clinician (one who is accustomed to taking time with the client to provide a context for experience), than to rely on medically trained individuals who may mechanically plunge clients into new ways of functioning. On the other hand, clinicians who are more psychotherapeutically trained will need background training in the different physical systems to better understand how to apply the Interactive Light Technology to human and animal lives.

Stephen Larsen Discusses the Photonic Stimulator

We got our first Bales Photonic Stimulator in 2002. It was not inexpensive (about $6,500), and I wondered if it was an extravagance. I didn't really know how to use it but followed Len Ochs's instructions. Immediately we had some successes. Following Len's advice, I tried it on my jaw after extensive dental surgery. The surgeon spontaneously volunteered that he had never seen such fast healing. In short order, a friend with agonizing back spasms that had kept him immobilized for days was up and walking about after a single, thorough, treatment on the affected area.

Then, a participant in one of our dream groups complained that diabetes was in his family, his own feet now had serious circulation problems, and his doctor had told him, in his genteel way, that "if your feet don't get better, I'm gonna have to cut 'em off!" After two treatments, this man's feet were no longer blue and the feeling in them came back (and he was "allowed" to keep his feet!). At the same time, an art therapist in one of our training groups was depressed because a muscle

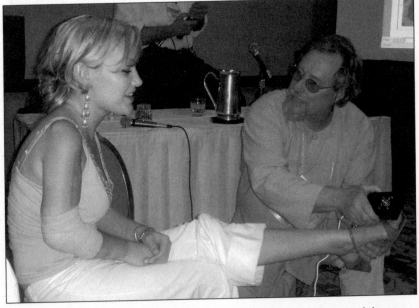

Fig. 12.2. *Stephen Larsen demonstrates, with Julie Beasley, the use of the new LENS Photonic Stimulator in a LENS Training Seminar at the Association for Applied Psychophysiology and Biofeedback, Austin, Texas.*

Courtesy of Julie Beasley; R. Larsen

spasm at the bottom of one foot kept her in agony. Before her (probably stress-induced) lameness, she had loved to walk long miles each weekend in the country. After a single ten-minute treatment with the photonic stimulator, she reported that she was again able to walk distances without pain.

These experiences gave our "magic wand" (the infrared light applicator) quite a reputation. Wary of placebo effect, I decided to try it out on horses and dogs. It worked equal wonders. Probably the most dramatic was with a fifteen-hundred-pound "killer" horse, who, since a bad head injury acquired on a botched steeplechase jump, had been very aggressive to his handlers. I couldn't approach the horse because of the possibility of being attacked by him, so, I held the body of the instrument, a couple of yards away, while the owner, acting like he was doing ordinary "grooming," applied the wand (with the LED) around his neck and head. After five minutes, the big guy sighed, put his head down, and let anybody who wanted to approach. The horse then preened his neck in the direction of the little glowing wand, as if he were saying: "More, more, give me more!" The owner reported that he continued to be much mellower after the treatment. Dogs with spinal injuries, and other traumas, also respond well, despite the disclaimer that dog hair is hard to penetrate with infrared light.

We have, however, also experienced overdose reactions. TBI and fibromyalgia patients were at times stiffer and more in pain after the treatments. The treated body parts sometimes warmed up or throbbed painfully. But ultimately, after a couple of hours, or rarely, days, they usually seemed better.

The overdoses have taught us that there can be enormous differences in the level of treatment required by different people. Some can take no more than a light brushing of a few seconds over all their limbs, or their finger and toenail beds, while others can take up to forty minutes of an intense, slow-moving application all over an afflicted area and feel much better for it. The same patient can respond well to *a lot of stimulation on one body part, and very little on another.*

These experiences testify to the importance of being aware of the several kinds of potential sensitivity that an individual client may have. This was stressed by Len Ochs in his advice to LENS practitioners who include photonic stimulation in their repertoire of treatments.

Adam, one of our teenage clients with ADD, who was helped in his concentration by the LENS, also was growing so fast that his feet and knees were always intensely uncomfortable (a well-known problem called Osgood-Schlatter's syndrome—or "growing pains"). During the course of our treatment, his feet did indeed expand from an impressive size 11 to an awesome 13. After the photonic treatments, given at the same time as his weekly EEG sessions, he would relay that the pain had disappeared almost completely, gradually building up again over the week—until the next treatment eased it again. In this way, he was able to get over most of the months the Osgood-Schlatter's lasted, with ameliorated pain. Adam came to call the photonic stimulator "The God Machine," and there could be no doubt that he definitely looked forward to its application on his afflicted (but always growing) lower extremities.

The LENS and the Interactive Metronome

We were first introduced to the Interactive Metronome (IM) by a master practitioner, Rodney Lindquist. For some time I had been looking for something to help with the processing problems of ADD and ADHD children and adults, which had to do with *planning, sequencing,* and *organizing.* Even in a brain that is balanced and regulated through the LENS, these important pacemakers may need to be fine-tuned. Since we live in a *temporal flux,* a flow of time, and all our activities are choreographed temporally, we need to be able to put things in their proper order, one after the other, for them to make sense or be practically useful. Rodney told us the Interactive Metronome would provide just the right kind of training for this.

He turned out to be 100 percent correct!

The Interactive Metronome was devised by James Cassily, a young rock and jazz musician who was looking for a way to help musicians "cook," that is play "in the zone." When musicians are in the zone, long, complicated pieces seem easy, and the audience is totally entranced. Some years of development resulted in the Interactive Metronome, a feedback device that lets one know, within *thousandths of a second,* whether one is on the beat or not. The brain relies upon such precise timings to coordinate its complex activities. Thus, this training seems to help a multitude of timing-related tasks.

Training first himself, and then friends and family, he noticed that the IM training, as it came to be called, translated not only to improved performance by musicians of whatever persuasion but also resulted in overall benefits *that were totally unexpected.* Cassily discovered that IM trainees were reporting astonishing improvement in a variety of things. They were organizing and prioritizing better. They were less impulsive, more able to pay attention. They were better coordinated.

Furthermore, as Rodney Lindquist had told us, the IM could be used diagnostically. Because the software could measure so precisely, we could literally see where people were on or off their "game." People with poor timing often muffed social cues; they approached, and organized tasks, poorly.

Injuries from TBI or "mild closed head injury" are relatively easy to spot with a simple five-minute diagnostic. Put on the training tasks, a very few repetitions for the head-injured can bring fatigue, as they try to get damaged circuits to work normally. The same thing happens with ADD sufferers whose attention wobbles when they are asked to hold to a repetitive precision task. Their errors, of being either anticipatory or tardy, are often up in the 500 millisecond range (compared to 30–40 milliseconds for normals).

People who have inner splits, "dissociative disorder," or "multiple personalities," as they sometimes are called, also have very high scores. It is almost as if each "subpersonality" has a different pattern within the nervous system (including different allergies, or addictions) thus "switching" between them can produce the processing-delays. The IM leaves no doubt that they are suffering from a neurological problem. The IM is also very good at measuring impulse-control and anger problems. In these cases, the scores are almost always heavily weighted in the "anticipatory" category: they jump the gun and keep jumping it!

Sam: A Case of Cerebral Palsy

The role that the IM can play in healing is well demonstrated by the case of Sam, a young man born with cerebral palsy. Though his parents had done an amazing job with the therapies and other remediations they applied, he was always a little precarious in school. Although he was very bright, he was shy and daydreamy. When he was transferred from a smaller to a larger school because his parents moved, he wilted.

Later, at a large university in Boston, Sam felt overwhelmed and fell apart, right in the middle of his senior year. Inattentive ADD, secondary to the CP, and severe anxiety problems were diagnosed. He was put on Prozac, which didn't seem to help much. Ritalin was tried, but discontinued because he got very anxious while on it. However, a few months of the LENS treatments restored Sam's functionality. While living at home, he was able to take a course or two at a time at a college that had a credit transfer option with his university, and get As in them! Finally, he finished his last course and was able to graduate. Still, he sat at home and played with the family's pets, didn't socialize much, and seemed to be slipping back again, in the eyes of his very attentive mother.

We decided to try IM. At first Sam, who was kind of weak-limbed and uncoordinated, was resistant. The results of the first session indicated he had some problems in sequencing and organizing but his scores weren't too bad. Asked to do longer training sessions, he complained vociferously and got obviously tired. But after about five or six sessions, he was doing 100 and then 120 repetitions of thirteen exercises, with very good scores!

One day, Sam's mother called our center to ask: "What are you doing?" She was unaware that we had added another biofeedback modality, the IM, to Sam's treatment. "He's much more social, and involved, thinking on his feet, and appropriate. This is amazing!" And Sam continues to make progress, both on the IM and in life. He often drives the ninety miles or so each way to his appointments, through hectic New York traffic and on the NY Thruway. Perhaps more importantly, Sam's sense of humor and social presence are palpable. As of this past year he has applied to several graduate schools in—of all disciplines—psychology. His goal, as he says, is "to help others, as he has been helped." (See www.interactivemetronome.com. and the Resources section).

LENS and Deep Vascular Relaxation

Deep Vascular Relaxation (DVR) is an efficient and simple way to dilate surface vasculature and to comfort oneself. Surface vasodilation is useful for reducing or eliminating migraines and other vascular pain (that is, pain of a throbbing nature) by increasing the blood volume in an area of the body away from the pain. Comfort is increased in relation to sadness, hurt, and anger, by directing increases in blood volume to the center part of the chest.

Blood flow is directed to a spot by noticing any sensation in that spot on the body's surface. Some years ago Len Ochs developed a set of suggestions to maximize the directing of blood flow so that people with migraines could gain relief. In brief, they are as follows:

- First attend to the sensation of the movement of the chest as you breathe.
- If warmth or tingling is observed, move the attention to the shoulders and notice what happens to the warmth.
- If the warmth spreads, successively move attention to the feeling of the presence of the next set of joints, increasingly further away from the chest, each time waiting for the warmth to spread.
- Moving the blood volume away from throbbing pain decreases that pain. Starting with the center part of the chest rapidly increases comfort by touching the heart with your own attention.*

We have found that DVR is useful as an adjunct to the LENS approach, not only for clients who suffer from migraines, but also for clients with a variety of other problems. It gives them a tool for increasing comfort should difficult times be encountered in between sessions.

The LENS and Nutritional Support

If we are to set the nervous system to work to repair itself, the raw materials, the "building-blocks," must be present for the healing process to really work. This means nourishment and support not only for neurons but also the scaffolding of glia that supports them, the many neurotransmitter pathways and channels through the brain, as well as the ability to synthesize neurotransmitters themselves. We have found that a number of vitamins and supplements, or "nutraceuticals," are helpful to this process.

As people begin neurofeedback or biofeedback, we say something

---

*The full instructions for this procedure are offered as a free informational service on Ochs's Web site, http://migrainehelpers.com. Much more information is available at the Web site, some for free and some for a fee.

like this: Suppose you had a team of excellent workmen lined up for a major reconstruction job—that would make your place look spanking-new. The workers arrive with their tools, and they are just as skilled as promised, but there are no building materials to work with. . . .

Our experience has been that if ADD kids aren't getting better with our treatments, or anxious, insomniac teenagers aren't responding, check their diets.

The SAD (Standard American Diet) is notoriously lacking in essential nutrients—from an agriculture that relies on inorganic, nitrogen (chemical-based) fertilizers, the dyes and preservatives added, to long shelf lives, to the processing and bleaching of natural grains such as wheat or rice. (Welcome to the wonderful land of empty calories!) Then there is the specter of genetically-modified fruits and vegetables, and hormonally-loaded meat and dairy animals—not to mention such suspected neurotoxins as aspartame, appearing in many commercial soft drinks, and that has been implicated in a bewildering variety of CNS symptoms, including hallucinations and seizures in airline pilots, who use the caffeine in such products to keep awake.

A healthful human diet includes organic fruits and vegetables, nuts, fish, and animal protein from animals raised without steroids and antibiotics, and slaughtered in humane ways. Since few people have access to a consistent intake of such nutritional substances, supplementation is usually required. Whenever possible, organically derived vitamins and supplements are preferred over synthetic vitamins.

The B vitamin family is probably the most important of the vitamins for the regulation of the nervous system. All parts of the "family" serve important purposes, but the B-complex vitamin should, of course, contain thiamin, niacin, cobalamin, and folic acid, along with pantothenic acid. (Life Extension has a good composite B vitamin, as does a company called Bio-Strath, based in Switzerland, whose extremely high quality formula has measurable effects on ADD in schoolchildren, and on stamina, focus, and performance in world-class athletes. Please see www.naturesanswer.com for more information; see also the Resources section.)

Omega 3 fatty acids (sometimes, in the best formulas, along with long-chain Omega 6s and 9s and usually based on fish and flaxseed oils), are as *good* for us as trans-fats (found in much American fast food) are *bad.* The presence of these more viable lipids allows for pliable neuronal cell walls and a more flexible nervous system—whereas the trans-fats found in much commercially deep-fried foods interfere with the permeability and pliability of neuronal tissue. The nervous system becomes brittle and unresponsive. The owner of the nervous system (say an American teenager who lives on "fast food") may become mentally sluggish, wildly volatile, or a combination of the above—and on a schedule probably not unrelated to the intake of food.

Vitamins C and E are more effective antioxidants (sponging up deleterious free radicals) when taken together than either alone. With the addition of beta-carotene, they form an extremely potent antioxidant combination. For the vitamin E to do its work across the cerebrospinal barrier, and take out dangerous free radicals that cause damage to brain tissue, it must contain gamma tocopherols as well as tocotrienols. Blueberries and strawberries are good natural sources of gamma tocopherols.

The use of SAM-e (S Adenosyl Methionine) can address many problems at one time. It is useful for depression, for osteoarthritis (affecting joint connective tissue), and liver problems. Extremely high doses of SAM-e (up to 4000 mg/day) can be very helpful for degenerative diseases such as Parkinson's or chronic conditions such as fibromyalgia. (See *Stop Depression Now,* Dr. Richard Brown's informative book on SAM-e.)[4]

The use of adaptogens such as Rosavin (Rhodiola Rosea) from the former Soviet Union can be immensely helpful in empowering the body's mitochondrial sources of energy, the fluctuations in which affect mood and the energy, which includes, of course, mental energy. The meaning of *adaptogen* is that if your motor is running a little fast, it helps you slow down. If you're too slow, it helps you speed up a bit. It helps you take things in your stride. Up until the last decade or so, the USSR was keeping Rhodiola (and associated compounds) as a carefully guarded secret, because it gave their athletes, astronauts, and military personnel an edge. (See also Dr. Richard Brown's book: *The Rhodiola Revolution.*)[5]

Recently, working with a nutritionist, we have started some of our patients on *glyconutritionals,* sugar-based nutrients that actually can help diabetics! Five of the sugars represented—mannatose, ambrotose, galactose, fucose, xylose, n-acetyl-glucosamine, n-acetyl galactosamine, and n-acetyl-neuraminic acid—are also found in mothers milk and are part of the explanation for why nursed babies are so healthy and immune.

The sugar molecules give a *cellular language* to the body so that it can identify and respond actively to the larger, more cumbersome proteins (amino acids) and fats (phospholipids.)

Glyconutritionals, usually in the form of aloe-derived monosaccharides, are especially helpful in all kinds of autoimmune problems, including irritable bowel and ulcerative colitis, as well as allergies and asthma, hives, shingles etc. In these disorders, in which people's immune systems literally attack their own body as if it were a dangerous invader, the discrimination of "self" versus "not-self," becomes crucial. The monosaccharides seem to help the body become more internally intelligent—which is also the goal of biofeedback. When the energy people have wasted attacking their own physiology is made available to them through this new self-efficiency, it flowers into all the things *they want to do* in life—the results are comparable to good neurofeedback, and definitely enhance them. Due to their more efficient operation, people have more energy for creativity and for pleasure. (More can be read at glycoscience.org.)[6]

LENS and the Art of Living (Sudarshan Kriya Yoga)

In 2001, the author was initiated into the discipline of *Sudarshan Kriya Yoga,* an international movement, also called *The Art of Living,* whose members follow the guru, Sri Sri Ravi Shankar. It involves very intensive breathing practices, asanas (postures), and meditation, along with a very effective program of community service, and mounting effective volunteer programs to help with disasters like 9/11 and the *tsunami.* The breathing practices, or *kriyas,* in particular, have profound effects upon brain chemistry and the induction of hypocapnia (based on the relationship O2 and CO2 in the blood) through hyperventilation. The method is also associated with theta states, and recovery of unconscious or repressed materials, as well as powerful catharses, or religious experiences—often experienced during the breathings.

Wanting to see what the physiology of the yoga practices were, I attached myself to a HeartMath *Freeze-Framer* (a biofeedback device) while doing the *kriya,* a full rapid breathing workout. It showed that the effect on the heart was profound. Instead of seeing the familiar sine waves of entrainment, I saw jagged, rapid, high amplitude waves. After the *kriya,* as I sat there breathing normally, my heartbeat gradually calmed down.

As I settled into the more familiar breath pattern for HeartMath, about six breaths per minute, diaphragmatically controlled, extremely high amplitude sine waves began to make their appearance. As I quieted more, the familiar Heart Rate Variability waves appeared, extremely regulated. I felt peaceful, but centered.

Soon after this experience I had an insight: Aha! The rapid breathing of the kriya yoga practice is a *disentrainment* process. Like the LENS, it stimulates and makes things chaotic for a while. Then the intrinsic health and wisdom of the body is reasserted, and the person returns to *an enhanced normalcy,* in which energy is flowing, but the person is calm and mentally clear.

Dr. Richard Brown, our colleague mentioned earlier, is an Art of Living instructor who has made referrals to us, which has enabled us to see dozens of people benefit from the kriya yoga practices, integrated into a wellness program that includes neurofeedback/biofeedback and nutritional support. Sometimes Dr. Brown will refer patients to us for LENS or HeartMath *before they do the kriya,* so that their nervous systems will be in balance when they do the more strenuous practices. (The initial beginner's practice is an obligatory five day, five hours a day intensive, involving a number of practices, but centered on the breathing. There are also advanced courses. See www.artofliving.org)

LENS and Qi Gong

Qi gong is an ancient Chinese energy practice. It is actually the root, not only of traditional Chinese medicine but also of *tai chi chuan, kung fu,* and various other Oriental martial arts. The practice includes meditation, visualization, and extremely slow movements, coordinated with breathing. The goal is *to be able to move the subtle energies of the body* volitionally, and as the occasion warrants.

Dan was a very depressed man in his midthirties, who had been hospitalized several times and placed on every possible medicine, singly and in combination. He was also what we call a "flatliner," someone whose brain wave amplitudes were *very low,* and with little energy.

We had done over forty sessions on Dan without much improvement at all, although he had been able to get off all medications. One nice day, feeling frustrated with his lack of progress, and on a hunch, I invited him onto my deck to try some qi gong. He took to it immediately, and at his next session, a week later, reported he had been doing it every day. Almost imperceptibly at first, we saw his depression lift. Then he found a qi gong teacher and began taking classes and practicing more intensively. Within three months his depression had lifted completely, and a two-year follow up found Dan doing well in graduate school.

More recently, a patient too sensitive to respond to the LENS—he improved slightly, then plateaued on the lowest of treatments—responded instantly when taught some elementary qi gong exercises. Again, he practiced every day and continued seeing undeniable improvements.

Recently, *Time, Newsweek,* and *National Geographic* have all looked at what it takes to age gracefully. Outstanding among the world's cultures are the Georgians (from an Eastern area of former USSR) who drink coffee, wine, sometimes smoke tobacco, but also eat lots of almonds and apricots (very little if any refined flour or bread), in addition to walking up and down steep hillsides every day, do hard physical labor, and take Rhodiola Rosea. Another is the Chinese, who can be seen in parks all around China—and particularly Okinawa, doing *tai chi* and *qi gong,* at the break of day. Clearly there is benefit to controlled diaphragmatic breathing and slow movements. Studies show that elders who take up *tai chi* have improved balance, are less likely to fall, are more flexible, and have enhanced productivity in general.

LENS and Open Focus

Open Focus is a method developed by one of the senior brain wave researchers in the country, Dr. Les Fehmi. Based on his considerable knowledge of Zen and meditation practices, he developed Open Focus as an art of meditation that *can be utilized every day, any time, in everyday life.* It is a technique of opening awareness softly to include the felt presence of the body in time and space, in its surroundings. In this technique, relaxation and focus are equally supported and maintained.

Fehmi associates Open Focus with *good alpha,* synchronized across the hemispheres and lobes of the brain, and an effortlessness of functioning, which seems entirely comparable to the effects of the LENS. Jim Robbins, in *A Symphony in the Brain,* says that Fehmi's protocol induced in him one of the most profound states of his life, and that the effortlessness and ease of functioning accompanied him for days after the experience. For him, it was one of the unmistakable proofs that neurofeedback *works*. My wife Robin and I have had similar experiences, training with Fehmi and his wife Susan Shor at their Princeton Biofeedback Center. During our first in-depth training, we both had an almost identical dream the same night and noticed ourselves in unusual, well, synchrony—Fehmi's hallmark—a rather delightful resonance with each other.

At Stone Mountain Center, we have taught people Open Focus techniques, and had them listen to Open Focus tapes at home, for many years. Open Focus is another discipline of consciousness that can be learned on biofeedback machines, and then used spontaneously in all kinds of different life situations. The author is also convinced that when clinicians practice Open Focus techniques, their sensitivity to all kinds of useful signs and clues from their clients is enhanced. (See www.openfocus.com. and the Resources section.)

Is there a kind of *lingua franca* for the brain, an alphabet, the key to its *generative grammar* as Noam Chomsky calls it? Psychotherapy looks for ways to talk to the psyche, so there is less inner disharmony; neurofeedback uses its grammar of EEG *frequency* to talk to the nervous system, so it becomes more calm and yet resilient. We hope we have shown you how the LENS may indeed facilitate this latter goal of CNS quieting—thereby also aiding all dimensions of our psyche—and even our capacities for transcendence and optimal performance.

In the next chapter we take a few conceptual leaps—but perhaps you are ready for them now, with the talk of energy fields and esoteric practices like yoga and qi gong. The bold premise of our next chapter is that the recent work with the LENS comments on the entire paradigm of how we conceive of mind, body, energy-body, and spirit.

SPECULATIONS ON PHYSICS, ENERGY PSYCHOLOGY, CHAOS THEORY, AND MAGNETITE IN THE BRAIN

Stephen Larsen, Ph.D., and Evelyn Soehner, M.A.

In their earliest manifestations, some novel phenomena appear weak, ill-defined, and hardly more significant than the background noise against which they stand out. The Wrights struggled to stay airborne for a few seconds, as Marconi strained to hear the first wireless radio transmission, or Joseph Niepce peered to discern the faint image of the first photograph. All were threshold phenomena initially. Equally, these embryonic phenomena are feeble and vulnerable to early extinction, just as living embryos are precarious and defenseless. The nailed boot of scientific derision alone may be enough to trample the life out of such delicate seedlings.

RICHARD MILTON IN *ALTERNATIVE SCIENCE*

In his paradigm-challenging book, quoted above, Milton does an incisive job of showing how important discoveries are often made by visionary amateurs, working in home laboratories or workshops, rather than in established and powerful research institutions. This also seems to be the case with biofeedback in general, and the LENS in particular. No large business or funding sources have (yet) identified the economic value of biofeedback methods to themselves, and so they have overlooked the immense potential benefit they hold for humanity.

That hasn't, however, stopped men and women of integrity, usually clinicians, from continuing to help people, and carefully documenting the effects of what they do, *in the best application of the scientific method to their limited economic and institutional situations*: studying single cases or a few cases at a time. As we have seen, much of the LENS work—after a brilliant combining of electronic, computer programming, and clinical skills—has been developed by clinicians treating themselves, their families, their friends, and their clients. The phenomenon is so robust that experimental evidence will ultimately accumulate, for the reasons mentioned throughout this text, until some graduate student will not be able to resist such a plum, ripe for picking. Such a study has the potential of making an academic reputation (or ruining it, if the old-paradigm thought-police turn their radar on it!).

In the meantime, LENS practitioners are often scoffed at by conventional scientists, neurologists, psychiatrists, and even our own neurofeedback peers. Probably what most bugs scientific materialists, and even *neurofeedback fundamentalists* about the LENS is that they can't figure out how wisps of information, carried on waves in the radio frequency range, at extremely weak levels, can have *any effect* on the brain whatsoever. (They also don't understand how an effect can happen when the person isn't *trying to do anything*.) And yet the reality of what LENS clinicians encounter every day leaves us no doubt about what already shows up in the preliminary studies, and would show up in the larger ones, could they be funded: these tiny doses of textured energy evoke astounding and beneficial results!

One class of people who have no trouble at all reconciling the smallness of the LENS stimuli to their profound effects seem to be the quantum physicists, who are used to tiny bundles of energy appearing unexpectedly: muons, mesons, neutrinos, positrons, charmed quarks, and the like. Physicists, unlike social scientists, are introduced to the principle of *paradoxicality* (the idea, for example that light can be made of waves or particles, depending upon the method used to investigate it) at a fairly early point in their education.

These people have trained themselves to know that we live in a seething sea of energy, only the smallest portion of which is available to our senses or even to our most refined instruments, and that the manner of observing the energy continuum changes it, as in Heisenberg's *uncertainty principle* in which it is established that the method used to probe a physical system or energy itself cannot be excluded from the finding—the observer must be included! They also know that in dynamical chaotic systems, *tiny stimuli can have huge effects,* just as in the geophysical weather system, where, according to *chaos theory,* the butterfly's fluttering in Central America could cause the typhoon in Japan!

Throughout this book, we have been stressing the principle that, *when dealing with intelligent, resonant, self-rectifying systems, tiny stimuli produce large results.* But the converse is also true: *when dealing with intelligent, resonant, and self-rectifying systems, increasingly large or forceful stimuli freeze the system up.* This principle has evolved concurrently with the development of the LENS, and we offer it as a central, paradigmatic insight to perceptive physicians and pharmacologists, as well as occupational therapists, massage therapists, psychotherapists, and energy healers: *less is sometimes more.* Stimuli that don't mobilize massive resistance are more likely to initiate a positive resonance in the system, based more on invitation than coercion. Just imagine how we respond to an aggressive jerk on the arm, rather than a gentle or seductive pull!

Why should we think of the sensitive, self-rectifying subsystems *of which we are made,* as being different from the "I," the *metasystem that we are?* How can a self-respecting science, such as social science or psychiatry, systematically ignore chaos theory, paradoxicality, resonance effects, and the behavior of living dynamical systems, in its picture of humanity and its mental health or illness? Human beings are more complex than elementary particles—being made up of galactic formations of them!

In this chapter, we bring in the insights of some leading contemporary thinkers about the nature of energy and cosmos, to make the mechanisms of the mysterious LENS just a little more comprehensible. First, however, we shall take a historical look at how the current *chemistry*-based paradigm of Western medicine gained its ascendancy over a long-standing tradition of *energy*-based medical modalities.

The Politics of Energy and Matter (Physics and Chemistry)

Around the end of the nineteenth and beginning of the twentieth century, a kind of *paradigm coup* took place, in which one subcategory of a number of flourishing types of medicine took over and instituted what can be described as an *orthodoxy of healing*. This orthodoxy is called "the medical model," or sometimes "allopathic medicine" to distinguish it from its strongest rivals—"homeopathic medicine" and "naturopathic medicine"—which came to be portrayed, by the dominant paradigm, as "primitive," even fraudulent, prescientific models. The new medicine was based on modern chemistry. It dictated that all biologically active medicines should be prescribed by physicians, should be of pharmaceutically measurable proportions, and should be subjected to experimental trials on animals, and then on humans.

All other modalities were to be shunned, especially the *vitalist* approaches that talked about working with the *energy or structure of the body*, rather than its chemistry. From the manipulations of chiropractors or osteopaths, to the use of energy devices in connection with the body, any healing approaches based on *physics* were rejected. In the new medical realm *chemistry* was king.

Prior to this, the field of energy medicine had a historical momentum, dating back to Greek and Roman times, when physicians had systematically applied electric eels (of the *torpedo* variety) to emperors and common folk alike, for pain relief and to speed bone healing. In China, the ancient practice of qi gong—utilizing energy generated in the nervous systems of the healers themselves—evolved into meridian-based acupuncture, redirecting and balancing the patient's own *qi,* or "chi."

At the beginning of the twentieth century in America the Carnegie Endowment had made funds available to look into *electromedicine*. In fact, forays into the use of electricity for pain relief, healing, and bone knitting had been going on for some time. As far back as 1812, electrical currents were used to accelerate the healing of broken bones. In 1816 electro-acupuncture was evaluated and regarded as successful by Berlioz, shortly followed by Sarlandier's work, which confirmed the principle: DC (direct current) electricity runs through the body through corridors that offer less resistance (greater conductance), and have effects on health. In the early 1900s Frazee was showing that electrostimulation through aquarium water helped salamanders regenerate limbs.[1] I remember finding an old electrical stimulation apparatus in my grandfather's house, which he used for his arthritis (you held onto handles, put a plate on the affected area, and got someone to turn a little crank).

But 1909 saw the publication of *The Flexner Report*; based on superficial and already prejudiced criteria, it dismissed the *entire field* of energy healing as "without merit." It said, in effect, that "energy medicine" didn't exist. This, of course, then became the official opinion of the American Medical Association, the guild that serves physicians and promotes their interests. At around the same time, in an attempt to "modernize medicine," the Chinese emperor forbade acupuncture and Traditional Chinese Medicine (TCM), in favor of the Western medical model. But the traditional practitioners of China, known as *barefoot doctors,* had also studied Taoism and knew how to "play ball on running water." They just went right on practicing, inconspicuously, and millions of people continued to be helped by their methods over the three decades until the "People's Revolution," when Maoism became the main political force in China, and the "peoples medicine" (TCM) was back, again, big time.

Meanwhile, the West didn't fare so well. The American Medical Association, backed by the burgeoning pharmaceutical companies, tried to make their coup complete. In nineteenth-century America a cornucopia of folk diagnostic and healing methods had been popular, including medical intuitives, dowsing, pendulums used over the body (*radiesthesia*), but also prayer, and "laying on of hands," as well as methods of electrostimulation. All of these types of healing were declared to be *quackery*.

The to-be-excluded methods also included chiropractic and osteopathy (*physics-based* modalities involving the physical manipulation of bone structure and connective tissue to facilitate the flow of the natural energies of the body).

But practitioners in these two guilds made a formidable organized and legal comeback over the early part of the twentieth century, proving to legislative bodies that their methods were beneficial to people, and were also based on science. They successfully advocated for the position that doctorates in their professions should entitle practitioners to at least some of the privileges granted to medical doctors.

Some of the other modalities, however, fared less well: laying on of hands, pendulum usage or "dowsing" of any kind over the person's body, diagnosis by medical intuitives, psychic reading or healing, and *radionics* (homeopathic-like preparations infused by vibrations in a

BIZARRO/By Piraro

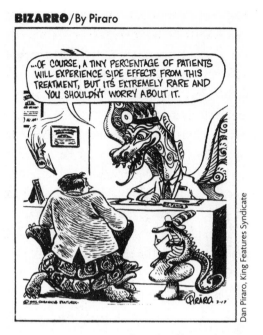

Fig. 13.1. A commentary on the side effects of medication

machine) were proscribed by the medical profession's Rules of Ethical Conduct: if it were discovered that a practitioner had used them, it could lead to professional disgrace, disbarring or even arrest.

Casualties of the paradigm coup abound on every side, so that *iatrogenic* illness (and death) has become an epidemiological fact of our time. Thus it is whenever fixed ideas, or a "hidden agenda," prevails, and the free and open inquiry that is the true hallmark of science is attacked.

In essence, the chemical fundamentalists are ignoring the implications of modern physics. The chemical-pharmaceutical paradigm is as leaky as it is lethal, as fragile as it is formidable. There is no question that it works, and also at times saves life, as well as improving the quality of life for some people. But its manner of use, and the *unconscious* physics-based paradigm behind it—if it doesn't work *use more, and then more force*—is Newtonian. So is a science that only relies on the *nomothetic*, the responses of large numbers of subjects in an experiment, rather than observing the unique *ideographic* effect of *a particular medicine on a particular, unique* psyche/soma (a person).

Nomothetically informed medicine, consciously or unconsciously held, misses the boat of personal treatment totally. Patients come in one at a time, not in diagnostically assigned groups. People live as people, not categories, and need to be understood, not castigated, even when they don't respond well to medicines that seem to work fine for others—or are treated at doses that work fine for 80 percent of the population—but not the neurologically sensitive 20 percent.

In all fairness, the electrical devices that the Flexner report evaluated in 1909 were relatively crude, because of the primitive state of electronics at that time, and most energy healers could only claim clinical, not experimental, successes. The century-old Flexner dismissal, whose influence still prevails, was long before the exquisite and amazing discoveries in solid-state circuitry, and the ability to measure, pulse, titrate, diffuse, or concentrate, electrical currents and fields in all kinds of ways never previously imaginable.

Some of the technical devices made possible by the amazing discoveries of modern physics—such as X rays, the EEG, CAT scans, MRIs, PET scans, chromatography, lasers, and electron microscopy—*are* certainly employed by modern medicine. But *for diagnostics only!* In the realms of healing, the energy devices of physics are curiously lacking. Still, one of the few energy procedures that falls within the scope of modern medical practice is a curiously medieval one: ECT or electro-convulsive therapy, in which a powerful electrical current is run through the brain until the person convulses (in recent times the grosser aspects of the seizure are controlled by anticonvulsant medication—now, *that's* progress).

Energy Medicine

The understanding of our multidimensional nature and the application of subtle energetic medical approaches will allow medicine to evolve beyond its present-day need for drugs and surgery to less traumatic and more natural systems of healing. In addition, the recognition of our relationship to these higher frequency energy systems will ultimately lead to a fusion of religion and science as scientists begin to recognize the spiritual dimension of human beings and the laws of expression of the life-force. The trend of "holism" in medicine will ultimately move physicians toward the recognition that, for human beings

to experience health, they must enjoy an integrated relationship
between body, mind, and spirit.

RICHARD GERBER, *VIBRATIONAL MEDICINE*[2]

Once again the music is changing, and the exiled healing modalities are now coming back, dancing and slinking like tai chi masters through the cracks in the cultural paradigm: Acupuncture, Shiatsu, Ang-ma (originally from China), Qi Gong, Ayurveda, Reiki, Foot Reflexology, Thought-field Therapy, "post-Reichian" therapies such as Bioenergetics (even though Reich was imprisoned and died in jail for talking about Cosmic Orgone Energy). Many physicians writhe with agony and disdain as their clients casually talk about visits to their Reiki master or medical intuitive (while still visiting the medical doctor for good measure).

A new reincarnation called "Energy Medicine" seeks to provide an umbrella of common legitimacy to them all. Attempting to define the field, Edgar Wilson writes: "At its most primitive level, energy acts through electromagnetic potentials generated across cell membranes and at tissue interfaces producing excitability, rhythmicity, and conductivity through directed ionic potentials of the DNA-governed molecular substrate."[3]

One representative of these possibilities is the TENS (Transcutaneous Electrical Nerve Stimulator) machine, a prototype of which had existed during the 1850s, but disappeared with the paradigm coup. It was reintroduced to the public market in the 1970s (after a period of sixty to seventy years during which the public suffered without a potentially helpful tool, due to prejudice). During the 1980s and '90s the government, through the FDA, tried to revoke the licenses of manufacturers of electro-stimulation devices such as the TENS and force them to take their machines off the market. But the manufacturers fought back and held the government to a stalemate. At last TENS was placed into a peculiar, "grandfathered" realm, which it shared with the far-more-extreme ECT. (I guess if running *big* currents right through the brain is ok, then running much *smaller* currents through other selected areas of the body might be ok!)

The innovation that has made the electro-stim principle used in the TENS a much more useful tool for addressing all kinds of problems was the discovery of the *current of injury*, a much tinier current than TENS technology used, *based on the body's own electricity*. Beginning in the 1950s, Dr. Robert Becker's work, through his book *The Body Electric* and other publications, showed how vast was the neglect of the energy domain in medicine. His discovery relates paradigmatically to the theme of this book, in that electro-stim technology also found that *less is more*: the more delicate, refined currents of *alpha-stim* worked better and kept their usefulness much longer than those of the larger, coarser TENS.

Meanwhile, not all the world was as committed to the new pharmaceutical fundamentalism as America. In the 1960s Russia was doing serious experimentation on telepathy, telekinesis, and healing. (Even a socialist society can find a use for its mystics and shamans.) After visits there, American investigators such as Dr. Stanley Krippner brought back from "behind the Iron Curtain" an electronic device used to affect the brain. Called the "Electrosone," it used a pulsing sinusoidal wave of 100 Hz frequency, but a power of only 1.5 mA (milli-Amperes).

It was used to induce a pleasant state of relaxation, deep reverie, and freedom from pain, known as "electrosleep" for lack of a better word. It had been used in the USSR to induce dreamlike states of reverie, susceptibility to hypnosis, and perhaps psychic, or even healing, abilities. The same device had been sold in Japan and used to provide a state of deep relaxation and recuperation between runs, for drivers of the *Shinkansen,* the bullet trains that run up and down at super high speeds over much of Japan. (They wanted their engineers refreshed and back on the job ASAP! American investigators noted that it seemed to work.)

The machine used two electrodes over the back of the neck or occiput, and two over the eyelids (like the early versions of the LENS). Some users complained of "overstimulation," and discomfort, so the frontal locations were changed to just above the eyes, which seemed better. American subjects reported the same experiences as did the Russians: The "electrosleep" machine wasn't a sure-fire sleep-inducing device (though it did that for some), but it did provide general relaxation. It seemed to help people free themselves from anxiety or depression, and perhaps sleep better overall. The name evolved into CES, or Cranial Electrical Stimulation, and used the same technology as microcurrent stimulation for muscle and nerve pain in other parts of the body. CES is now recognized by the FDA as a drug-free treatment for anxiety, depression, and insomnia.[4] Even though much weaker than TENS, *and hence much less likely to do damage,* CES still had to "fight for its life" to be included in the same grandfathered category as ECT.

The accumulated scientific studies now show that both the CES and LENS stimulation modalities have unmistakable benefits. But it is very important to note the differences between them. CES uses a fixed external stimulus of .5–1.5 mA, vibrating at 50 Hz or 100 Hz. Although small, this electrical current is still massive compared to that of the brain's own microcircuitry. To my way of thinking, its beneficial effects are probably due to the effect of the stimulation in opening pathways, as well as provoking a self-rectifying response in the brain as it attempts to process, and recover from, an alien stimulus (the CES energy). (This disruption itself is still millions of times smaller than that given by electroconvulsive therapy, suggesting that CES could be beneficially used to give gentle but repeated treatments before ECT is ever used. It might save a few million brain cells and would be *much cheaper.* If necessary, ECT could still be used as a last resort.)

The stimulus used in LENS is as many million times weaker than CES as CES is than ECT! No electrical current is introduced into the brain. Rather, as we know, some very weak radio waves, much tinier than what goes right through our heads when we use any cell phone, stir some receptors in the brain *with a pattern of its own energy,* at an offset. If this insignificant something has any power, it is *due to the principle of resonance in dynamical systems.* Any effects of the treatment that become perceptible to the conscious mind of the experiencer—say through a feeling of well-being or even the wiredness or tiredness of an "overdose"—reflect a vast magnification of the original insignificant stimulus.

As the *intensity of the stimulus* cannot explain the *intensity of the response, another variable must be at work.* This could only be explained by the unique configuration of the fed-back stimulation, tailored to the individual, and its ability to evoke resonance within the *chaotic dynamical integrity* of the brain and body. Biofeedback and neurofeedback could perhaps be regarded as energy medicines, although some within the field may take exception to this designation. They differ from the other energy approaches in one specific way: in the biofeedback paradigm, only *the person's own information is fed back to them in some form.*

The efficacy of the principle is undeniable and is clearly demonstrated by my daily experience. As a LENS therapist, I sit the same distance away from the crystal clock that emits the pulsed radio waves of treatment as my patients do. Although I sit there all day long, with as many as fifteen patients, I feel nothing. At the end of the day I sit in the chair myself and one of my clinicians treats me. After about three hundred treatments I am still very sensitive. I take only one second of treatment—and I feel the effects for hours and days. *Our own patterns* resonate within us awesomely!

The LENS occupies a unique and fortunate position among biofeedback methodologies. Because of its passive nature, behaviors on the part of the subject that can operate as confounding variables in biofeedback experiments, such as trying too hard, or not trying hard enough, are eliminated. That makes it easy to do double-blind studies in which subjects have no clue about whether they are in the experimental or control group. It is our belief that the LENS paradigm can thus help the entire field of biofeedback achieve greater legitimacy and recognition than it now enjoys.

When biofeedback achieves its own critical mass, as did chiropractic, it will be increasingly hard for the medical establishment to denigrate its efficacy, as they now do, often relegating it to "experimental procedures." LENS contributes to the possibility that the physics or energy-based paradigm will immeasurably enlarge the medicine of the twenty-first century.

Science Comes of Age

I can't help but find the image of a fumbling teenager an apt metaphor for our contemporary science when I consider announcements such as the following in national media: "Doctors astounded to note that MRI studies actually have a therapeutic—or contrastingly, disturbing—effect on the patient." Astonishing! Exposing an exquisitely sensitive electro-biochemical system to a *very* strong magnetic field actually affects it! In fact, many of our head-injured patients have reported how awful they feel after MRIs, in part because of the physical discomfort and the confinement, but also because of something they can't quite put their finger on. Injured and sensitized as they are, they just don't feel right, sometimes for days after the treatment.

But there are positive signs that medical science may be coming of age, albeit slowly, indicating that in this new century energy medicine approaches will find their way back into our lives, to our benefit. The year 2004 brought to us a comprehensive new textbook on Bioelectromagnetic Medicine assembled by a talented international group of scholars and published by Dekker.

Here is their online description of the book:

> Over the last two decades, progress in MRI, PET, SQUID, and other sophisticated imaging techniques have revolutionized medical diagnosis. Similar advances in bioelectromagnetic therapy now promise to replace drugs and surgery for many disorders. The sudden surge of interest in this rapidly emerging modality has produced a plethora of spurious products making worthless claims that make it difficult to distinguish between true and false claims of efficacy. *Bioelectromagnetic Medicine* provides the tools and skills to make such evaluations and distinctions by:
>
> - Thoroughly explaining the biologic effects of magnetic and electromagnetic fields and the importance of dosimetry in determining clinical efficacy and safety;
> - Presenting examples of cutting edge breakthroughs supported not only by rigid clinical trials but also by solid basic science research;
> - Tracing the origin and evolution of transcutaneous electrical nerve stimulation (TENS), cranioelectrical stimulation (CES), vagal nerve stimulation, (VNS), repetitive transcranial magnetic stimulation (rTMS) and other proven therapies by pioneers and authorities responsible for their discovery and development;
> - Identifying promising new approaches based on research advances in the U.S., Europe, Eastern Europe, Russia, and Pacific Rim countries.
>
> The 86 internationally recognized contributors to *Bioelectromagnetic Medicine* have strived to insure that it will remain the gold standard in the field for many years. Its 50 chapters and thousands of references dealing with every aspect of this topic make it an essential guide for physicians and all health care professionals, biophysicists, physiologists, biochemists and other basic scientists, as well as students and anyone interested in non-invasive and authoritative alternative medicine approaches.[5]

One of the methods mentioned in *Bioelectromagnetic Medicine*—repetitive transcranial magnetic stimulation, or rTMS—was developed by a leading researcher, Dr. Ralph Hoffman of Yale's Psychiatric Institute, as a treatment for schizophrenia. In rTMS powerful magnets are used to help schizophrenics who hallucinate voices, but for whom medications have failed to provide relief. The treatment does not exactly feel subtle, being "kind of like having a woodpecker knock on your head once a second for sixteen minutes." The woodpecker-like sensation is caused by the contraction of scalp muscles to the powerful magnetic field, pulsing once a second. On a subjective rating scale regarding the hallucination of voices, subjects given the full sixteen-minute treatment (but not lesser amounts) lowered their score from "10" (the worst) to an average of 3.8 points (more moderate). The effects last for a couple of days and then the treatment has to be repeated.

At the time of this writing, a *Time Magazine* article (March 21, 2005), "Resetting the Brain," brings rTMS to the public attention as a new treatment for major depression, with the caveat that it is a "flaky sounding treatment." (Why? Because it comes from physics rather than chemistry, uses energy rather than drugs?) The author explains that the doctors who use it do not really know how it works but suggest that the strong magnetic field induces "electrical currents along neuron pathways." One of the doctors cited even sagely reminds us that the *brain is an electrochemical organ*—so why shouldn't rTMS work?

The article praises the noninvasiveness of the procedure, which unlike psychosurgery, ECT, or psychopharmaceuticals, does not invade or disrupt the neurons, just stimulates them. But once again the old paradigm prevails: the article stresses that *powerful* magnets are needed to "reboot" or "reformat" the neural pathways in the pathological sections of the brain.

But our own findings indicate that *weak* electromagnetic signals do the same, or perhaps perform even better. The article says that patients treated with rTMS may need the woodpecker-like pulses "for one hour, five times a week, for six weeks."[6] That's thirty hours, or 1800 minutes, or 108,000 seconds of treatment. If, on the other hand, we postulate what would be a generous course of twenty LENS sessions, and an average length of treatment time of a very generous ten seconds (actual practice averages are about fifteen sessions and maybe four seconds each treatment), that's a total of two hundred seconds, or a little over three minutes of treatment total! (Of course the comparison is unfair, because the LENS signal is exquisitely attuned to the person's own frequencies, whereas the rTMS, as far as I know, is generic: A pulsing magnetic field of a certain standardized intensity.)

More and more information is accumulating that magnetic fields can have a significant effect on the brain, even in such minute amounts as are involved in the LENS treatments. Biologists have explored such subtle energy phenomena as the awesome orienting abilities of migrating birds, or the invisible warnings that result in few or no wild animal victims of a *tsunami* (while thousands of heedless humans succumb). In her very interesting paper—presented at the the Association for Applied Psychophysiology and Biofeedback national conference in 2002 and also included here—Evelyn Soehner shows convincing evidence of a commonality that exists between migrating creatures and humans: the presence of *magnetite*, a ferromagnetic material, which is found throughout the brain, but with greater concentrations in the pineal gland.

Could this vestigial remnant of our biological ancestors—who had to be able to read subtle energies to survive—be connected with the ability to respond to the LENS? We don't know yet, but her paper explores the way in which a very subtle intervention—small dynamic nudges of electromagnetic information, which correspond to the fluctuations of the human system—could be instrumental in producing a therapeutic result.

The Therapeutic Role of Bioelectromagnetics[7]
Evelyn Soehner, M.A.

All living creatures have electromagnetic components that play a part in governing their structure and physiology. Electricity and magnetism are intimately involved in the sensing and communicating systems of living organisms. The idea of a global interactive electromagnetic field within organisms is based on a new biophysical view of life. This view calls us to look at the human body as an electromagnetic organism that contains informational systems or structures. The atomic structure as having an electrical nature has, in fact, been proposed to establish the energetic foundation of life itself.

How do electromagnetic field (EMF) information interactions contribute an important role in biological processes?

One example of the process of energetic interaction with electromagnetic fields is *photosynthesis*, which involves the conversion of light to chemically stored potential energy for plant life. Light consists of a stream of tiny particles, or photons, carrying energy but not mass. Photosynthesis is nature's direct energy conversion, whereby radiant energy is converted to an easily usable form with an intermediate heat engine. The result is an increase in the energy stored in the plant. Some of the light energy is converted to chemical bonding energy, which the plant uses, and which any animals eating the plant obtain, for their survival. As an example of the process of information interaction, the same plant also converts sunlight into information, which it uses to monitor environmental changes in light and to regulate physiological processes.

In the last decade, biologists have discovered that electroreception is present in many mammals. One example is the blind mole-rat, a solitary, subterranean rodent that digs and inhabits a system of branching tunnels, which it never leaves. Scientists have discovered that the blind mole-rat must be able to orient efficiently through its use of the magnetic field of the earth, which it detects through the magnetite in its brain. Crystals of magnetite have been found in the brains of amphibians, birds, salamanders, fish, turtles, and lobsters. Magnetite is a form of iron oxide that was used for early compasses under the name of "lodestone."

The loggerhead turtle also uses magnetic fields for navigation purposes. This turtle navigates an extremely long (eight thousand miles) path in the Atlantic Ocean using only the warm water currents. It stays within these currents (because if it ventured out of these warm water gyres, it would die) by using the electromagnetic fields of the ocean itself. Another species that utilizes magnetic material for navigational purposes, the homing pigeon, has magnetoreception mechanisms, which involve the sensory detection of weak voltages induced by movement through the Earth's geomagnetic field. The homing pigeon *Cher Ami* was flown by the United States Army Corps in World War I, at Verdun France. He delivered, before he was shot down, a message that was instrumental in rescuing 194 members of a lost battalion. He was (posthumously) awarded the French Cross for his heroism.

So what is important about the magnetic material found in these creatures? And how does it apply to human functioning?

It was discovered in 1992 that human beings have magnetite crystals in their brains as well. The quantity ranged from a minimum of five million up to a hundred million single-domain ferromagnetic crystals per gram in the human brain. The large numbers of crystals allow effects at low-level electromagnetic field exposures and facilitate the interaction with electromagnetic fields. Recently, some new crystal-receptor formations were identified in the human pineal gland. They bear a striking resemblance to the calcite crystals that form the otoconia on the maculae of the human inner ear, which have been demonstrated to be extremely responsive to electromagnetic fields.

Nature is inherently parsimonious. Why do we have magnetite and crystalline receptors in the human brain? What role could they possibly play?

The brain, heart, eye, and the musculoskeletal system and other organ systems all generate electromagnetic fields. Bioelectromagnetic intercommunication of the heart and brain has been demonstrated. Electric fields are bio-activators of multicellular processes. For example, the electric fields from the sino-atrial node probably control the entire vascular tree, because the heart by itself cannot possibly do all the work of pumping blood around the body.

A growing body of research has accumulated concerning the biological effects of electromagnetism. The allopathic model is made of atomic structures composed of systems, organs, cells, molecules, and atoms. We need to include the subatomic interaction of protons, neutrons, electrons, muons, pions, and others that are energetic, to expand the medical model.

To begin the story, we look back to the nineteenth century when an enormous extension of knowledge of electricity and magnetism was accrued due to a mathematical formulation by James Clerk Maxwell. He found that the velocity of electromagnetic waves is 186,000 miles per second, which is also the velocity of light. Maxwell's theory was that light waves were electromagnetic in nature, thus connecting the phenomena of cosmic radiation, sunlight, the microwave, and radio and television frequency waves. Maxwell developed a theory of electromagnetism, which argued that energy—in the form of electromagnetic fields—is preeminent over mass, and that these fields permeate space.

In 1900, Max Planck came up with an equation in physics that predicted the correct spectrum of black-body-radiation. For his equation to work, the increasingly accelerating electrons in hot bodies must be released in minute packets of light energy, which he termed *quanta*. Each quantum of light carried one energy packet. How could the existence of light packets coexist with the theory of light waves proven by Maxwell's equations? Albert Einstein solved this problem by confirming Planck's observations and suggesting that light waves were a stream of quanta packets, called *photons*. In 1904 he proposed the *photoelectric effect*: the intensity of light is driven by the number of photons, and the energy of light is determined by the photon energy and hence the frequency of light. Einstein won the Nobel Prize in 1921 for his work on the photoelectric effect.

Later, Richard Feynman developed the theory of *quantum electrodynamics*, revealing the wave-particle duality of both matter and energy. Photons could be both emitted and detected as particles, but they travel through space as waves. These waves of photons fall into a measurable range, or spectrum, of electromagnetic radiation or light energy. The frequency times the wavelength is equal to the speed of the electromagnetic energy. If the frequency of light is high, the wavelength will be short, and if the frequency is low, the wavelength will be long. Electromagnetic frequencies range in speed from cosmic Y rays, through nuclear Y rays, X rays, visible light, infrared, microwave, and radio waves, ranging over many orders of magnitude. The entire spectrum of these frequencies are all electromagnetic radiation and move at the speed of light—thus the generic name for all these radiations has become *light*.

Classical thermodynamics is the study of energy flow, specifically the motion of atoms in gases under the influence of heat. It is the branch of the physical sciences that deals with the study of heat. In particular, thermodynamics (from the Greek words meaning "movement of heat") is concerned with the relationship between heat and mechanical energy and the conversion of one into the other.

Classical thermodynamics describes the laws governing the conversion of heat into energy so that the heat energy absorbed at every stage has time to spread through the system. The usefulness of classical thermodynamics is limited in that it is mandatory only for systems that come to equilibrium. It is applicable to closed systems where no matter is exchanged, even though energy exchanges occur, and for isolated systems where neither energy nor matter is exchanged with the surroundings. The model of classical thermodynamics does not incorporate the processes of irreducible complex structures that can't be understood through simple causal relationships.

Living systems are open systems.

Only open, living systems have simple states that lead to complex behavior. In a living system, such as the human brain, all of the domains perform their various functions autonomously, yet when coupled together, they generate a flow of patterns and cycles that function in coherent phase together and demonstrate coherent oscillatory activity. Even though cells interact only with their closest neighbors, long-range correlations and larger patterns emerge from the local couplings.

Local information is able to propagate through the whole lattice, creating structures that cannot be understood solely in terms of the properties of the individual cells. This appears to happen because of the dynamic organization of the cells (which involve emergent properties acting to resolve the complexity of cellular activities into patterns of coherence).

The interconnection of neurons in cells, with neurotransmitters bridging the gaps (synapses) between them, is the most studied, but far from the only, form of electrical activity within the brain. In fact the subtle electromagnetic fields that come from such electron flows, and their effect on other neurons, has been almost ignored. For a single neuron, effects may seem insignificant, but when many neurons fire simultaneously the cumulative wave energy plays a significant role in the operation of the brain.

SQUID (superconducting quantum interferometric device) magnetometers, which monitor the electrical activity of the brain, have revealed an amazing series of coherent changes in oscillation that can sweep over large areas of the brain in milliseconds. Molecules such as proteins, nucleic acids, and cellular membranes are affected by a particular electrical field across them. They are packed densely together, representing a special solid-state system of interacting electric forces. They vibrate at various frequencies and build into a collective mode of oscillating and radiating waves, which are called *coherent excitations*.

When we study the activities of the most microscopic matter, the photon, we leave the laws of classical physics behind and encounter *quantum mechanics*. This school of thinking, which revolutionized physics at the beginning of the twentieth century, helps us understand energy properties such as *coherence*. Quantum coherence is a description of many things joining together in a unified phase, such as the coherent light emitted from a laser, in which all portions of the optical wave are vibrating in unison. A coherent field implies a relationship between one emission and another, happening in phase, and a state of order across an entire spectrum. This kind of coherence involves a pure state that includes inseparable, nonlocal interactions.

Coherent oscillations of electromagnetic forces, which have been demonstrated to resonate over long distances, are considered responsible for some aspects of cellular organization in the brain.

The human central nervous system is a complex system that weaves unified meaning out of diverse threads. Neurons fire in collective rhythm and display oscillatory behavior in various brain areas. Synchronized electrical discharge-firing by neurons acts as an information gate in the brain. Incoming electromagnetic signals are interpreted and integrated into coherent patterns, as the photons are decoded into waveforms of specific frequency and amplitude, which represent a kind of order. The neurons respond to these waveforms, firing when stimulated by their patterns, and changing when changes in the patterns sweep through the receptors.

Electromagnetic fields affect not only the brain but the entire organism through the exchange of energies.

The organism receives and converts energy into what it needs to survive by means of energetic and informational interactions. The predominant molecular and intermolecular forces in living systems are electric. Cells and living organisms have been demonstrated to be highly sensitive to electric and magnetic fields. It is believed that this sensitivity is due to the dipolar nature of molecular and intermolecular interaction. Electric currents in the form of electrons or protons flow along membranes.

The absorption of a single photon could excite hundreds of membrane-bound molecules simultaneously, as the photic stimulation arrives at the cell membrane.

Based on the evidence that electromagnetic properties are produced within the body and are present in the central nervous system, an externally applied electromagnetic field may bring about a change by stimulating a resonance between the external and the internal oscillations. The body's cells have diameters of around ten to twenty microns. So waves of this length will vibrate them, in the same way as an opera singer can vibrate a distant glass with a specific note. During the LENS neurotherapy, for example, a *resonance* between externally applied electromagnetic fields and the brain's excited endogenous electromagnetic fields is created. Low frequency, low intensity waveforms are able to exert subtle influence on neural activity because there is an emission and absorption spectra match.

The human body is an electrochemical instrument of exquisite sensitivity. Its orderly function and control are regulated by oscillatory electrical processes of various kinds, each characterized by a specific intensity and frequency, such as those found in the human brain. These are close in range to those arising from the equipment. They recognize each other. The strength of the potential energy arises through the energy match between the receptor and the applied field. Thus, the effects arise from an *oscillatory similitude* between the electromagnetic field application and the living organism, via the living organism's ability to recognize certain field characteristics.

Researchers testing electromagnetic fields that have been applied to biological material have observed a range of frequencies and intensities that are consistently effective in healing. The field effects are specific to a particular power intensity and frequency window. (The effective intensity of one ten-millionth of a volt is implicated in the interaction between cells.) This is the very same level of intensity found in the control of human biological rhythms, the level of the EEG in brain tissue, and the level associated with navigation in fish, turtles, animals, and birds. Interestingly, this is also the intensity (as determined by Lawrence Livermore Laboratory) of the field emitted from the microprocessor driven EEG encoder used in the LENS system.

Weak ionizing pulsed electromagnetic fields such as specific light wavelengths have specific effects on tissues in the body. Recent research indicates that electromagnetic fields (EMFs) may bias the movement of cell structures and can alter the environment in which cells grow and move within the body. EMFs have been demonstrated to produce a broad array of impacts on the central nervous system, even though the energy imparted was far too low to have energetically driven the changes. The person's metabolism furnished the energy, while the applied EMFs were primarily eliciting the change.

Central nervous system dysfunction may be regarded not only as a functional abnormality, but as a disturbance of a communications network between elements in the body that are capable of coherence as well as resonance.

Resonance occurs in the field of electromagnetism, biology, and physics. Any system that has a range of oscillation frequency can become synchronized to frequencies close to its own. Extremely small signals are capable as acting as regulators and may play a decisive role in the restructuring of the system.

A disturbance of communication in the central nervous system may be brought back to a state of homeostasis, by mean of change in energy by interaction with an applied electromagnetic field. Open systems, such as the human body, behave sensitively to *electromagnetic conversations*. The essence of vitality can be seen as the mind-body's dynamical adaptability to stimuli creatively breaking through to new levels of order. *Very small stimulus input can effect a tremendous range of responses*. Engaging a new view of psychophysiology that incorporates the emerging science of bioelectromagnetics will greatly extend our understanding of physical and psychological reality. In this new science, moving toward an interactive, self-organized, and unified view of life, the behavior of the human central nervous system may be more accurately accounted for. Through a review of the puzzles and mysteries inherent in any investigation of biological phenomenon, important evidence has been provided to suggest a hypothesis for understanding the efficacy of the LENS.

The Holographic Brain and the Binding Problem

In his presentation of the concept of the holographic brain, Karl Pribram showed that all mechanical models of brain processing were clunky compared to the living, thinking, feeling thing. For Pribram, the physical brain was merely the choreographer for an exquisite dance of energy, pulsing throughout, wave front intersecting wave front, to produce the vibrant hologram of our living experience. These pulses, studied in various inflections throughout this book, carry the names alpha, theta, delta, and beta, but they are much more than that. They are the waves on which the boat of consciousness rides, and that carry it this way and that: clearly *the different frequencies of brain waves not only relate to different types of consciousness* but how thoughts and images move through the brain.

As neurology is now waking up to the power of this "symphony in the brain," it chooses its usual tools—surgery and the implanting of pacemakers *in the brain itself*—to work with the new discoveries, rather than following the intriguing leads offered by neurofeedback. As writer Rob Stein described it in a *Washington Post* article:

Known technically as "deep brain stimulation," the approach has been used on tens of thousands of patients with Parkinson's, as well as patients with two other movement disorders, essential tremor and dystonia. Encouraged by the success and safety of the treatment for those disorders, researchers began exploring its potential for other conditions.

Modeled on heart pacemakers routinely implanted in people's chests to automatically regulate heart rhythms, brain pacemakers were first developed in the late 1980s to treat Parkinson's, a devastating brain disorder in which victims inexorably lose control of their muscles.

In a painstaking six-hour procedure, surgeons drill two small holes into a patient's skull. Then, using computerized scans and electrical monitoring of the firing of nerve cells to precisely guide them, they carefully thread two electrodes, each about the diameter of a piece of spaghetti, to specific areas on each side of the brain, depending on the nature of the disorder.[8]

But this approach has raised hackles in other quarters. The *Washington Post* goes on to say that:

> Nevertheless, the research arouses fears of reviving the reckless use of brain surgery, about the wisdom of poking around in what some consider the font of a person's humanity, about oversimplifying mental illness as a purely biological problem, and the temptation to move too quickly to try out new technologies. "Any time you start messing with the brain and start treating it as, quote-unquote, just another organ, we're going to have questions of the propriety of doing this kind of thing," said Raymond De Vries, a medical sociologist at the Institute for Advanced Study in Princeton, N.J. "This is the brain. This is the seat of who we are."

If the procedure improves the quality of life for patients with Parkinson's and dystonia, it must have value. The method now is being experimentally applied to depression; while anxiety and OCD wait in the wings as likely candidates. And it may have some beneficial effects (the brain being an electrochemical organ). But paradigm blindness and the need for *powerful treatments* for serious illnesses have classical neurology overlooking the gentler technologies such as neurofeedback and LENS. (The same mindset that offers expensive and hazardous surgeries, also likes powerful machines with huge energy fields.) These approaches fit the dominant paradigm, but at the very least, it couldn't hurt to try the gentler approaches *first*.

The following quotes from a different *Washington Post* article (March 5, 1995) not only address the rationale for the drilling and implantation procedure but also implicitly validate the LENS:

> "The brain is an electrical organ with circuitry that carries messages. It's like having an orchestra playing a symphony, with various areas playing different parts. They have to play together," said Ali R. Rezai, director of functional neurosurgery at the Cleveland Clinic Foundation in Ohio. "In some cases, some parts aren't playing in synchrony. You hear chaotic music. That's what's happening—it's chaotic activity. We can get in there and modulate that chaotic activity."

Scientists do not understand exactly how electrical stimulation may work. The brain uses tiny electrical and chemical impulses to transmit messages. The external stimulation may either turn on or amplify—or perhaps turn off or diminish—certain electrical signals, ameliorating the system.

Consciousness, Chaos Theory, and "The Binding Problem"

The author of the article quoted above uses "chaos" in the conventional sense, as something "bad," where orderly principles are lacking, while we are introducing "chaos theory" from the new physics, as in where there is hidden order in the complexity of what seems to be apparent "chaos."

Despite amazing advances in physics and brain science, we are still trying to understand the amazing thing called "consciousness" that we each experience every day. One aspect of this has been the subject of yelling controversies for years in neuroscientific circles. It is known as "the binding problem": how does the encounter between the apparent chaos in the brain and the chaos outside the brain *bind* into our coherent experiences of the world?

The controversy is so heated because it pertains to nothing less than accounting for the physiological basis of human consciousness itself. Over the last decade or so, Dr. Rodolfo Llinas at New York University and his colleague, Dr. Urs Ribary, have isolated a magnetic field at 40 hertz constantly sweeping the brain from front to back every 12.5 thousandths of a second. Llinas believes this could be the brain's binding signal that integrates auditory, visual, and motor signals into our experience of the world.

Tiny amounts of radio stimulation could tweak such a dynamic active field, producing much larger changes. The change could be as global and quick as "everything seems brighter," which we have heard dozens, if not hundreds, of times as people finish their session. Or "my mood just changed." Or "the pain in my back (or its interpretation by the brain) is less." These changes are so subtle that they are hard to fit into the cookie-cutter world of experimental validation, but they are real, because they are where we live.

The familiar brain wave ranges are colors on the artist's palette of the self, occurring alone or overlapping and blending, to produce the colors and intricate textures of the world in which we live. What is certain is that the lightest touch can indeed release the finest displays of consciousness, because it is left free and unimpeded. The flexible, comfortable, brain supports the spread peacock's tail of consciousness.

As I mentioned earlier, Len Ochs says he didn't begin thinking in new-paradigm ways about the method he was developing until he read James Gleick's influential book: *Chaos: Making a New Science*. In it Gleick does a marvelous job of showing how new ideas in science grow, allowing them to bypass hidebound old orthodoxies. Gleick points out that when passionate investigators study living systems and how matter and energy really flow, the old boundaries between disciplines weaken. Not only that: their discoveries have the appeal demonstrated by the gorgeous curlicues and sea-horse tails of Mandelbrot's "fractals," which immediately attract the eye because they are more like natural processes or living things than staid old Euclidian geometry.

Scientists from many fields—such as physics and mathematics, geology, meteorology, metallurgy, aerodynamics, biology, and specifically the subfields of genetics and embryology—have started talking together, creating a symphony in science itself, giving rise to incredible new languages, paradigms, and discoveries. Gleick called this new science *chaos*, which I envision as swirling like a strange attractor (the nucleus, or heart of the fractal) between the disciplines.

Speculations on Physics, Bioelectromagnetics, the Holographic Brain, and Chaos Theory

Being inspired by the discovery of chaos theory—and the lives and insights of Mandelbrot, Lorenz, Ruelle, Smale, May, Swinney, Libchaber, Hubbard, and many other wonderful contributors who risked their reputations and careers to defy and yet exceed the scientific orthodoxies of their time—I began to ask, *Where is psychology's contribution to chaos theory?* It's not hard to find the chaos in human doings; that's easy, just pick up a newspaper, or go to a meeting of some sort, from a faculty room to the floor of the Senate, and you will certainly *experience chaos!*

I also know, from my lengthy internship with Joseph Campbell, that ambiguity, or paradoxicality, is unbearable for humans, leading them to embrace almost any belief system that offers to bring order out of chaos. The field of mythology is a study of human belief systems down through the ages, providing a paradoxical array, such as in the concept of God as being: male, female, old, eternally young, single, multiple, kindly and loving, or wrathful and judgmental, and so on.

The early days of psychology were filled with orthodoxies from the Pavlovian to the Freudian. But gradually the historical playing field began to morph, more toward holism and chaos theory. Think of Gestalt Therapy, which tries to use a few words or gestures to bring a pattern-shift and new insights to the patient, or Ericksonian hypnosis, which uses subtle tricks and verbal sleight of hand, to precipitate a hypnotic trance or engineer a cure. Carl Rogers thought that a warm and supportive environment—rather than any deliberate therapeutic intention of the therapist—would cause *an intrinsically healthy system to reconfigure in a healthier way.*

Stanislav Grof's LSD-assisted therapy showed how the ingestion of a few millionths of a gram (micrograms) of Lysergic Acid Di-ethyl-amide could precipitate a recapitulation of the birth experience, encounters with ancestral figures, or transpersonal experiences. (Grof later developed a method called *Holotropic Breathwork*, which used hyperventilation and programmed music to trigger similar therapeutically valuable eruptions of psychodynamic material from people, in the supportive atmosphere of weekend intensives. See *Realms of the Human Unconscious* and his other books.)

However, I was dismayed to realize that such an extraordinary interdisciplinary twentieth-century collaboration as chaos theory had, for the most part, left out—and been left out by—psychology. After all, isn't the human being the acme of all complex, dynamical systems in the universe—at least the ones we know about? But I would submit the LENS as a genuine contribution from the social sciences, or the healing arts, to chaos theory. Because of the incredibly small nature of its stimulus and the fact that its specifications are derived from the patient's own nervous system, it falls into the category of *initial conditions* in a dynamical system, as formulated by physicists versed in chaos theory.

The role of initial conditions is illustrated by the example Gleick gives of German physicist Peter Richter who had a "pet dynamical system," a well-oiled double-pendulum, in his laboratory. He would set it spinning randomly, but "The dependence upon initial conditions was so sensitive that a stimulus so small as 'the gravitational pull of a single raindrop a mile away,' could mix up the motion within fifty or sixty revolutions, about two minutes."[9] Chaos theorists would thus have no difficulties with the energy-dilutions LENS works with: intensities of *nanowatts*, billionths of a watt per square centimeter, and exposure times of a second or two.

Although we don't yet have large-scale experiments that document the physical efficacy of such events, the *qualitative research*, that is, a careful keeping-track of the clinical effects of what we do on *individuals* (*self-contained dynamical systems*), dozens of times per day, in offices around the country, is overwhelmingly positive. And without a doubt, the healthier the living, dynamical system, the more such an entity seems to be nonviolent to others, creatively or socially productive, existentially content, and quite simply, *more fun to have around*. The implications of this data should be no less world-shaking for science (especially behavioral science and medicine) than Mandelbrot's folding of surfaces or Libchaber's studies of fluid dynamics were for the fields of physics and meteorology respectively. Not to mention its implications in a context where humanity as a whole sometimes seems like it is "redoubling its effort, when it's forgotten its aim."

A couple of years ago, I was having lunch with Dr. Tom Fink, the clinical psychologist mentioned earlier, who started out being very skeptical about what his wife, Evelyn Soehner, was reporting about her experience of the LENS work. But he has since become a staunch advocate (though not a practitioner) of the method. I asked him for an overall appraisal of what he had seen.

"If this were a sane or a fair world," he said, "in which real contributions to science or healing were really recognized, rather than certain vested interests furthered, I think Len Ochs would get the Nobel Prize!"

The Seat of the Soul

A year or two ago I began conversations on the problem of consciousness with my friend Jay Gunkelman, who probably has thought more about it more deeply even than most people in the field of neuroscience. This year (2005), he was able to present his thoughts in a "tour-de-force" presentation of the subject at the ISNR (International Society for Neuronal Regulation, Denver, Colorado). His presentation was too complex to go into all the details, but I found myself in awe at his conclusions: Consciousness, and our experience of the world, is not found, simplistically, in any of the known brain wave ranges, though they invariably influence it with their color and texture. It is instead to be found in the intersection of the (apparent) chaos that is the living EEG, with the DC currents that are found throughout the connective tissue of the body, and in the neuroglia—the so-called "scaffolding cells" we have referred to in other places in the text.

"Consciousness," he says, "is too quick for ordinary neural transmission," it moves at the speed of light, not meters-per-second, as in even fast axonal transmission, and it moves through microtubules in the glia and connective tissue (as Dr. James Oschmann also asserts in his books on Energy Medicine). In the body, these energies are familiar to practitioners of acupuncture; they are fluctuations of DC or direct current potentials, rather than the AC, alternate current, of brain waves. Consciousness, says my forward-thinking friend, is the interface between the DC of our basic energy field, and the AC of the rhythmical brain waves. (Jay's contact info is found in the resource section. If you need a 19-channel QEEG done, he's your man!)

Jay's speculation reminded me of some elegant words of the poet Novalis on "the seat of the soul," with which I will conclude this chapter: "The seat of the soul is there, at the interface, where the inner world and the outer world meet." (Translation by Robert Bly in *News of the Universe*.)

14

THE LENS WITH ANIMALS

Improving the Behavior, Temperament, and Flexibility of Horses, Dogs, and Cats

Stephen Larsen, Ph.D., Sloan Johnson, M.A.,
Robin Larsen, Ph.D., and Carla Adinaro, A.R.I.A.

But where are the animal studies?

PANEL OF DOCTORS AT THE RUSH MEMORIAL HOSPITAL TO
DR. MARY LEE ESTY, AFTER SHE REPORTED HOW FNS (THE
PREDECESSOR OF LENS) HAD ALMOST TOTALLY CURED A
CHRONIC (THIRTY-YEAR) UNRESPONSIVE FIBROMYALGIA CASE
THEY HAD BEEN VERY FAMILIAR WITH, ALONG WITH
ACCOMPLISHING OTHER WONDERS WITH TBI AND
FIBROMYALGIA PATIENTS

We wouldn't even think of treating animals until the method
(the LENS) had been thoroughly tested out on humans first!

STEPHEN LARSEN ADDRESSING THE ASSOCIATION FOR
APPLIED PSYCHOPHYSIOLOGY AND BIOFEEDBACK
IN FORT LAUDERDALE, 2004

"Where *are* the animal studies?" is, of course, a very good question, one that this chapter addresses in a preliminary way. This question is important for two reasons. One relates to the possibilities of sharing the benefits of LENS as widely as possible, including with our animal friends. If the method is biologically effective, *it should work with animals* as well as with humans. The second is because everything about the LENS—its invisibility and subtlety, rarified action, and so on—can be seen as pointing to *placebo*. But, unlike belief-susceptible humans, *very few* animals are overly impressed by having wires attached to their heads and being made to sit (or stand) still!

Those of us who have treated animals have found it *very instructive* to compare the human responses to treatment with the animal responses: we learn more about the functioning of the CNS (central nervous system) by interspecies analogy. Like humans, animals such as cats, dogs, and horses *can be neurotic*. In most cases, it is humans who have made them so, and in whose eyes they then appear neurotic.

They bark ceaselessly, even when there is no intruder. They *balk* mindlessly at the sight of *that mailbox*, as they are coming down the driveway for the hundredth time. They shake with anxiety as the vet's station wagon approaches. They disappear at the first sight of a suitcase ("You're going to leave me, I know it!"). They stumble or are uncoordinated; they suddenly bite someone who reminds them of someone else, or is merely of the same gender. Their emotional lives and limbic system—the "old mammalian brain"—are virtually identical with ours: rage, jealousy, territoriality, but also affection, nurturance, affiliation or herd mentality, and dominance hierarchies are emotions and behaviors held in common. They even cop moods, as anyone who has neglected a horse, or left a dog or a cat alone in an apartment all weekend knows. Thus the furry soul mirrors the human soul and shares the disorders.

They also have central nervous systems that are almost identically patterned with ours, albeit with smaller outer brains or cerebral cortexes. In fact, the similarities are so great that a significant amount of veterinary EEG research has been driven by its usefulness to human seizure disorder. As a result, the EEGs of animals have been rendered on human-shaped cortical templates.[1] (See color insert page 8.)

As with much human neurological encephalography, veterinary study is concerned with seizures and their foci, and the propagation of wave forms as they perfuse through the cortex.[2] EEG speeding up or slowing down means similar things in animals and in humans, and the *power spectrum* of an animal at any particular location is not so very different from that of a person: lots of delta means sluggishness, lots of high beta means hypervigilance. QEEGs in animals or people can direct surgical interventions or help prescribe psychotropic drugs, which have similar, but by no means identical, action in animals and in humans.

LENS Benefits for Furry Friends

The similarities between the central nervous systems and emotional life of dogs, cats, horses, and humans provide clear indications that LENS offers the same benefits to animals as to humans. In fact, LENS offers potentially earthshaking possibilities for veterinary neurobiology and neuropsychology, and the treatment of traumatized and temperamentally anxious or nervous animals. It's more lasting than drugs—to which veterinary creatures are often more sensitive than humans—and much nicer, because the creature is not dopey, but rather *more like its* (hopefully lovable) *self*. One area of particular interest has to do with learning. The larger human cortex seems to provide the essence of our Darwinian advantage. Hornless and fangless, flatfooted creatures that we are, our secret weapon seems to be an almost endless ability to learn.

Of course animals *do* learn, although imperfectly from our human point of view. Around the turn of the twentieth century, psychologists observed that animals' learning was simpler but *paradigmatic of human learning*. If we keep them captive, and jumping to our stimuli of various sorts, as with Skinner's rats and pigeons, they show us much of how human nervous systems and physiologies respond. The mechanism, says Pavlovian and Skinnerian psychology, is identical: *Classical conditioning*—as in salivating dogs, or "operant," *reinforcement* and *extinction* (reward-based) paradigms in rats or pigeons—should tell us how to do *behavior modification* with humans. Animals and humans both *generalize,* that is, they learn about the world through comparing stimuli with other stimuli.

Some kinds of animal learnings, however, seem almost impossible for the animals to unlearn, even under the *extinction* criteria Skinner proposes. Animals *generalize* quite easily, which often includes a *limbic*, subcortical component. They fear not only the *something (aversive stimulus)* that brought about their pain; they also fear the environment in which it was inflicted, including incidental *discriminative stimuli*—such as a colored light, an odor, or a sound—that had nothing to do with the *punishment* or *negative reinforcement*. Unless an animal has received extensive obedience training, its ability to discriminate and inhibit, the hallmark of higher learnings and behavior, is very weak. The difficulties that this can present are well illustrated by the following story.

About twenty years ago, a pleasant and bright young woman teacher whom I shall call Lucy came to me for psychotherapy. She was working on a classical problem that turned out to have an unusual twist. She had had an abusive boyfriend and, in an emotional episode in which he physically began to strike her, she told him they were through. During the scuffle, Lucy's little dog, Ruffie, tried to intervene and save *his mistress*, the most important, even godlike, being in the world. The rough boyfriend kicked the little guy across the room, smashed some furniture, smacked the woman some more, and left—thank God—for good!

We had some therapeutic work to do, to get Lucy to even think about entering into another relationship. After a limited period of mourning and processing, she assayed a new one, with a much nicer, mellower, guy. Unfortunately, on the first date, when Lucy tried to bring her boyfriend home, Ruffie (who probably had indulged himself in some kind of doggy Bruce Lee fantasy of what he would do *next time*) emerged from under the couch, all fifteen pounds of him, eyes blazing, growling with shrill fury, and savaged the new boyfriend. The gentle boyfriend, now traumatized (and subject, perhaps, to the same Pavlovian dynamics as Ruffie, and *generalizing* in his own turn), left the girl with such a ferocious guardian, and went on to greener pastures. After all, as Skinner says, *an organism is an organism*, be it a planaria, a rat, or a human.

Lucy tried to explain to Ruffie, "No, Ruffie, this one is not like the other one. Bad Ruffie, you've just driven off my boyfriend!" Unfortunately for my beleaguered client, the pattern happened again, and again, with other relationships. The problem came to dominate her therapy. She loved Ruffie and wouldn't think of giving him up, but she was young and eligible and wanted a boyfriend!

I suggested various systematic *desensitization* procedures, like muzzling Ruffie when a boyfriend initially showed up, and having the boyfriend feed and pet Ruffie. We tried these measures, with mixed results. Such traumatic responses as Ruffie had are hard to extinguish; Ruffie's growling that accompanied these friendly overtures left no doubt that, muzzled or not, Ruffie did not like *anything about these mean human males*.

Unfortunately these events all happened a decade before I knew of the amazing ability of LENS to defuse heated-up reflexive patterns and generalizations in animals. Now our experiences clearly indicate that the

LENS treatment, *followed by behavior modification or extinction protocols,* might become very useful to animal trainers and pet owners alike.

In addition to exhibiting anxiety and trauma-induced generalization, animals suffer from several other problems that could be helped by the LENS. They certainly experience auditory-processing problems as illustrated in the Gary Larsen cartoon where the owner is saying, "Sophie, I really want you to stop getting on the couch! Do you understand, Sophie?" and what Sophie hears is "Sophie, blah blah blah blah, Sophie, blah blah."

Animals, like people, can have poor coordination (*ataxia)* or clumsiness (*dyspraxia).* Animals can also show poor executive functions—timing, sequencing, and organizing—so that, for example, an otherwise bright dog may be unable to do complex obedience trials, or an athletically capable horse may prove too anxious or distractible for *dressage,* an exquisitely choreographed set of movements in which rider and horse are synchronized exactly.

As for cats, they never even pretend they are going to cooperate with anything, but their social responses to other cats, unexpectedly macho rodents, people, relocations, or other stress situations can be quite telling!

Like humans, horses have abundant opportunities for head injuries. A random backfire or horn blast can cause them to rear up in a trailer, or shy and fall on pavement, hitting their heads. The same can happen if they rear in a stall. Horses also fall, in a variety of mishaps, some quite serious, as in a missed steeplechase jump or water-obstacle, or stumbling in a boulder-strewn creek bed in an eventing course or a cross-country ride. Some are traumatized by harsh trainers or jockeys, immature or sadistic owners, motor vehicle accidents, or attacks by other dominant horses or predators, such as when uncontrolled domestic dogs or feral dog packs drive a panicked horse into a devastating collision or fall.

Dogs (and housecats) fall out of cars or are in cars that have accidents. Many, sad to say, are simply abused by their owners (occasioning such organizations as the ASPCA). Over many years, I have had ample opportunity to practice homeopathy on animals. In a rural setting, with a veterinarian available only after many phone calls have been made, and who still has to travel a distance, homeopathy often was the *first recourse.* It is astonishing how effective homeopathy has been in stopping convulsions caused by rhododendron poisoning, in curing fevers, abating colic, easing foal-birth, even combating infections.

In the last decade or two, this unlikely treatment has blossomed in veterinary circles into a quasirespectable sideline of veterinary medicine, as have acupuncture, shiatsu, and Linda Tellington-Jones's brilliant "T-Team," a way of handling and manipulating animals that is sensitive to body signals, which constitute a language readable by the discerning trainer or therapist.[3] In all of the above modalities, animals often respond beautifully and quickly to gentle remedies, showing that these *medicines perfected on humans also work well on animals.*

Animals respond similarly to the LENS, as the case studies shared in this chapter demonstrate. Larger scale trials, or more controlled studies, could indeed follow, but the author *does not doubt the outcome.* In an intelligent, responsive system, the size of the stimulus doesn't seem to matter: a tiny dose does wonders for a big animal. Horses, for example, are vegetarian, live outdoors, are relatively uncomplicated and not afflicted by Judeo-Christian or Existential guilt. They do just fine with tiny doses of homeopathy, acupuncture needles, or the LENS.

LENS Case Presentations with Animals

The animals who have been studied, and whose cases are presented in this chapter, are "socialized," sometimes called "domestic" animals, who live and interact with humans. They live in domestic, outdoor or barnyard, environments, not in cages, so it could be argued that they are less *controllable*, in the scientific sense. But I would answer back that these habitats are perhaps more genuine and natural than the Skinner box or other laboratory environment, and thus the *animal behaviors that are elicited are "truer,"* in a different sense.

Unlike laboratory animals in experimental trials, these animals are not "sacrificed" at the end of the project so that their physiognomies can be examined—nor would their owners like the idea at all! In fact, these are not *experimental animals*, but *patients in treatment.* But they *are* animals, and their responsive and operant behavior can be examined as minutely as any laboratory behaviorist would require. Blood, saliva, and urine samples can be taken, and their immunological responses measured. Their blood pressure, digestion, and activity levels can also be measured.

To do meaningful *before* and *after* evaluations, we need, above all, *skilled observation* by humans with whom the animals interact. In this chapter we have been lucky enough to get the testimonies of professional animal handlers, trainers, and riding instructors on changes they have observed in these cases. These cases provide some of the most interesting comparisons we can have between the animals' experiences and those reported by humans undergoing the same procedures. In this way, the animal cases can and do *enlarge our science.*

Not only were our animal patients not tortured or in any way hurt in these procedures, rather, their well-being was enhanced, sometimes in ways that were rewardingly obvious to "their humans." Operating from a value base that regards the four-footed and the winged ones as *our brothers,* the LENS and photonic stimulation treatments were given in the context of *a working relationship,* a kind of *partnership* wherein the animals were being helped as well as studied.

The first case we will hear about is described by Sloan Johnson, a California practitioner who was trained by Len Ochs, and sometimes fills in for him, if he is traveling. She is also, as will become obvious, an animal lover.

Shaka the Horse
SLOAN JOHNSON, M.A.

Shaka, a sixteen-year-old horse, was labeled as "a fine pet, but not a show horse" when my client acquired him at fifteen. The horse had had multiple owners, some more skilled at owning and training a horse than others. His current owner reported that the horse had had a few "bad riders." At four years old Shaka had been involved in an accident while being towed in a trailer and came away with a pronounced two-inch lump between the left frontal and left temporal lobe of the head, which remains to this day. The horse exhibited various problems, such as depression, hypervigilance, inability to learn, and clumsiness. His owner agreed it might be worthwhile to try neurofeedback.

During the first treatment, Shaka was disinterested in what we were doing but seemed annoyed at the application of the electrodes, which was manifested by fretting. Immediately after the annoying treatment, though, the horse seemed far more happy and relaxed. The next day the horse and the owner had a session with the trainer. Afterward I received a call from the woman who owned Shaka, saying that: "The trainer's mouth was hanging open," at the difference in the horse's behavior. The trainer had thought the horse must have received an injection of liquid glucosamine and chondroitin for joint health, because "instead of taking ten shuffling steps as usual, the horse took seven, longer, more graceful, steps." The trainer also provided further details:

> Shaka had been locked up in his body. It was hard for him to go forward without shuffling. He would sequentially pick up, and stab, his front feet. He would say "No" before he even knew what you were asking him to do. Now he seems to be listening, and sort of game: "Yes, I can do that!" He used to have a lot of resistance and tension. He now has better use of his legs. He's more graceful. He seems less arthritic.

When I came to do the second treatment, Shaka seemed almost eager for it. He let me put on the electrodes with little opposition; after treatment, he was so relaxed that when the owner went to put the bit in, she had her whole hand in his mouth before he even noticed, which was uncharacteristic behavior for him. He even let her fuss around, cleaning his teeth, without seeming to notice or care. He now has a gleam in his eye and seems much happier. The mood improvement has been there ever since the first treatment.

The owner says he's "much softer and more reasonable with requests for action." She also says he's calmer and seems to like the treatment. Now, whenever I come, Shaka is very accommodating and receptive. When I finish, the horse seems very relaxed and happy. We've finished a three-site per treatment map and are now starting the regular treatment schedule. We are thrilled with the improvement and hope it continues.

Della the Dog

SLOAN JOHNSON, M.A.

Della is a nicely raised and trained nine-year-old German shepherd. For most of her life, she and her owner lived on a large rural property, and her owner often worked at home. Della got to frisk and frolic nearby. At five or six years of age, however, Della's owner accepted a job in a nearby city, and Della and she moved to an apartment there. Having begun the new job, Della's owner was now gone for eight hours at a time; quite a switch of lifestyle for Della!

After a few months of this, Della began to exhibit signs of depression, which manifested in separation anxiety and even a sort of random anxiety, in which she was skittish and afraid of simple things such as the bathroom door. She developed many physical problems as well: frequent colds, immune system problems, and kidney and liver problems. This psychological buildup culminated on the day that she couldn't stand it any more. She tried to follow her owner to work—by jumping out of a second-story window! She landed hard, incurred some major structural damage, and hit the left side of her head. She wore a cast on her front right paw for three weeks. After this sad event, the "life" left Della's eyes, and she was consumed by an evident anxiety and fear.

Fortunately, we were able to intervene in what was clearly a descending spiral for this dog. We did both the LENS and the photonic stimulator and, as a result, her energy and attitude improved and she is now doing very well. Her immunoglobulins have come up nicely in testing. Her anxiety is almost unnoticeable, and her right paw is almost back to normal, thanks to the photonic stimulator. She rarely gets sick now, as compared to two colds per month that she was experiencing before (which provides an interesting comment on human immunological function and stress!). But most dramatically, Della's anxiety has diminished to the point of her being once again "a normal dog." Her owner still lives in the apartment, and Della's life is still not the same as it was out in the country (where a dog can take a breath of the fragrant forest air), but her owner lavishes lots of love on Della and takes her for long walks, which they both love! (See color insert page 8.)

Dizzy the Displaced Cat

STEPHEN LARSEN, PH.D., WITH ROBIN LARSEN, PH.D.

Dizzy was a large, formidable orange cat whose owner came to live with a man who occupied a cabin on our farm just a short distance from our house. From the start, our cats Arlecchina and Ni, a tough couple of calico mousers, had it in for Dizzy, especially if he transgressed into their territory. Arlecchina and Ni, mother and daughter, were very affectionate with each other, but on the subject of Dizzy they were of one accord. We would find him cowering in various places about the carport after having suffered some abuse from Arlecchina or Ni or both. Dizzy was a peripheralized, neutered, neurotic male, and hence an ideal candidate for a trial of the LENS.

It was not easy to get Dizzy to cooperate with the treatment. Robin had to hold him in her lap and pet him a lot, until I finally could attach the electrodes. Dizzy *did not like the electrodes.* As he sat there, his claws extending more and more into Robin's thigh, the two house cats, seeing the prize target of their animosity sitting on their mistress's lap, assembled outside on the window-ledge. I got a glove and a claw-absorbing towel for Robin's thigh. Throughout the treatment, the two cats displayed their animosity by a baleful stare of ominous intensity, accompanied by a low rumbling growl, in stereo (even we were scared).

Fortunately, a large plateglass window separated them from the rest of us. Dizzy emitted his own rumbling growl. Robin endured, and we finished the treatment: one second at C4 and one second at C3 (both hemispheres of his brain). Dizzy was released outside, and we will not speculate about what punishment he subsequently may have endured. But he probably mostly skulked in the woodpile, thinking we all were crazy.

Nothing remarkable was observed for about a week, but then I noticed Arlecchina on her own territory (our porch) hissing and yowling at something formidable and backing away. I was sure it must be Morgan, the big black cat who keeps the rats out of the barn, or even an intruder from the outside. But no, it was Dizzy, now stalking Arlecchina. Over the two months or so that remained until Dizzy was taken to his new home by his owner, this reversed dominance pattern never broke: *The stalked had become the stalker,* and Dizzy's own fierce stare showed he had learned his lesson well, perhaps from his hostile watchers, in his *one and only neurofeedback* treatment. (See color insert page 8.)

Moondog, the Ancient, the Lovable

Stephen Larsen, Ph.D., with Robin Larsen, Ph.D.

When we first got Moondog, a tailless Australian shepherd, no one could have imagined a cuter puppy for our eleven-year-old daughter Gwyn. Silver-blue brindled, silky of fur, Moondog was as joyful as her mistress, healthy and full of life. (She was named after an eccentric blind poet named *Moondog,* whom we used to know in Greenwich Village, where he would declaim strange Anglo-Saxon rhymes while wearing a bearskin and a Viking helmet. He was wonderful and has since become internationally celebrated.) Oddly, our own little Moondog's eyes failed to develop completely, and we soon realized she was largely blind.

She was blissfully unaware of her handicap, though, and whenever Gwyn and I (Stephen) would go off for walks in the mountains, Moondog would merrily accompany us, along with two older dogs. We would scramble over boulders and steep rocky places, and I remember her astonishment as she watched the two old dogs decline to climb a boulder or scramble on a ledge. She herself was everywhere, bounding and just enjoying herself.

A sheepdog without sheep, her self-appointed mission on a horse farm became to get the horses to behave. Unfortunately, forty-five pounds versus one thousand pounds makes for an unequal contest. Sometimes we would drag Moondog out from under the hoofs of horses stampeding into the barn—horses don't like things that keep them from their food—astonished she could still be alive. Head, and probably spinal, injuries accumulated (which still did not deter her from thinking that horses were sheep).

We don't think Moondog was prepared for old age in any way. She was the paragon of vibrant and energetic *dogginess*, until about the age of twelve, when some complication from the old spinal injuries inflicted by the horses came into play. She seemed to have lost control of her back legs and her front and rear legs seemed to walk in different directions. The poor creature was visibly dismayed and puzzled by her uncooperative back end, and by this inconvenient handicap that prevented her from running freely about the farm. She became depressed and despondent.

Sometime in her twelfth year, we were having a training program for neurofeedback professionals at our center. One of the participants wanted to see if LENS neurofeedback would work with animals. Moondog was selected. We all sat around the computer screen and looked at her brain waves, which looked rather like human ones, similarly distributed throughout the frequency and amplitude ranges. Her power spectrum, to our initial surprise, favored the higher frequencies—from SMR up to high beta—with a frantic little white bar, representing the dominant frequency, zooming quickly back and forth. It looked like the brain of a hypervigilant person.

"The cunning and hypervigilant brain," I intoned, "of the sheepdog."

Everyone laughed. Moondog, proudly sitting in the treatment chair, electrodes on her head, smiled.

Moondog received a second of treatment at each of C3 and C4. Within an hour or two of treatment, every one of the ten or so students—not to mention teachers—had noticed some differences in our dog. Her gait was smoother; she walked more normally. Back legs followed front legs as she assayed a version of the familiar doggy trot. She was more cheerful and lively.

It has been almost three years since then. After a period of occasional treatments, we began a more regular program about two years ago. Moondog gets LENS neurofeedback maybe once a month, and some photonic treatment for her spine and hind end. Some of our clients are startled to see a dog sitting patiently in the waiting room, then going in to treatment when called (don't worry, we change the electrodes for dogs!). She is now fifteen and still going. She gets lots of petting, especially at the feed store and the hardware store. Moondog looks at the horses, and smiles her doggy smile, but does not try to herd them. (Even though I know that in her heart of hearts, she still thinks they are sheep.)

When the coyotes come to sing across our meadow at night, Moondog still wants to join them, as she always did (and become their supper). She seems to have all kinds of (dream) animals visiting, having visibly active adventures during her REM sleep. Most important, even though she is approaching the same end as the rest of us mortals, Moondog has left all signs of depression behind her and gives every appearance of being a happy old dog-person.

Dancer the Horse
DRESSAGE INSTRUCTOR CARLA ADINARO

When I first met Dancer, I saw a handsome dark bay Morgan gelding with a worried facial expression and body-stance. He was also very quick to startle or spook. Carrie (his co-owner with Claire) would ride him in a lesson with me and he seemed tense and quick. He wanted to trot too fast, canter too fast. He seemed frantic and unable to think slowly and figure out what Carrie and I wanted. Instead, he seemed to jump to conclusions, hoping that he was guessing correctly.

We spent a lot of time reassuring him that our goal was relaxation and rhythm. We wanted him to move and think more slowly and mindfully. We tried to show him that, whether or not he made a mistake, we would not lose patience with him. Sometimes we would get glimpses of him becoming more relaxed and thoughtful, with a steadier rhythm during all his gaits.

Carrie and I were working on the first tier of the training pyramid of dressage: rhythm and relaxation. Without this basic, the next tier of suppleness cannot be taught. After suppleness is learned, the next step is to teach the horse to seek and accept contact with the bit by stretching the neck and back into the rider's hand. Once this is established, the next step is to teach the horse impulsion or RPMS. The horse needs to go forward with thrust from the hind legs. Once the horse has mastered these steps, he needs to learn to be straight in movement, the hind feet following the front feet, hoof prints on straight lines, circles, and so on. The last step one asks for is collection, where all the preceding steps and skills are utilized to develop carrying power in conjunction with thrust.

This makes for an athletic warhorse, bullfighting horse, dressage competitor (the ballet of horsemanship), powerful jumper, or simply an incredible horse to ride. This technical list of equine skills shows that what we were asking of Dancer was so basic and easy that it should have been a fifteen minute to one hour lesson—repeated, of course.

But every week we found that we had to start *back at square one* and progressed only a little. Was he just stubborn? Was he too worried to think clearly? Were we being clear in our instructions? I knew he wasn't stupid.

Then in one lesson, there was a marked improvement. What I saw was, in fact, more than "marked"; it was a *vast* improvement. Dancer was trying more obviously to listen to Carrie. He was more contemplative and not so tense. I assumed we had had a breakthrough in our training. But I later found out that earlier that week Robin and Stephen had done a demonstration neurofeedback session on Dancer.

As winter was coming and we had no indoor ring, I only taught Carrie on Dancer a few more times, during which time Dancer was given another treatment or two. In those sessions he was in a mental state that was focused, relaxed, and much more educable. I was really pleased, believing that, had we been able to continue on, Dancer would have kept learning, responding to the slightest nuances of the skilled rider's body language, in place of: *kick to go, pull to stop and turn*—crude mechanisms that some people mistake for the skill of riding.

Later I had the opportunity to teach his other owner, Claire, on Dancer. Claire is a college student with all the grace of youth and the instincts of a natural rider. She was just learning this "dressage thing" on a horse that had undergone a subtle change. Dancer was much quieter and more receptive, and Claire was learning new skills, on what seemed like a new horse!

The last time Dancer received a neurofeedback session was during a training for professionals. He was tense, with the wires, computer, electrodes and all, along with lots of people crowded around him. One could see the tension in the worried and peaked eyebrows, the lips slightly turned down, the nostrils tense and elongated, and the rigid neck and back. But immediately after the treatment, he heaved a big sigh, relaxed his body, and became more content. (See color insert page 8.)

The Future of LENS Research with Animals

Lens is an ideal modality for experimental exploration for animals or humans because of its brevity and the passivity of the subject. I propose that our animal treatment data be extended into the realms of experimental research. Instead of following the trajectory of common biological and social science, however, let's *not* make a bunch of rats, cats, or dogs sick, poisoned, drugged, or lobotomized, then divide them into experimental and control groups, so we can see if the experimental group treatment works as opposed to the control. What a lot of misery, for a lot of creatures, for a little knowledge!

There is already a vast pool of candidates who would benefit from LENS treatment, such as the abundant population of neurotic animals, many of which can be found in dog pounds or animal shelters, greyhound tracks as well as other racetracks, and rodeos (these are only some of the more *visible* environments wherein these animals reside). Zoos also have captive populations of *neurologically suffering animals*, which can be seen in their demeanor, repetitive pacing, shaking the bars of the cage, or other frustrated responses to captivity.

We would like to see the creation of an independent panel of experts, who would rate animals on various behavioral dimensions such as restlessness, anxiety, stereotypical movements, hypervigilance, even quality of sleep. Physiological markers such as pulse rate and blood pressure, as well as immunoglobulins or hormones, could also be tested. *Only the panel* would have to be "blinded" as to whether or not the (brief, invisible) treatment was administered. Data could be collected, and then the group *not* given treatment could also be treated (and more data collected).

Veterinary energy medicine is the medicine of the future. Animals show us how exquisitely sensitive is the living, sensitive, uncomplicated CNS—without human rationalizations and defense mechanisms. Animals given LENS treatments show us how *intelligent, self-regulating systems* respond to tiny and subtle stimulation.

They likewise teach us to *do less and see what happens. If this doesn't work,* then *try a little bit less. Then reduce the stimulation further.* Only at this point, *do we try more.* Or we try the same but *more frequently,* which gives the organism time to respond to the treatment. Then we can go up a little in intensity, vary the stimuli up and down, *or try another treatment.* If there is an inveterate neurological condition, more treatments may be needed. But judging from some recent cases, animals seem to need about a third of the treatments humans do to produce a lasting amelioration (three to five treatments in uncomplicated cases).

With animals as with humans, the LENS works well with other subtle modalities; in combining the LENS with the gentle methods of veterinary massage, acupuncture, and homeopathy, among others, we can learn much from our animal companions about sensitivity and responsiveness.

15

POSTSCRIPT: THE TAO OF LENS

Positive Psychology and Optimal Performance[1]

Stephen Larsen, Ph.D.

Chao-Chou asked, "What is the Tao?"
The master [Nan-chüan] replied: "Your ordinary consciousness
is the Tao."
"How can one return into accord with it?"
"By intending to accord you immediately deviate."
"But without intention how can one know the Tao?"
"The Tao," said the master, "belongs neither to knowing nor to
not knowing. Knowing is false understanding; not knowing is
blind ignorance. If you really understand the Tao beyond doubt,
it's like the empty sky. Why drag in right and wrong?"

Buddhist to hot-dog vendor: "Make me one with everything!"

Having been exposed to the obviously life-enhancing qualities of neuro-feedback training, especially the LENS, through the stories in this book, you, dear reader, may now wish to experience those benefits for yourself. But that may give rise to the question: *Does a person have to have some or all of the problems mentioned in the earlier chapters of this book to benefit from the LENS treatment?*

The answer is absolutely, "No." LENS can help everyone experience a holistic improvement in their quality of life, particularly in regard to balancing of functionality, fostering the ability to respond to the enormous stresses of modern life, and optimizing one's full potential. Most of us have a combination of some highly accomplished features and some less-accomplished features of personality.

As Freud put it in *The Psychopathology of Everyday Life*, most people don't come all the way out of the infantile condition and probably shade into dysfunction or neurosis somewhere. Some people function beautifully in this modality but are unevolved in that one. Some have fine intellectual, but little emotional, intelligence; others have the inverse problem. Some are stellar extraverts, who grace any social occasion, but lousy introverts, who are bored when alone or left to their own devices. Others are very self-reliant when left to themselves but have social anxiety with groups. The LENS can help us *even out our functionality*; it seems to facilitate emotional and cognitive agility, aiding our capacity to respond effectively to a variety of situations.

Modern life puts stresses on us that are unexampled in all of human history. At least some instances of chronic fatigue or "burnout" are likely just human incapacity to keep up with such a demanding environment. Generically, the legendary flexibility fostered by the LENS training is enormously helpful, aiding us to respond successfully and gracefully to such demands.

Recently, there has been a renewed recognition of the value of *positive psychology* and *optimal performance*, whether in the workplace or for personal growth. We don't have to model our psychology on the failures, as in the Freudian *neurosis* model. Recognizing that, at our best, humans are pretty amazing creatures, we can learn from, celebrate, and cultivate more successes. At the top of his pyramid of human capacities, Abraham Maslow put *self-actualization*, that is, the full realization of the capacities inherent within the self.[2] Unlike the old stereotypes of the neurotic artist or the geek scientist, Maslow found that the highest self-actualizers he studied were well-rounded, motivated, life-affirming, often sociable, humanitarian people, who usually had a good sense of humor, besides! They demonstrate that there is a way of being human that is fulfilling, functional, flexible, and fun. LENS has shown—in my own experience as well as that of others—that it can be extraordinarily helpful in fostering greater access to these optimal ways of being.

Beyond Remediation

The power of LENS in all these areas has been demonstrated by the experiences of a few dozen people (among the hundreds) who have been treated at our center. This subpopulation was already high-functioning when it started but was looking for more improvement. It includes professional athletes and martial artists, computer programmers, doctors and professors, musicians and artists, practitioners of Zen and other mindfulness traditions. Although neurologically speaking they each already had a "well-oiled machine," LENS was able to add fine-tuning. In almost every case, they found their day-to-day functioning improved, particularly in respect to three factors that we label the "Three Fs": Force (mental and physical energy), Focus (directing and sustaining attention), and Feeling (mood and affect).

The results of LENS training with some high-functioning people:

- A computer programmer told me after a couple of weeks of treatment, "I've experienced a gradual reduction of that chatter in my head. It was always standing between me and what I would be doing." He acknowledged that he felt clearer in every way and moved more easily from task to task.

- Several clients found themselves suddenly resolving what had seemed to them and others to be "character flaws," such as disorganization and carelessness. When they realized these problems were neurological, they were also able to become less guilty and self-blaming.

- Some found they had more energy and clarity for their spiritual practices; they were able consistently to do them, whereas before, they could never quite "get it together" to practice.

- A concert pianist found his runs and arpeggios were not only improving, but he could also imbue them with more emotional coloration. He said his music had more "texture and life," and that those who listened to him remarked on how the vibrancy had come back into his playing.

- A writer found that his "writer's block" had dissolved, and words were coming much more easily. He found he could visualize the structure of his paragraphs at the same time as he focused on the sentences and words.

- A lecturer said it felt like his whole presentation was at his fingertips:

when he lectured there were no fits and starts, just a smooth moving from topic to topic. He felt more capable of mesmerizing his audiences with eloquence.

- An elementary school teacher found herself more tuned in to the children, better able to experience where they were coming from and to handle their demands gracefully.
- A businessman said he could see future possibilities in ways that had previously eluded him. Because he had organized his own details at work so well, he was able to look at "a bigger picture."

All of the experiences cited also include another important feature of LENS training: while it effects significant change, it does not do so by altering a person so that they become a stranger to themselves or others. Rather, the effects seem to be guided by the "self-similarity" principle identified by chaos theory. This principle is found throughout nature in simple binary processes that reproduce themselves, creating the organic forms of which Nature is made. Similarly, as human beings mature, they also become very "similar to themselves."

The negative instances are the curmudgeon who becomes more antisocial, the miser more stingy and miserly. But the positive possibilities can be seen in the examples of people whose personal obsessions flower into genius, whose private ideas turn into cosmic theorems, whose peculiar idiosyncratic art inspires generations, such as: Einstein becoming more Einstein-like, Mother Theresa more Mother Theresa-like, Charlie Chaplin more "Chaplinesque." People grow in a way that is somehow true to their essential pattern, producing something inimitably unique, yet that also benefits humankind. This is *self-actualization* indeed. LENS appears to have the capacity of speeding up this kind of *self-similarity*. Acting as a subtle catalyst, it helps people to turn into themselves more exquisitely, and there is something wholesome, and something basically "right" and intrinsically splendid about the process and the results.

The Tao of the LENS[3]

The *Tao Te Ching*, the book containing the wisdom teachings of Lao-tzu, tells us that in order to become successful as human beings, we must study the nature that is all around us. Take the water. Water overcomes obstacles by flowing around them. Also called "The Watercourse

Way," the experience of the Tao is most often referred to as "Flow" by those who dip into it.[4] The bliss-bestowing capacity of being in a state of "flow" has been remarked by people engaged in athletic competition; modern sports psychologists—realizing the stunning performances that can be given by people in such a state—seek to evoke it. The experience of flow is also reported by people engaged in music, dance, acting, and public oratory; it can probably be found to attend any creative or therapeutic act in which there is a feeling of unity, of being "at-one" with All there Is. In such a state the self is experienced as transparent, effortless, graceful; there is no obstacle between thought and enactment.

But what if, instead of feeling oneness, we feel, as Woody Allen says, "At two with everything"? Daily life may be a nightmare of fits and starts, noble intentions, but impoverished performances. We bungle this and overreact to that. We wax far too optimistic for our own good, then feel defeated and lapse into a dark, paralyzing pessimism. We make impossible generalizations from our experience—"I'll never, ever, do that again!"—and violate them the next week, because they were ridiculous in the first place.

Then we look around us and see that everyone else is in the same sorry state, more or less. The world is a theater full of blunders, some great, some small. Cartoonist Robert Crumb caught the atmosphere: "Back in Grimesville, time lurches on!" The news tells the story: people all over this good Earth communicate poorly, overreact, cling to nasty attitudes, and act unfairly to each other.

"Our life story," said the great American psychologist Jerome Bruner, "is the vicissitudes of intention." We intend *this,* but the unexpected happens, and we get *that.* Put more succinctly by John Lennon: "Life is what happens while you are making other plans." And life keeps lobbing those old curve balls at us: divorce, financial failure, tragedy, negotiations with insurance companies, meetings with the IRS. Each takes their toll. Other people may refuse to see us as radiant and wonderful, and we take on their negative vision of us or even begin to act it out.

Modern life puts additional stresses on us in the form of multiple information-processing tasks that our ancestors never dreamed of, along with the demand that we be able to switch quickly from task to task, such as: balancing our budgets, acquiring technical and computer literacies, achieving political correctness, single-parent child rearing, driving in traffic, negotiating international airports, staying fit and healthy in a toxic world, and nourishing our souls in an (often) cultural wasteland.

These difficult demands verge on the impossible, especially when we are out of harmony with ourselves. Somehow, on the threshing floor of existence—with our own lives in the balance—the ancient Taoist flexibility may be more than a nice idea: it may be a way of survival, an ancient tool for finding harmony in unharmonious places. An innate flexibility may help us cope with the factuality of unexpected or unwanted events, and the simultaneous, ongoing, niggling demands for detailed high-performance that contemporary life seems to require.

The experiences of our clients—from those struggling with the most damage to the highest functioning—attest to the capacity of the LENS training to provide everyone with at least a taste of the experience of flow and flexibility, and sometimes far more.

As I sit in front of the computer screen and watch the *dominant frequency* bar of a client's EEG move easily between the ranges, I know that the person in front of me is gaining more flexiblity. Growing in their capacity to avoid interior stuckness, they are learning to "play ball on running water" (a metaphor from Taoism and Zen).[5] I don't know of any other biofeedback treatment that measures this ability to slide smoothly between the brain wave ranges, as a desideratum.

Yet we have seen again and again that this correlates to greater fluidity in meeting life's challenges: People get more pragmatic, and more appropriate, as well as more flexible, with the LENS training. The LENS takes the sting out of negative affective states and helps a person to process things more dispassionately. Unlike Prozac and other drugs, it does not seem to do this at the cost of numbing a person's affective, or *feeling* tone; it just removes some of the bitterness or compulsion out of negative emotions.

People who begin functioning at a much higher level keep doing things that make them still better—they play their musical instruments, do *tai chi*, or *Pilates*. They solve kinesthetic problems in their sports or other motor skill performance. They study more because they retain more. They try new activities because they're less afraid of failure. And best of all, without any particular agenda, *life around them flourishes*, as it did around the rainmaker in one of Carl Jung's favorite stories, an old Taoist story from ancient China.

There was a region where people would quarrel openly, the dogs snarled and bit each other, there was filth in the streets, and the courtyards were cluttered. Then there was a great and terrible drought—no rain fell for months. The crops were dying, the animals were distempered and ill.

Finally, at a town meeting, full of bickering among the desperate townspeople, someone suggested: "Get the Taoist, the Rainmaker!" Many mocked the idea, but no one had a better solution.

A messenger was sent, in haste, to the Taoist's eyrie, high in the misty mountains.

He finally arrived, an old bearded man with a rucksack and a staff, taking his time, walking around the town and surrounding area. Finally he made a simple request: a small, poor hut where he could sit alone. By the third day, people were beginning to grouse and complain—but then the rains began! They moistened the fields and quelled the awful dust; they filled the watercourses and the wells. The people were astonished.

They came to the old man, where he still sat in his hut, meditating. "How did you do it? You must be a great magician, you changed nature, you changed the world itself!"

"Not really," said the Taoist gently. "When I first came here, I felt a great disharmony. Nothing was in resonance with anything else. I understood why the dogs bit each other. The whole world seemed angry. I even felt that way myself. I didn't like that, so I sat down to put myself in harmony. It took me longer than I expected: three days. But when I found my own harmony, then it began to rain."

The people were still astounded and begged him to stay there.

The old man just shrugged his shoulders. "All I know is that now I feel better." He picked up his bag and went back to the mountain. (The author's own retelling of Carl Jung's story.)

The beneficial impact of the old Taoist in this story provides helpful insight in understanding the positive role that sensitivity can play when a person is aided in using it rather than being victimized by it, as expressed by Len Ochs to the author:

There is no honored place for sensitivity per-se in our culture; outside of the arts, sensitivity has generally been something to be avoided and feared, because the people who are sensitive are wild cards. They are their own people; they depend on their own intuitions; they do not listen to other people; they cannot be pressured as much, and so on and so forth. But these people often are comfortable with their own sensitivity. In psychology, we all have started clinically with the reality of illness and dysfunction in others and then, axiomatically, in ourselves. Thus our sense of optimal functioning is based on what we *don't want* either our clients or ourselves to be: rigid, locked in, hysterical, or dissociative. But as the LENS enables people to recover from illness and rigidity, they shade more toward optimal functioning and health. This treatment brings a new freedom and depth to their lives. Ease of functioning is something people can evaluate for themselves, if they have even a modicum of self-reflective awareness. They are also able to express how far short of their own expectations they have fallen and *that* in itself is a really important faculty. I have the ultimate respect for the sensitivity of people; it shows their ability to know what is good for them and what is not.

I hope LENS is a tool that will deepen our awareness and our discernment, and improve our capacity to use our sensitivity. It could contribute to the evolution of people as being more functional and kinder, more compassionate and smarter, all of which depend on sensitivity. When sensitive, bright people really get better, the sky is the limit.

Finishing Up

When I asked Len what he thought needed to be included in this culminating chapter, he said "Finishing up."

"What?" I asked.

He explained, "Over the years, I have had many people come into treatment who were capable, but self-sabotaging. They seemed to have what it takes, yet they could never really make it all work and bring their projects to conclusion. After the LENS training they could."

I asked why he thought that was so.

"It has to do with their improved flexibility and greater access to a wider range of their own functionality. Instead of being blocked about what they really want to do, they just do it."

As he spoke, one of my cases immediately came to mind.

Frank is one of my favorite people: funny, talented, and smart. But some years ago, he was blocked on finishing the dissertation for his Ph.D. at NYU. He had completed everything else necessary for obtaining the degree. Frank's academically high-functioning family was fully behind him, but he seemed stuck in the mud and had been that way for *eight years* before he came to give LENS a try. Here's his story, told in his own words:

From the time I finished my coursework, until the time I handed in my final dissertation draft in September of 2000, more than eight years passed. I had been struggling for a long time with writer's block and high anxiety around the project, but following the death of my wife, Joan, my emotional state became extreme. For more than a year I could not remember anything I read, a dire circumstance for a graduate student who is being told at every opportunity to "finish up" before his whole dissertation committee retires—or dies!

As a now single parent, with a growing son in elementary school, living in an isolated area, where I had to drive five miles for a quart of milk, I had my hands full. I was determined to complete my task, yet doubted seriously that I could. I was completely committed, and yet very fearful of what the cost would be, even if I succeeded. I was utterly ambivalent.

I spent days and weeks stewing in anxiety. I lived in dread of telephone calls from my thesis advisor, because I would make commitments to her, and be unable to fulfill them. I suffered from *alopecia areata* (an autoimmune disease that causes hair to fall out in patches), as well as other physical symptoms of stress. I found myself awakening at three in the morning. I would often spend time simply arranging objects in my house, unable to sit still and write. This restless state ebbed and flowed, depending on the circumstances. But even in the good times, when I was able to write, often the writing took the form of disjointed notes that were not leading to completion.

I believe the biofeedback (the LENS) did indeed help me and that the good effects were due to more than placebo. For one thing I definitely felt physical effects. I would feel more relaxed immediately after the session. (I had to be very careful driving home because sometimes I would be drowsy.) I think that my underlying tiredness, from the insomnia, was coming to the surface as my hypervigilance was moderated by the biofeedback. The tension and anxiety I had been suffering were exhausting, but I had not felt them as such, rather I felt always "wired." (Underneath I was tired.)

After each session I would look at the graphs of my brain waves and watch them morph. I began to feel calmer. Little by little, the cycle of sleeplessness, anxiety at my lack of progress, the periods of great straining to yield a verbal *gnat*, and my unnecessary time-filling errands in and out of the house began to change. Over time I actually began to make progress on my writing, and could see the progress. I began to think about what I was doing, and to plan. The waters that had threatened to overwhelm and drown me subsided.

I found myself working longer and longer. The project began to take shape, and the texts began to find their form. Chapters emerged. Friends of mine commented that I now was speaking of the task in a way that led them to believe I might finish "the damn thing." I had begun to feel less "determined," by circumstances, and more *determined to act*—it was as if my action now mattered. The obstacles went from daunting to "merely something I was going to handle"—because I knew I was going to finish.

And I did.

(Dr.) Frank Boyer, March 2005

Finally the day came when it was all done! Frank told his family, and they all cheered! Then all he had to do was to "defend his thesis" to, by now, a somewhat disgruntled, fragmented, committee. (As seems inevitably to happen, some faculty *had* died or moved on, and others had taken their place.) But defend that long-gestated baby he did, articulately, "fiercely, like any mother," and, as he reported back, with verve and humor. He felt grounded and in control. The committee was impressed.

Frank came in later that summer for a social call—no more treatments needed. "*Doctor* Boyer I presume?" I asked in a made-up accent.

He smiled broadly and shook my hand: "*Doctor* Larsen, I presume."

Frank's case can be seen as a demonstration of the immense freeing of behavior that can take place when a person experiences what Joseph Chilton Pearce calls "unconflicted behavior." In his compelling book linking brain and behavior, *The Biology of Transcendence*, Pearce says that in this unconflicted state things that might otherwise be blunted by anxiety or sabotaged by fatalistic depression suddenly seem touched by grace and flow supervenes.[6] Another explication of the meaning of "unconflicted behavior" in the context of the LENS training can be seen in the following story.

A mother of a sixteen-year-old boy with ADD brought him to us for treatment. She had "hired" him to clean out the courtyard behind their Manhattan brownstone every year for four years. It had always ended in the same dismal failure, the mother not wanting to pay for such a lousy job, and yet desperately wanting to reinforce positive behaviors in her son.

During the course of the intake interview and CNS Questionnaire, I learned that her son Chet had been delivered by forceps, and when born, had two huge hematomas. The residual effect was two permanent cone-shaped bumps on his head. When we did the mapping of his brain waves, everything looked pretty good at most sites. But when we got to the vicinity of the injury, the moderate delta frequency activity jumped dramatically, creating high amplitude waves of delta and even theta, indicating that whenever Chet tried to focus or concentrate (requiring beta waves), he would be experiencing a truly conflicted brain state. But his chart also showed a beautifully flexible, low amplitude strip at a site right next to the damaged region.

I asked his mother, "What does Chet do really well, physically?" The mother beamed with pride and said he was as good in tennis as he was bad in school. He was a champion in the making, in fact. This was a very good sign and led me to the decision to treat the good sites that were right "next-door" to the sites of his birth-related injuries.

After only eight treatments the huge delta-theta waves began to diminish noticeably. His mother called up, overjoyed. She had been able to pay her son for a courtyard she could be proud of. It was organized— and tidily completed in the course of a weekend. Two days later Chet reported that he had been able to sit down for four hours and complete all his back homework. (The longest he had previously been able to concentrate had been about fifteen minutes.) The elegance and skill that he had already developed in tennis crossed a few neuronal pathways and lodged in the areas that controlled his academic abilities—and his ability to clean courtyards! Some months later, he completed a creative architectural project that was the envy of all his classmates; and that his teacher called "outstanding," marveling not only at the vision Chet had put into it, but at his perseverance and ability to complete things.

Gateway to Transpersonal Experience

During his later years, Abraham Maslow—one of the founders of the Human Potentials Movement in American psychology—started the "Transpersonal" movement. When self-actualization is fairly complete, he said, there come those moments of "self-transcendence" spoken of in the mystical literature of the world. If Maslow and some of his successors— such as Ram Dass, Stanislav Grof, Jean Houston, and Ken Wilber—are correct, "losing the self" and "finding the self" are one and the same thing. Paradoxically, participation in a greater (universal–eternal– transpersonal) life is the deepest affirmation of one's own selfhood.

Certain therapeutic modalities, such as Alcoholics Anonymous, are based on contact with a "higher self." As Carl Jung put it to Bill W., one of the founders of AA, "Only Spirit can free you from spirits (alcohol)." Researchers and practitioners of neurofeedback such as the Greens, Peniston, Fahrion, Kelly, White, and others have explored the capacity of training that specifically encourages the production of particular brain waves (alpha and theta) to give their clients access to therapeutically useful transcendent experiences. The LENS has no such overt agenda of seeking a brain wave state that opens the door to transcendent experiences. Nonetheless, we who are experienced clinicians have found that it indeed may do so at certain stages of the process. And for those clients who are open to this dimension, it can be a profound and life-enhancing experience.

The abbreviated story given below gives us a privileged access to one of these experiences. You have already met the protagonist in previous chapters: he is Joe Rock, the Vietnam Veteran who experienced immense trauma during the war and then relived much of it in the course of his treatment.

As we continued to work with Joe, his recollections of traumas began to thin out and the quality of his life continued to improve. He had fewer flashbacks, night sweats, and nightmares to cope with. But it was time to remap and re-offset. The more gentle map was accomplished in a couple of sessions, but then came time to do the offset, a process that at first can sometimes precipitate temporary discomfort—or even in the reactive patient, rather dramatic reactions. I asked him if he was ready (and tough warrior that he was) he said, "of course."

With some trepidation I began the offset, watching him carefully as the ten-minute procedure of stimulation began. He sat absolutely still. In the second half, tears began to roll down his cheeks. I paused the session and asked if he was okay. He nodded silently, so we continued.

When we were done, he sat with eyes closed for awhile; when he finally opened them he looked at me like a man emerging from a dream. He told the following story—which contrasts strongly with the traumatic memories we had become used to. During the course of the session he suddenly felt as if "a wise old man" was standing over him, someone like the figure Gandalf in *Lord of the Rings*. Kindness and love emanated from this figure, and he communicated telepathically with Joe, telling him to "relax and watch carefully." Joe felt enfolded in the being's cloak, like wings wrapped softly over him. He felt himself rising suddenly, and for quite a while. He said he felt like he took a ride up his own spine.

Then the cloak or wings was pulled back and Joe "saw" himself standing with the being on a mountaintop with a breathtaking view. Down below he saw his life spread out as if it were a landscape. He saw the suffering, obstacles, and limitations, and yet that there was a purpose behind it all. He seemed to see much deeper into the meaning of his life, that it was all "okay," and that a new period would now be beginning for him, and that was why he wept. Even when he opened his physical eyes, he said he could still feel the presence of the being, and the awesome love and wisdom radiating from him. The emotions persisted for days, and Joe noticed he was calmer about everything. His scores on the subjective symptom rating were noticeably lower.

Weeks passed, and his discomfort with his situation at home started to mount once again, as did his subjective rating scores (from 4s and 5s to 6s and 7s). Joe felt that he needed a "retreat" and an offer for one came from a kindly friend, a fellow veteran, who had a log cabin up in the Adirondacks. He invited Joe up for a week.

During Joe's sojourn with his friend among the peaks and pines near Lake Placid, the friend proposed an outing to Whiteface Mountain. There are many hard ways to get up Whiteface and all involve climbing, but—fortunately for those disinclined to such efforts—there is also a roadway to the top. Amazingly, there is also an elevator that goes up the center of the mountain for a couple of thousand feet to the very summit.

Taking the elevator requires traveling into the center of the mountain via a little electric train that goes through a tunnel. As Joe sat in the center of the mountain, waiting for the elevator, he looked down the long tunnel with the bright spot of outdoor light at the end. Then, with great emotion, he thought: "There is a light at the end of the tunnel." He said it to his friend, and before he realized what was happening, he was laughing and crying at the same time. Soon the elevator came to lift them up the channel in the center of the mountain. Joe was in quite a state.

When he got to the top he ran out under the open sky, oblivious of the startled tourists, and yelled: "Great Spirit, here I am standing here before you, a broken man in need of healing. I ask your help." He was shaking and crying. Suddenly there were winds buffeting the mountaintop, and people took cover as the two vets stood there—arms raised to the sky. Then, Joe reported—eyes flashing with the intensity of the moment—they noticed a strange thing: the winds seemed to come first from the East, then the South, then the West, and finally the North. Then his friend screamed against the wind: "Joe, look!" Two magnificent bald eagles were circling the mountaintop.

When Joe came into therapy the following session, his scores of insomnia, nightmares, anxiety, and rage attacks had dropped from 7 or 8 to 1 or 2. There had been healing on those winds. As Joe told me the story, we both remembered his vision in the session several weeks before. I think we both had goose bumps. My inner Jungian leaped to the fore, noting the similarities between the energy he had felt moving up his spine, the axis the yogis call the *Sushumna,* and Joe's journey up through the center of the mountain, and the presence of the four winds of the Native American Medicine Wheel, coming from each of the directions.

I also pointed out that in shamanic initiation the person faces an overwhelming challenge—such as the many meetings with death Joe had experienced in the war and relived in our sessions—and how facing one's fears can lift one out of one's usual fog. It can result in an encounter with something *other*, particularly a transpersonal other or others, such as the wise figure, and the bald eagles. The whole experience in some way recharges and renews the self, making one stronger.[7]

Joe's eyes were wide with amazement as I told him all of this. He was realizing that his story fit into a grand archetypal one, that the universe was offering him a new meaning. But what was most important for Joe was the *experience*, as Joseph Campbell would say, even more than the meaning. Like the young Native American warriors on a vision quest, he felt a sense of belonging, and a sense of the sacredness of all life. Though I have been a psychotherapist for about forty years, I think this moment with him was one of the absolute highlights of my career. My client brought me up to the mountaintop of initiation with him, and we both, for a little while, had the eyes of eagles.

The story of the rainmaker teaches us that "If you seek for it, it will not come. But if you expect nothing and purify your heart, it comes!" I am actually rather proud that transpersonal experience is not an explicit

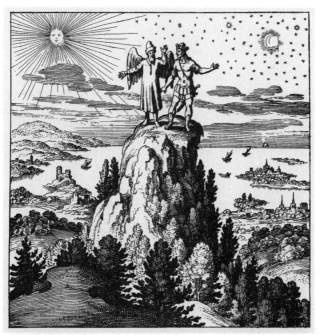

Fig. 15.1. Hermes shows the King's son the world from the mountaintop.

goal of the LENS process, but that sometimes, like an unannounced and holy guest, it comes. In my experience, not so different from Maslow's insight, it comes best when you have balanced the brain, soothed the body, and prepared the soul.

Here is a nice little story that illustrates the kind of effortless freedom the LENS training can foster for everyone: One snowy winter's day in New York State, a five-year-old girl begged her mother for permission to follow her father's snowplow down their half-mile long driveway. With some trepidation, her mother let her go, all bundled in her snowsuit, running after the plow on her little short legs. At the end of the driveway was a hill her mother never could have imagined her running up, but up she went, seemingly effortlessly. She caught up to her dad and rode triumphantly home in the plow, having completed a minihero's journey.

On her return, her mother marveled at her run up the hill.

"Oh, I didn't really do it," said the little girl, "Mother Nature carried me!"

Moving gently, from state to state, like clouds on a moonlit night, relaxed, calm, confident, in our training, our self-education, we sense the depths of the psyche; eyes and ears open, mind lightly poised, taking on the reflections of experience like a mirror, flowing like water. Thus may we receive instruction, and a little "lift" from Mother Nature, learning to move through our lives in Tao.

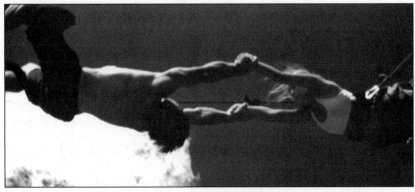

Photo S. Larsen

Fig. 15.2. The sky is the limit: Merlin Larsen catches Claire Woolger on the high flying trapeze at Stone Mountain Farm (June 2002).

NOTES

Introduction: Flexible Brain, Quiet Mind

1. James Pennebaker, Ph.D., *Writing to Heal: A Guided Journal for Recovering from Trauma and Emotional Upheaval.*
2. James Gleick, *Chaos: Making a New Science,* 90.

Chapter One: The LENS in Clinical Practice

1. Details of crime from *The New York Times,* 7/20/96.

Chapter Two: A Brief History of EEG Neurofeedback

1. Robin Larsen, ed., *Emanuel Swedenborg: A Continuing Vision;* Emanuel Swedenborg, *Spiritual Diary,* trans. G. Bush, J. Smithson, and J. Buss; Emanuel Swedenborg, *The Universal Human and Soul-Body Interaction,* ed. and trans. George F. Dole, introduction by Stephen Larsen, preface by Robert H. Kirven; see "The Soul and the Abyss of Nature" by Stephen Larsen in the first reference, and index entries on "Brain," "Tremulations," and "Cerebellula" in the other works.
2. Jim Robbins, *A Symphony in the Brain: The Evolution of the New Brain Wave Biofeedback,* 16.
3. C. G. Jung, *Experimental Researches, The Collected Works of C.G. Jung.*
4. See *Biofeedback: Advances in Neurofeedback and Neurotherapy* 28, no. 3 (Fall 2000). The issue is dedicated to Hans Berger (1873–1941).
5. W. G. Walter, "An Automatic Low Frequency Analyser," *Electronic Engineering* (June 1943): 9–13; and "The Electrical Activity of the Brain," *Scientific American* (June 1954): 54–63.
6. F. A. Gibbs and J. R. Knott, "Growth of the Electrical Activity of the Cortex," *Electroencephalography and Clinical Neurophysiology* (1949): I 223–229.
7. R. Fried, "What's in the Brain That Ink May Character Which Hath not Figured to Thee My True Spirit—Shakespeare," *Megabrain Report: The Journal of Mind Technology* 2, no. 4 (1994): 52–57.
8. J. V. Basmajian, *Biofeedback, Principles and Practice.*
9. Barbara B. Brown, *Stress and the Art of Biofeedback,* 125.

10. Karl Pribram, "The Neurophysiology of Remembering," *Scientific American* 220 (1969): 75; Karl Pribram, *Languages of the Brain.*

11. B. B. Brown, "Recognition of Aspects of Consciousness through Association with EEG Alpha Activity Represented by a Light Signal," *Psychophysiology* 6 (1970): 642; and "Awareness of EEG-Subjective Activity Relationships Detected Within a Closed Feedback System," *Psychophysiology* 7 (1971): 451.

12. A. Kasamatsu and T. Hirai, "Science of Zazen," *Psychologia* 6 (1963): 86–91.

13. Scott Lukas, "Brain Electrical Activity as a Tool for Studying Drugs of Abuse," *Advances in Substance Abuse* 4, no. 1 (1988).

14. E. Green and A. Green, "Biofeedback and States of Consciousness," in *Handbook of States of Consciousness.*

15. P. A. Norris, "Clinical Psychoneuroimmunology: Strategies for Self-Regulation of Immune System Responding," in *Biofeedback Principles and Practice for Clinicians,* third ed., ed. J. V. Basmajian.

16. T. Budzynski, "The New Frontier," *Megabrain: The Journal of Mind Technology* 2, no. 4 (1994): 58. Presented at the Fifth International Conference of The Psychology of Health, Immunity and Disease, sponsored by the National Institute for the Clinical Application of Behavioral Medicine (NICABM), Hilton Head, SC, 1993. Published while Budzynski was at The Center for Behavioral Medicine, University of West Florida, Pensacola, Florida. The same "trauma" of kissing a dead relative was recovered by Chris Sizemore, the actual patient in "Three Faces of Eve." In her case it led to the multiple personality or dissociative disorder that Eve (Chris) developed.

17. For more on mixing the LENS and psychotherapy see Chapter 12: "The LENS and other Modalities." Sebern Fischer and Seb Streifel have helped professional bodies such as AAPB educate themselves as to the ethics of "mixing therapeutic modalities." See Archive at AAPB.org, and WinterBrain, www.futurehealth.org/98 Brain Abstracts.

18. Budzynski, "The New Frontier."

19. Ibid.

20. Ibid., 59.

21. J. F. Lubar and M. N. Shouse, "Use of Biofeedback in the Treatment of Seizure Disorders and Hyperactivity," in *Advances in Child Clinical Psychology,* 204–51.

22. J. F. Lubar, *Neurofeedback,* pamphlet (Amsterdam: Biofeedback Foundation of Europe, 2001), www.bfe.org, mail@bfe.org.

23. J. F. Lubar and J. O. Lubar, "Neurofeedback Assessment and Treatment for Attention Deficit/Hyperactivity Disorders (ADD/HD)," in *Introduction to Quantitative EEG and Neurotherapy,* 103–43; J. F. Lubar, "EEG Biofeedback and Learning Disabilities," *Theory Into Practice* 24 (1985): 106–11.

24. Budzynski, "The New Frontier," 61. See also AAPB Newsletter: Interview with Margaret Ayers. Abstracts of her work also available from Ayers at Psychoneurophysiology, 427 Canyon Drive, Suite 105, Beverly Hills, CA 90210.

25. Budzynski, "The New Frontier," 61.

26. Siegfried Othmer, *Megabrain Report: The Journal of Mind Technology* 2, no. 4 (1994): 24.

27. J. Isaacs, "The Church of Brain Wave Training, Wherein the Author Is Converted and Sees the True Path Forward," *Megabrain Report: The Journal of Mind Technology* 2, no. 4 (1994): 14.

28. Ibid., 18.

29. E. Peniston, "EEG Alpha-Theta Neuro-Feedback: Promising Clinical Approach for Future Psychotherapy and Medicine," *Megabrain Report: The Journal of Mind Technology* 2, no. 4 (1994): 40.

30. Ibid.

31. Ibid., 42.

32. M. Kelley, "Brain Wave Biofeedback for Substance Abuse: The Development of a Navajo Alcohol Abstinence Empowerment Program," *Journal of Transpersonal Psychology* 2 (1991): 1–26.

33. N. White, "Alpha-Theta Training for Chronic Trauma Disorder, a New Perspective," *Megabrain Report: The Journal of Mind Technology* 2, no. 4 (1994): 50.

34. J. Hardt, "A Tale of Self-Discovery," *Megabrain* 2, no. 4 (1994): 16.

35. Hardt's *Biocybernaut Institute*, to the best of my knowledge, is still found at 1052 Rhode Island St., San Francisco, CA 94106.

36. L. Fehmi, "The Megabrain Interview," *Megabrain Report: The Journal of Mind Technology* 2, no. 4 (1994): 30–39. Fehmi notes in the article that this was also intended for publication in a forthcoming book by Joe Kamiya. See also Fehmi and Fritz, "Open Focus: The Attentional Foundation of Health and Well-Being," *Science*, Spring 1980, and "Attention and Neurofeedback Synchrony Training: Clinical Results and their Significance," *Journal of Neurotherapy* 5 (1/2) (2001).

37. See also chapter 12: "LENS and Other Modalities," where Fehmi's Open Focus work is documented.

38. J. P. Rosenfeld, "EEG Treatment of Addicitons: Comment on Ochs, Peniston, and Kulkosky," *Biofeedback* 20, no. 2 (1992): 12–17.

39. W. B. Plotkin, "On the Social Psychology of Experiential States Associated with EEG Alpha Biofeedback and Behavior"; W. B. Plotkin and K. M. Rice, "Biofeedback as Placebo: Anxiety Reduction Facilitated by Training in Either Suppression or Enhancement of Alpha Brain Waves," *Journal of Consulting and Clinical Psychology* 49, no. 4 (1981): 590–96.

40. J. Cowan, "Alpha-Theta Brain Wave Biofeedback: The Many Possible Theoretical Reasons for Its Success," *Megabrain Report* 2, no. 4 (1994): 32.

Chapter Three: The Development of the LENS Approach (Stephen Larsen)

1. M. R. Rosenzweig, "Experience, Memory and the Brain," *American Psychologist*, April 1984; M. R. Rosenzweig, "Brain Changes in Response to Experience," *Scientific American*, February 1972.

2. M. Diamond, "A Love Affair with the Brain," *Psychology Today*, November 1984.

3. James Oschman, *Energy Medicine in Therapeutics and Human Performance*, 220, 221.

4. E. L. Bennett and M. C. Diamond, "Effects of Differential Environments on Brain Anatomy and Brain Chemistry," in *Psychopathology of Mental Development*.

5. Budzynski, "The New Frontier," 62.
6. Ibid. Budzynski cites and summarizes the work of Carter and Russell; he also discusses the discovery process of Len Ochs in the same article.
7. Len Ochs, "New Light on Lights, Sounds, and the Brain," *Megabrain Report: The Journal of Mind Technology* 2, no. 4 (1994): 48.
8. Ibid.
9. *Megabrain Report* 2, no. 3 (Spring-Summer 1994).
10. Ibid.
11. Robbins, *A Symphony in the Brain*, 87.
12. Ochs, "New Light on Lights, Sounds, and the Brain," 48, 52.
13. Ibid., 52.
14. Ibid., 3.
15. 1993 Dialogue between Dr. Len Ochs and the author.
16. Ibid.
17. Ibid.
18. James Gleick, *Chaos: The Making of a New Science*.
19. 1993 Dialogue between Dr. Len Ochs and the author.
20. Ibid.
21. Ochs, "Thoughts," 5.
22. Ibid., 15.

Chapter Four: Traumatic Brain Injury (TBI) and Spinal Injury and the LENS

1. Robbins, *A Symphony in the Brain*, 82.
2. *The TBI Homepage, For Survivors and Caregivers* (The National Brain Injury Association, 105 Alfred Street, Alexandria VA 22314; tel. (703) 236-6000; www.tbihome.org).
3. Clearly a cloudy sensorium, aphasias and agnosias, ataxias and dyspraxias (types of clumsiness), or even mere depression or agitation can make a person more "accident prone," but there seem to be other as yet unaccounted variables in these histories of multiple traumas that make people susceptible to many accidents, even ones out of their own control, uncanny as it seems! (One patient, after the sudden death of her daughter, began to have auto accidents—four in two years. In one, a car coming the opposite way veered straight into her, causing a collision, and in another she was hit from behind at 40 mph while sitting at a traffic stoplight in an open area. Naturally it is helpful if these patients can also be helped with psychodynamic or insight-oriented therapies.)
4. Robbins, *A Symphony in the Brain*, 15.
5. A. Ommaya, "Head Injury Mechanisms and the Concept of Preventive Management: A Review and Critical Synthesis," in *Traumatic Brain Injury: Bioscience and Mechanics*.
6. J. S. Delaney et al., "Concussions during the 1997 Canadian Football League Season," *Clinical Journal of Sport Medicine* 10 (2000): 9–14.
7. Esselman and Uomoto, 1995, cited in M. Lezak, "The Walking Wounded of Head Injury: When Subtle Deficits Can Be Disabling," *Trends in Rehabilitation* 3, no. 3 (1988).
8. Lezak, "Walking Wounded"; Ommaya, "Head Injury Mechanics"; C. Brown,

"Biomechanics of Whiplash Injury," Annual Meeting Proceedings, American Academy of Pain Management (2001).

9. Alan J. Watts, *Low Speed Automobile Accidents—Accident Reconstruction and Occupant Kinematics, Dynamics and Biomechanics.*

10. See www.stonemountaincenter.com, Articles, for a posting of this paper, "The Tao of Neuroscience: Len Ochs's Magic Lights and the Realization of Cortical Flexibility," also delivered at "Winter Brain" (www.Futurehealth.org) in Palm Springs, in 1998 (www.Futurehealth.org/98 Brain Abstracts).

On more than one occasion while treating the bodily effects of head injury we have seen knots or spasms in the body come to the surface, intensify, and then disappear. A woman in her thirties with (congenital) Cerebral Palsy had a spasm that she experienced as a tight painful knot in her thigh that never diminished. She had tried muscle relaxers, massage, Feldenkrais, all to no avail. After the seventh FNS treatment, she was riding a bus somewhere in New England, when the pain of the spasm began to intensify. She felt terrified, alone on a trip, handicapped, and with this awful pain. Fortunately, after a while it subsided a little, and to her astonishment, shifted its location. Over the next few days it intensified and shifted several times, and then was gone totally. That was over twelve months before the time of this writing and the problem has not returned. She credits the FNS with relieving her of a pain she carried for over thirty years.

Chapter Five: Healing the Mind of Childhood

1. Daniel Goleman, *Emotional Intelligence: Why It Can Matter More Than IQ.*

2. Dr. Cripe can be reached at Crossroads Institute, Cave Creek, Arizona, or ctcripe@att.net or ctcripe@direcway.com. Glen Doman's interesting work in sensory integration can be googled with his name.

3. Thom Hartmann, *ADD Success Stories; Focus Your Energy; Healing ADD; Beyond ADD.*

4. Thom Hartmann, *Attention Deficit Disorder: A Different Perception,* 17. Hartmann Lists Hallowell and Ratey's criteria as well as the DSM criteria.

5. Edward Hallowell and John Ratey, *Driven to Distraction.*

6. Thom Hartmann, *ADD Success Stories; Healing ADD.*

Chapter Six: The Twilight Zone

1. Piedad Bernikow, "Missing Links: Unexplored Facts About FM and Accidents Which May Hold the Key to Recovery," *Fibromyalgia Frontiers* 9, no. 2 (2001): 1–9.

2. M. Melton, *The Complete Guide to Whiplash.*

3. Mueller, Donaldson, Nelson, and Layman, "Treatment of Fibromyalgia Incorporating EEG-Driven Stimulation," *Journal of Clinical Psychology* 57, no.7, excerpt from pages 947–49.

4. Bob Flaws, "Fibromyalgia—The Western Understanding," *Traditional Chinese Medicine World* 4, no. 1 (2002): 11.

5. Mueller, Donaldson, Nelson, and Layman, "Treatment of Fibromyalgia Incorporating EEG-Driven Stimulation," 934.

6. Coderre, Katz, Vaccarino, and Melzack, "Contribution of Central Neuroplasticity to Pathological Pan," *Review of Clinical and Experimental Evidence* 52 (1993): 259–85; Cited in Mueller, Donaldson.

7. Donaldson, Sella, and Mueller, "Fibromyalgia: A Retrospective Study of 252 Consecutive Referrals," 116–27.

8. Mueller, Donaldson, Nelson, and Layman, "Treatment of Fibromyalgia Incorporating EEG-Driven Stimulation," 933–52.

9. Ibid.

10. Mueller, Donaldson, Nelson, and Layman, "Treatment of Fibromyalgia Incorporating EEG-Driven Stimulation," 933–52; Donaldson, Sella, and Mueller, "Fibromyalgia: A Retrospective Study of 252 Consecutive Referrals," 116–27.

11. Sacheti, Szemere, Bernstein, et al., "Chronic Pain Is a Manifestation of the Ehlers-Danlos Syndrome," *Journal of Pain and Symptom Management* 14, no. 2 (1997): 88–93.

12. Primary Sjogren's involves lacrimal glands (eyes) and other salivary glands such as the parotid. Secondary Sjogren's is when the above symptoms are accompanied by a disease affecting the body's connective tissue. This is about 50 percent of the total Sjogren's population. Clearly Sheila fell into this category. One can find out more about Sjogren's at www.sjogrens.com/whatis.htm or wwwdir.nidcr.nih.gov/sjogrens/sjogrenindex.htm.

13. "Lyme Disease, the Unknown Epidemic," *Alternative Medicine* (May 2001): 84, 85.

14. Ibid. The spirochete *Borrelia burgdorferi* is named after the discoverer, Dr. Willy Burgdorfer of the U.S. Health Service. Drs. Allen Steere and Steven Malawista and their colleagues at Yale University were the among the first to describe the clinical characteristics of the disease in the mid-1970s. See also www.vrp.com/art/1370.asp and www.vrp.com/pdf/JulyNews2004.pdf.

Chapter Seven: High Anxiety, Deep Depression

1. Mihaly Csikszentmihalyi, *Flow: The Psychology of Optimal Experience*.

2. Daniel Goleman, *Emotional Intelligence*.

3. Each year, since 1999, Rob Kall has included an "Optimal Performance" section in his annual "WinterBrain" neurofeedback conference. I have presented something on the LENS method, in one or another of its inflections, in several of them. (See the online archive of www.Futurehealth.org).

Chapter Eight: The Divine Madness

1. M. B. Sterman and L. Friar, "Suppression of Seizures in an Epileptic Following Sensorimotor EEG Feedback Training," *Electro-Encephalography and Clinical Neurophysiology* 1 (1971): 57–86.

2. Robbins, *A Symphony in the Brain*, 46, 47.

3. Ibid., 48–9.

4. Ibid., 77.

Chapter Nine: Life Hurts

1. Anna Wise, *The High Performance Mind*.

2. Arthur Janov, *The Primal Scream.*
3. M. A. Tansey, "Righting the Rhythms of Reason: EEG Biofeedback Training as a Therapeutic Modality in a Clinical Office Setting," *Medical Psychotherapy* 3 (1990): 57–68.

Chapter Ten: Brain Attack

1. Steve Baskin, Ph.D., "Biobehavioral Considerations in Diagnosis and Treatment of Primary Headache Disorders," Invited Presentation at AAPB NorthEastern regional meeting, Winter 2005. Abstract available at www.AAPB.org.
2. Ibid. Baskin cites statistics that show "medication rebound" headaches are harder to cure than other types.
3. Green, Green, and Walters, "Voluntary Control of Internal States," *Journal of Transpersonal Psychology*, no. 11 (1970).

Chapter Eleven: Alternative Approaches to Evaluation and Treatment Using the LENS Perspective

1. S. B. Sells, ed., *The Definition and Measurement of Mental Health;* M. B. Smith, "Mental Health Reconsidered: A Special Case of the Problem of Values in Psychology," *American Psychologist* 16 (1961).
2. R. L. Spitzer, "On Pseudoscience in Science, Logic in Remission and Psychiatric Diagnosis," *Journal of Abnormal Psychology* 84 (1975): 442–52.
3. Ochs in conversation with the author, 2004.
4. Dr. Esty in conversation with the author, 2002.

Chapter Twelve: The LENS and Other Modalities

1. C. G. Jung, *Memories, Dreams, Reflections,* 247–48.
2. J. M. Schouten Dekker, E. G. Klootwijk, "The Zutphen Study: Heart-Rate Variability from Short Electrocardiographic Recordings Predicts Mortality from All Causes in Middle-Aged and Elderly Men," *American Journal of Epidemiology* 145, no. 10 (1997): 899–908.
3. Len Ochs's essay on the clinical use of the Photonic Stimulator by psychologists derived from a reply to Dr. Lynn Brayton, a LENS clinician, on our professional's *list serve.* At the time of this writing the mad-genius-driven OchsLabs has come up with its own version of the Photonic Stimulator, called the PS-1, an elegant, portable device, which is available from www.ochslabs.com.
4. Richard Brown, Teodoro Bottiglieri, and Carol Colman, *Stop Depression Now: SAM-e, the Amazing New Treatment.*
5. Richard Brown and Patricia Gerbarg, *The Rhodiola Revolution.* A supplier of high quality Rhodiola is Ameriden International. See www.ameriden.com.
6. The person who first educated us on glyconutrients, and our own personal supplier is Yvonne Cable (845) 657-7010. She also has access to educational information, and schedules for seminars on the subject.

Chapter Thirteen: Speculations on Physics, Energy Psychology, Chaos Theory, and Magnetite in the Brain

1. Daniel Kirsch, *The Science Behind Cranial Electrotherapy Stimulation*, 5–7.
2. Richard Gerber, M.D., *Vibrational Medicine*, 42.
3. Edgar Wilson, M.D. Unpublished paper in author's collection on Energy Medicine. See also Oschman: *Energy Medicine in Theraeutics and Human Performance* in Bibliography; and ISSEEM (The International Society for the Study of Subtle Energy and Energy Medicine). A conference is held once a year. See www.explorepub.com/events/06_23issseem.html. See also the work of Dr. Bruce Lipton: www.bruceliptoncom/cellular.php.
4. Kirsch, *The Science Behind Cranial Electrotherapy Stimulation*.
5. Paul Rosch and Marko Markov, *Bioelectromagnetic Medicine*, 850.
6. Christine Gorman, "Resetting the Brain: Can a Pulsing Magnet Really Change a Personality?" *Time Magazine*, March 21, 2005, 58, 59.
7. Evelyn Soehner, M.A., "The Therapeutic Role of Bioelectromagnetics," Association for Applied Psychophysiology and Biofeedback National Meeting (Las Vegas, Nevada, 2002).
8. www.washingtonpost.com/wp-dyn/articles/A34883-2004Mar5.html.
9. James Gleick, *Chaos: The Making of a New Science*, 230.

Chapter Fourteen: The LENS with Animals

1. Probably the world's most accessible collection on veterinary encephalography—the EEGs of many kinds of animals—has been assembled by the University of California at Davis. See www.vetmed.ucdavis.edu. Cornell University has also made available important information on animal EEGs through their veterinary college.
2. See the work of Terrell A. Holliday and Colette Williams at the Veterinary Medical Teaching Hospital, School of Veterinary Medicine, University of California Davis. Several excellent articles on veterinary encephalography have been made available online by Dr. Holliday at www.neurovet.org, with helpful references and further links. See www.neurovet.org/Hyperlinksofinterest.htm. The authors are particularly grateful for Dr. Holliday's generous posting of equine and canine EEG electrode placement maps.
3. For more information on Linda Tellington-Jones's work, and links to the international network that has grown out of it, see http://tteam-ttouch.com/.

Chapter Fifteen: Postscript: The Tao of LENS

1. The basis for this chapter is a paper originally presented by Stephen Larsen as "The Tao of Neuroscience: Len Ochs's Magic Lights and the Realization of Cortical Flexibility," Special Session, the Sixth Annual Winter Conference on Brain and EEG, February 1998, sponsored by Future Health (see resources).
2. Abraham H. Maslow, *Toward a Psychology of Being*, 2nd ed.
3. In the beginning was the Tao. It is sometimes translated as "Way." In the Tao, things are not wrong, they are the Way that they are. It is said that the larger one can imagine the Tao to be, the more likely one can harmonize or integrate

within it. It is a spiritual principle without a theology or the representation of anthropomorphic gods.

4. Alan Watts and Chung-liang Al Huang, *Tao, the Watercourse Way.*

5. *Playing Ball on Running Water* is also the title of a book on the Japanese therapies *Naikan* and *Morita* by David Reynolds.

6. Joseph Chilton Pearce, *The Biology of Transcendence: A Blueprint of the Human Spirit,* 15.

7. Stephen Larsen, *The Shaman's Doorway;* Joseph Campbell, *The Flight of the Wild Gander: Explorations in the Mythological Dimension,* 157.

BIBLIOGRAPHY

"Abstracts from the 5th World Congress on Myofascial Pain and Fibromyalgia." *Journal of Musculoskeletal Pain* 9, Suppl. no. 5 (2001): 116–27.

Alhambra, M. A., T. P. Fowler, and M. D. Alhambra. "EEG Biofeedback: A New Treatment Option for ADD/ADHD." *Journal of Neurotherapy* 1, no. 2 (1995): 39–43.

Ayers, Margaret. "Electroencephalographic Neurofeedback and Closed Head Injury of 250 Individuals." *National and Head Injury Syllabus, Head Injury Frontiers* (1987), 380.

Basmajian, J. V. *Biofeedback, Principles and Practice*. Baltimore, MD: Williams and Wilkins, 1989.

Bennett, E. L., and M. C. Diamond. "Effects of Differential Environments on Brain Anatomy and Brain Chemistry." In *Psychopathology of Mental Development*, edited by Zubin and Jervis. New York: Grune & Stratton, 1967.

Bernikow, Piedad. "Missing Links: Unexplored Facts About FM and Accidents Which May Hold the Key to Recovery." *Fibromyalgia Frontiers* 9, no. 2 (2001): 1–9.

Brown, Barbara B. "Recognition of Aspects of Consciousness Through Association with EEG Alpha Activity Represented by a Light Signal." *Psychophysiology* 6:642 (1970).

——. "Awareness of EEG-Subjective Activity Relationships Detected Within a Closed Feedback System." *Psychophysiology* 7:451 (1971).

——. *New Mind, New Body*. New York: Harper & Row, 1974.

——. *Stress and the Art of Biofeedback*. New York: Harper & Row, 1977.

Brown, C. "Biomechanics of Whiplash Injury." Annual Meeting Proceedings. American Academy of Pain Management, 2001.

Brown, Richard P., M.D., Teodoro Bottiglieri, and Carol Colman. *Stop Depression Now: SAM-e, the Amazing New Treatment*. New York: Berkley Books, 1999.

Brown, Richard P., M.D., and Patricia L. Gerbarg, M.D. *The Rhodiola Revolution: Transform Your Health with the Herbal Breakthrough of the 21st Century*. New York: The Rodale Press, 2004.

Bruner, Jerome S. *On Knowing: Essays for the Left Hand.* Cambridge: Belknap Press of Harvard University Press, 1962.

Budzynski, T. "The New Frontier." *Megabrain: The Journal of Mind Technology* 2, no. 4 (1994).

Campbell, Joseph. *The Flight of the Wild Gander: Explorations in the Mythological Dimension.* New York: The Viking Press, Inc., 1951.

"Cerebral Asymmetry, Emotion and Affective Style." In *Brain Asymmetry,* edited by R. J. Davidson and K. H. Hugdahl. Bradford Books. Cambridge: MIT Press, 1995.

Chabot, R. J., and G. Serfontein. "Quantitative Electroencephalographic Profiles of Children with Attention Deficit Disorder." *Biological Psychiatry* 40, no. 10 (1996): 951–63.

Chabot, R. J., H. Merkin, I. M. Wood, T. L. Davenport, and G. Serfontein. "Sensitivity and Specificity of QEEG in Children with Attention Deficit or Specific Developmental Learning Disorders." *Clinical Electroencephalography* 27, no. 1 (1996): 26–34.

Childre, Doc, Howard Martin, with Donna Beech. *The HeartMath Solution,* 281. San Francisco, CA: Harper/SanFrancisco, 1999.

Coderre, Katz, Vaccarino, and Melzack. "Contribution of Central Neuroplasticity to Pathological Pain: Review of Clinical and Experimental Evidence." *Pain* 52 (1993): 259–85.

Cork, Randall C. et al. "The Effect of Cranial Electrotherapy Stimulation (CES) on Pain Associated with Fibromyalgia." *The Internet Journal of Anesthesiology* 8, no. 2 (April 2004).

Cowan, J. "Alpha-Theta Brainwave Biofeedback: The Many Possible Theoretical Reasons for Its Success." *Megabrain Report* 2, no. 4 (1994): 29–35.

Crane, Adam, and Richard Soutar. *Mindfitness Training.* San Jose and New York: Writers Club Press, 2000.

Csikszentmihalyi, Mihaly. *Flow: The Psychology of Optimal Experience.* New York: HarperCollins, 1991.

Dekker, J. M., E. G. Schouten, P. Klootwijk et al. "The Zutphen Study: Heart-Rate Variability from Short Electrocardiographic Recordings Predicts Mortality from All Causes in Middle-Aged and Elderly Men." *American Journal of Epidemiology* 145, no. 10 (1997): 899–908.

Delaney, J. S., et al. "Concussions During the 1997 Canadian Football League Season." *Clinical of Journal of Sport Medicine* 10 (2000): 9–14.

Demos, John N., M.A. *Getting Started with Neurofeedback.* New York: W. W. Norton & Co., 2005.

Diamond, M. "A Love Affair with the Brain." *Psychology Today,* November 1984.

Donaldson, S., G. Sella, and H. Mueller. "Fibromyalgia: A Retrospective Study of 252 Consecutive Referrals." *Canadian Journal of Clinical Medicine* 56 (1998): 116–27.

Echemendia, R., and Julian L. "Mild Traumatic Brain Injury in Sports: Neuropsychology's Contribution to a Developing Field." *Neuropsychology Review* 11, no. 2 (2001).

Fehmi, Lester G., Ph.D. "The Megabrain Interview." *Megabrain Report: The Journal of Mind Technology* 2, no. 4 (1994): 30–39.

Fehmi, Lester G., Ph.D., and George Fritz, Ed.D. "The Attentional Foundation of Health and Well-Being." *Science*, Spring 1980.

Fehmi, Lester G., Ph.D., and J. T. McKnight, Ph.D. "Attention and Neurofeedback Synchrony Training: Clinical Results and Their Significance." *Journal of Neurotherapy* 5(1/2) (2001): 45–61. The Haworth Press, Inc.

Flaws, Bob. "Fibromyalgia: The Western Understanding." *Traditional Chinese Medicine World* 4, no. 1 (2002).

Fletcher, D. J., and Tom Klaber. "Lyme Disease, the Unknown Epidemic." *Alternative Medicine*, May 2001, 80–92.

Frank, Jerome D., and Julia B. Frank. *Persuasion and Healing: A Comparative Study of Psychotherapy*. With a foreword by Norman Cousins. 1973. The Johns Hopkins University Press, 1991.

Fried, R. "What's in the Brain That Ink May Character Which Hath not Figured to Thee My True Spirit—Shakespeare." *Megabrain Report: The Journal of Mind Technology* 2, no. 4 (1994): 52–57.

Gardiner, Harold. C., ed., Richard Whitford, trans. *The Imitation of Christ*. Garden City, NY: Doubleday, Image Imprint, 2005.

Gerber, Richard, M.D. *Vibrational Medicine*, 3rd edition. Rochester, VT: Bear and Co., 2001.

Gibbs, F. A., and J. R. Knott. "Growth of the Electrical Activity of the Cortex." *Electroencephalography and Clinical Neurophysiology* 1 (1949): 223–29.

Gleick, James. *Chaos: Making a New Science*. New York: Viking Penguin, 1987.

Goleman, Daniel. *Emotional Intelligence: Why It Can Matter More Than IQ*. New York: Bantam Books, 1995.

Gorman, Christine. "Resetting the Brain: Can a Pulsing Magnet Really Change a Personality?" *Time Magazine*, 21 March 2005, 58, 59.

Green, Elmer, Alyce Green, and D. Walters. "Voluntary Control of Internal States: Psychological and Physiological." *Journal of Transpersonal Psychology*, no. 11 (1970): 1–26.

Green, Elmer, and Alyce Green. "Biofeedback and States of Consciousness." In *Handbook of States of Consciousness*. New York: Van Nostrand Reinhold, 1986.

Grof, Stanislav. *Realms of the Human Unconscious*. New York: E. P. Dutton, 1976.

Hallowell, Edward, and John Ratey. *Driven to Distraction*. New York: Pantheon Books, 1994.

"[Hans Berger (1873–1941): Issue Dedicated To]." *Biofeedback: Advances in Neurofeedback and Neurotherapy* 28, no. 3 (Fall 2000).

Hardt, J. "A Tale of Self-Discovery." *Megabrain* 2, no. 4 (1994): 14–28.

Hartmann, Thom. *Attention Deficit Disorder: A Different Perception*. With an introduction by Edward M. Hallowell, M.D., with a foreword by Michael Popkin, Ph.D. Grass Valley, CA: Underwood Books, 1993, 1997.

———. *Focus Your Energy: Hunting for Success in Business with Attention Deficit Disorder*. New York: Pocket Books, 1994.

———. *ADD Success Stories: A Guide to Fulfillment for Families with Attention Deficit Disorder; Maps, Guidebooks, and Travelogues for Hunters in This*

Farmers' World. With a foreword by John J. Ratey, M.D. Grass Valley, CA: Underwood Books, 1995.

———. *Beyond ADD: Hunting for Reasons in the Past & Present*. Grass Valley, CA: Underwood Books, 1996.

———. *Healing ADD: Simple Exercizes That Will Change Your Daily Life*. With a foreword by Dr. Richard Bandler. Grass Valley CA: Underwood Books, 1998.

———. *Thom Hartmann's Complete Guide to ADHD: Help for Your Family at Home, School and Work*. Grass Valley, CA: Underwood Books, 2000.

———. *The Edison Gene: ADHD and the Gift of the Hunter Child*. Rochester, VT: Park Street Press, 2003.

Hawkins, David. *Power Vs. Force: The Hidden Determinants of Human Behavior*. Carlsbad, California: Hay House, 1995.

Hefferline, R. F. "The Role of Proprioception in the Control of Behavior." *Trans. NY Acad. Sci.* 20 (1958): 739–64.

Holliday, Terrill A., D.V.M., and Colette Williams, B.S. *Advantages of Digital Electroencephalography in Clinical Veterinary Medicine, 1*. Davis, CA: Veterinary Medical Teaching Hospital and Department of Surgical and Radiological Sciences, University of California Davis. www.neurovet.org.

———. *Clinical Encephalography in Dogs*. Davis, CA: Veterinary Medical Teaching Hospital and Department of Surgical and Radiological Sciences, University of California Davis. www.neurovet.org.

Isaacs, J. "The Church of Brainwave Training, Wherein the Author Is Converted and Sees the True Path Forward." *Megabrain Report: The Journal of Mind Technology* 2, no. 4 (1994): 12–19.

Janov, Arthur, Dr. *Primal Scream*. New York: Doubleday, 1970.

———. *The Primal Scream: Primal Therapy: The Cure for Neurosis*. New York: Perigee, 1999.

———. *The New Primal Scream: Primal Therapy Twenty Years On*. Abacus, 2000.

Johansen, Ruthann Knechel. *Listening in the Silence. Seeing in the Dark: Reconstructing Life After Brain Injury*. Berkeley and Los Angeles: University of California Press, 2002.

John, E. Roy. "Principles of Neurometrics." *American Journal of EEG Technology* 30 (1990): 251–66.

Joseph, R. *The Right Brain and the Unconscious: Discovering*. New York: Plenum Press, 1992.

Jung, C. G. *Memories, Dreams, Reflections*. Recorded and edited by Aniela Jaffé, translated by Richard Winston and Clara Winston. 1961. New York: Random House, Vintage, 1963.

———. *Experimental Researches*. The Collected Works of C.G. Jung. Princeton: Princeton University Press, 1973.

Kamiya, J. "Conscious Control of Brainwaves." *Psychology Today* 1 (1968): 57–60.

———. "Autoregulation of the EEG Alpha Rhythm: A Program for the Study of Consciousness." In *Mind Body Integration: Essential Readings in Biofeedback*, E. Peper, S. Ancoli, and M. Quinn, eds., 289–98. New York: Plenum Press, 1979.

Kasamatsu, A., and T. Hirai. "Science of Zazen." *Psychologia* 6 (1963): 86–91.

Keifer, C. K., and J. Cowan. "State/Context Dependence and Theories of Ritual." *Journal of Psychological Anthropology* 2, no. 5 (1979): 53–83.

Kelley, M. "Brainwave Biofeedback for Substance Abuse: The Development of a Navajo Alcohol Abstinence Empowerment Program." *Journal of Transpersonal Psychology* 2 (1991): 1–26.

Kirkpatrick, Sidney D. *Edgar Cayce, an American Prophet.* New York: Riverhead Books (Penguin Putnam), 2000.

Kirsch, Daniel. *The Science Behind Cranial Electrotherapy Stimulation.* Edmonton, CA: Medical Scope Publishing Co., 2002.

Larsen, Robin, ed. *Emanuel Swedenborg: A Continuing Vision.* New York: The Swedenborg Foundation, 1988.

Larsen, Stephen. *The Shaman's Doorway.* 1988. Rochester, VT: Inner Traditions, 1998.

———. "The Soul and the Abyss of Nature." In *Emanuel Swedenborg: A Continuing Vision.* New York, NY: The Swedenborg Foundation, 1988.

———. "Mending the Mind of Childhood." *Chronogram* (1997). (First in a Series of Three Articles).

———. "Mid-Life Metamorphosis." *Chronogram* (1997). (Second in a Series of Three Articles).

———. "Re-Magicking the World." *Chronogram* (1997). (Third in a Series of Three Articles).

———. "The Tao of Neuroscience: Len Ochs' Magic Lights and the Realization of Cortical Flexibility." Winter Brain Conference (Futurehealth.Org). Palm Springs, CA, 1998. www.stonemountaincenter.com/Articles.

Larsen, Stephen, Ph.D. "The Use of Flexyx Treatment Modality with Patients with Multiple Brain and Spinal Cord Injuries." *Futurehealth* (Winter Brain Conference) Feb. 2001.

Larsen, Stephen, Ph.D., and Robin Larsen, Ph.D., et al. "The LENS with Animals: Preliminary Observations." International Society for Neuronal Regulation, National Conference. Fort Lauderdale, FL, 2004. PowerPoint Presentation, with accompanying video.

Lezak, M. "The Walking Wounded of Head Injury: When Subtle Deficits Can Be Disabling." *Trends in Rehabilitation* 3, no. 3 (1988).

Linden, M., T. Habib, and V. Tadojevic. "A Controlled Study of the Effects of EEG Biofeedback on the Cognition and Behavior of Children with Attention Deficit Disorders and Learning Disabilities." *Biofeedback and Self Regulation* 21, no. 1 (1996): 35–49.

Lubar, J. F. "EEG Biofeedback and Learning Disabilities." *Theory into Practice* 24 (1985): 106–11.

———. "Electroencephalographic Biofeedback and Neurological Applications." In *Biofeedback: Principles and Practice.* 3rd ed., edited by J. V. Basmajian, 67–90. Baltimore, MD: Williams and Wilkins Publishers, 1989.

———. "Neocortical Dynamics: Implications for Understanding the Role of Neurofeedback and Related Techniques for the Enhancement of Attention." *Applied Psychophysiology and Biofeedback* 2, no. 22 (1997): 111–26.

Lubar, J. F., and M. N. Shouse. "Use of Biofeedback in the Treatment of Seizure Disorders and Hyperactivity." In *Advances in Child Clinical Psychology*, edited by B. B. Lahey and A. E. Kazdin, 204–51. New York: Plenum Publishing Company, 1977.

Lubar, J. F., M. O. Swartwood, J. N. Swartwood, and P. O'Donnell. "Evaluation of the Effectiveness of EEG Neurofeedback Training for ADHD in a Clinical Setting as Measured by Changes in T.O.V.A. Scores, Behavioral Ratings, and WISC-R Performance." *Biofeedback and Self-Regulation* 20 (1995): 83–99.

Lubar, J. F., and J. O. Lubar. "Neurofeedback Assessment and Treatment for Attention Deficit/Hyperactivity Disorders (ADD/HD)." In *Introduction to Quantitative EEG and Neurotherapy*, edited by J. R. Evans and A. Abarbanel, 103–43. New York: Academic Press, 1999.

Lubar, J. O., and J. F Lubar. "Electroencephalographic Biofeedback of SMR and Beta for Treatment of Attention Deficit Disorders in a Clinical Setting." *Biofeedback and Self-Regulation* 9 (1984): 1–23.

Lukas, Scott. "Brain Electrical Activity as a Tool for Studying Drugs of Abuse." *Advances in Substance Abuse* 4, no. 1 (1988).

Mack, John. *Passport to the Cosmos: Human Transformation and Alien Encounters*. New York: Crown (Random House), 1999.

Maslow, Abraham H., *Toward a Psychology of Being*, 2nd ed. New York: D. Nostrand, Insight, 1968.

McCraty, Rollin, Ph.D. *The Energetic Heart: Bioelectromagnetic Interactions Within and Between People*. E-book. HeartMath Institute, 2003. www.heartmathstore .com.

———. "Mechanisms of Weak Electromagnetic Field Effects in Biological Systems." In *The Energetic Heart: Bioelectromagnetic Interactions Within and Between People*. E-book. HeartMath Institute, 2003. www.heartmathstore.com.

McGann, Jerome J. *Social Values and Poetic Acts: The Historical Judgment of Literary Work*. Cambridge, Massachusetts: Harvard University Press, 1988.

Melton, M. *The Complete Guide to Whiplash*. Olympia, WA: Body Mind Publications, 1998.

Milton, Richard. "Alternative Science: Challenging the Myths of the Scientific Establishment." Rochester, VT: Park Street Press, 1994.

Mueller, H., S. Donaldson, D. Nelson, and M. Layman. "Treatment of Fibromyalgia Incorporating EEG-Driven Stimulation: A Clinical Outcomes Study." *Journal of Clinical Psychology*, 57, no. 7 (2001): 933–52.

Norris, P. A. "Clinical Psychoneuroimmunology: Strategies for Self-Regulation of Immune System Responding." In *Biofeedback Principles and Practice for Clinicians*. 3rd ed., edited by J. V. Basmajian. Baltimore: Williams and Wilkins, 1989.

Ochs, Len. "EEG Entrainment Feedback." Annual Meeting of the AAPB, 1993.

———. "New Light on Lights, Sounds, and the Brain." *Megabrain Report: The Journal of Mind Technology* 2, no. 4 (1994): 48–52.

———. "Thoughts About EEG-Driven Stimulation After Three Years of Its Uses: Ramifications for Concepts of Pathology, Recovery, and Brain Function." Flexyx Publications, 1996; see also Web site, www.neurofunction.com.

———. Interview with Stephen Larsen in *Interview (3)*. Cassette tape recording 3, 2000.

———. Interview with Stephen Larsen in *Interview (4)*. Cassette tape recording 4, 2000.

———. Interview with Stephen Larsen in *Interview (5)*. Cassette tape recording 5, 2000.

Ommaya, A. "Head Injury Mechanisms and the Concept of Preventive Management: A Review and Critical Synthesis." In *Traumatic Brain Injury, Bioscience and Mechanics*, edited by F. Bandak, R. Eppinger, A. Ommaya. New York: Mary Ann Liebert Pub., 1996.

Oschman, James. *Energy Medicine in Therapeutics and Human Performance*. Philadelphia: Butterworth and Heinemann, 2003.

Othmer, Siegfried F. *Megabrain Report: The Journal of Mind Technology* 2, no. 4 (1994): 22–29.

Othmer, Siegfried, and Susan Othmer. "EEG Biofeedback for Attention Deficit Hyperactivity Disorder." *EEG Spectrum*, October 1992.

Othmer, Siegfried F., Susan Othmer, and Clifford S. Marks. "EEG Biofeedback Training for ADD, Specific Learning Disabilities and Associated Conduct Problems." *EEG Spectrum*, September 1991.

Othmer, Siegfried F., David Kaiser, and Susan Othmer. "EEG Biofeedback Training for Attention Deficit Disorder: A Review of Recent Controlled Studies and Clinical Findings." *EEG Spectrum*, June 1995.

Pearce, Joseph Chilton. *The Biology of Transcendence: A Blueprint of the Human Spirit*. Rochester, VT: Park Street Press, 2002.

Peniston, E. "EEG Alpha-Theta Neurofeedback: Promising Clinical Approach for Future Psychotherapy and Medicine." *Megabrain Report: The Journal of Mind Technology* 2, no. 4 (1994): 40–43.

Peniston, E. G., and P. J. Kulkosky. "Alpha-Theta Brainwave Training and Beta-Endorphin Levels in Alcoholics." *Alcoholism: Clinical and Experimental Research* 13, no. 2 (1989): 271–79.

———. "Alpha-Theta Brainwave Neuro-Feedback for Vietnam Veterans with Combat-Related Post-Traumatic Stress Disorder." *Medical Psychotherapy: An International Journal* 4 (1991): 47–60.

Pennebaker, James. *Writing to Heal: A Guided Journal for Recovering from Trauma and Emotional Upheaval*. Oakland, CA: New Harbinger Publication, 2004.

Plotkin, W. B. "On the Social Psychology of Experiential States Associated with EEG Alpha Biofeedback and Behavior." In *Biofeedback and Behavior*, edited by Legewie and Beatty. New York: Plenum Press, 1977.

Plotkin, W. B., and K. M. Rice. "Biofeedback as Placebo: Anxiety Reduction Facilitated by Training in Either Suppression or Enhancement of Alpha Brainwaves." *Journal of Consulting and Clinical Psychology* 49, no. 4 (1981): 590–96.

Pribram, Karl H. "The Neurophysiology of Remembering." *Scientific American* 220 (1969): 75.

———. *Languages of the Brain*. Monterrey, CA: Wadsworth Publishing, 1977 (NY: Brandon House, 1971).

———. "Interview." *Psychology Today*, February 1979, 71ff.

———. *Brain and Perception: Holonomy and Structure in Figural Processing*. Appendices in collaboration with Kunio Yasue and Mari Jibu. Hillsdale, NJ:

Stanford University and Radford University; Lawrence Erlbaum Associates, Publishers, 1991.

Reynolds, David K. *Playing Ball on Running Water: The Japanese Way to Building a Better Life*. North Yorkshire, U.K.: Quill, 1984.

Robbins, Jim. *A Symphony in the Brain: The Evolution of the New Brain Wave Biofeedback*. New York: Atlantic Monthly Press, 2000.

Rosch, Paul, and Marko Markov. *Bioelectromagnetic Medicine*, 850. New York: Dekker, 2004.

Rosenfeld, J. P. "EEG Treatment of Addictions: Comment on Ochs, Peniston and Kulkosky." *Biofeedback* 20, no. 2 (1992): 12–17.

Rosenzweig, M. R. "Brain Changes in Response to Experience." *Scientific American*, February 1972.

———. "Experience, Memory and the Brain." *American Psychologist*, April 1984.

Rossiter, T. R., and T. J. LaVaque. "A Comparison of EEG Biofeedback and Psychostimulants in Treating Attention Deficit Hyperactivity Disorder." *Journal of Neurotherapy* 1, no. 1 (1995): 48–59.

Russell, H. L., and Carter, J. L. "Cognitive and Behavioral Changes in Learning Disabled Children Following the Use of Audio-Visual Stimulation: The Trinity Project." The Annual Meeting of the Biofeedback Society of Texas. Dallas, TX, 1993, 1009.

———. "Challenge and Stimulation of the Brain Related to Quantitative Changes in Functioning." Unpublished paper, 1992.

Sacheti, A., J. Szemere, B. Bernstein, T. Tafas, T. Schecter, and P. Tsipouras. "Chronic Pain is a Manifestation of the Ehlers-Danlos Syndrome." *Journal of Pain and Symptom Management* 14, no. 2 (1997): 88–93.

Schoenberger, Nancy E., Samuel Shiflett, Mary Lee Esty, Len Ochs, and Robert Matheis, J. "Flexyx Neurotherapy System in the Treatment of Traumatic Brain Injury: An Initial Evaluation." *Journal of Head Trauma Rehabilitation* 16, no. 3 (2001): 260–74.

Sells, S. B., ed. *The Definition and Measurement of Mental Health*. Washington D.C.: Department of Health, Education and Welfare, Public Health Service, 1968.

Smith, M. B. "Mental Health Reconsidered: A Special Case of the Problem of Values in Psychology." *American Psychologist* 16 (1961).

Soehner, Evelyn, M.A. "The Therapeutic Role of Bioelectromagnetics." Association for Applied Psychophysiology and Biofeedback (AAPB), National Meeting. Las Vegas, Nevada, 2002.

Starlanyl, E., and M. E. Copeland. *Fibromyalgia & Chronic Myofascial Pain*. Oakland, CA: New Harbinger Publications, Inc., 2001.

Sterman, M. B. "Studies of EEG Biofeedback Training in Man and Cats." In *Highlights of 17th Annual Conference: VA Cooperative Studies in Mental Health and Behavioral Sciences*, vol. PP. 5060. Veterans' Administration, 1972.

———. *EEG Biofeedback Training in the Treatment of Epilepsy*. S. C. Padnes and T. R. Budzynski, eds. Roche Scientific Series, NC 6, 1977.

———. "Physiological Origins and Functional Correlates of EEG Rhythmic Activities; Implications for Self-Regulation." *Biofeedback and Self-Regulation* 21 (1996): 3–33.

————. *Atlas of Topometric Clinical Displays: Functional Interpretations and Neurofeedback Strategies.* New Jersey: Sterman-Kaiser Imaging Laboratory, 1999.

————. "Basic Concepts and Clinical Findings in the Treatment of Seizure Disorders with EEG Operant Conditioning." *Clinical Electroencephalography* 31, no. 1 (2000): 45–55.

————. "EEG Markers for Attention Deficit Disorder: Pharmacological and Neurofeedback Applications." *Child Study Journal* 30, no. 1 (2000): 1–22.

Sterman, M. B., and L. Friar. "Suppression of Seizures in an Epileptic Following Sensorimotor EEG Feedback Training." *Electro-Encephalography and Clinical Neurophysiology* 1 (1971): 57–86.

Swedenborg, Emanuel. *Spiritual Diary.* Translated by G. Bush, J. Smithson, and J. Buss. New York: The Swedenborg Foundation, 1978.

————. *The Universal Human and Soul-Body Interaction.* Edited and translated by George F. Dole. Introduction by Stephen Larsen, with a preface by Robert H. Kirven. New York: Paulist Press, 1984.

Tansey, M. A. "Righting the Rhythms of Reason: EEG Biofeedback Training as a Therapeutic Modality in a Clinical Office Setting." *Medical Psychotherapy* 3 (1990): 57–68.

Thompson, Michael, and Linda Thompson. *The Neurofeedback Book: An Introduction to Basic Concepts in Applied Psychophysiology.* Wheat Ridge, CO: The Association of Applied Psychophysiology and Biofeedback, 2003.

The TBI Homepage, for Survivors and Caregivers. www.tbihome.org.

Walter, W. Grey. "An Automatic Low Frequency Analyser." *Electronic Engineering,* June 1943, 9–13.

————. "The Electrical Activity of the Brain." *Scientific American,* June 1954, 54–63.

Watts, Alan J. *Low Speed Automobile Accidents—Accident Reconstruction and Occupant Kinematics, Dynamics and Biomechanics.* Lawyers and Judges Publication Co (800-209-7109). Sales@lawyersandjudges.com.

Watts, Alan, and Al Chung-liang Huang. *Toa, the Watercourse Way.* New York: Pantheon Books, 1975.

White, N.E. "Alpha-Theta Training for Chronic Trauma Disorder, a New Perspective." *Megabrain Report: The Journal of Mind Technology* 2, no. 4 (1994): 44–50.

————. "Theories of the Effectiveness of Alpha-Theta Training for Multiple Disorders." In *Introduction to Quantitative EEG and Neurofeedback,* edited by James R. Evans and Andrew Abaranel. San Diego: Academic Press, 1999.

Wise, Anna. *The High Performance Mind.* New York: Tarcher/Putnam, 1997.

GLOSSARY OF ACRONYMS

AAPB: Association for Applied Psychophysiology and Biofeedback, an organization whose mission is to advance the development, dissemination, and utilization of knowledge about applied psychophysiology and biofeedback to improve health and the quality of life through research, education, and practice.

ABA (study): A research design in which subjects are exposed to condition A, (the independent variable, for example) then B (nothing done, for example), then A the independent variable) again, to observe the effect of the different conditions on the dependent variable—effect or result.

AchE: Acetylcholinesterase is an enzyme that digests (erases) the neurotransmitter acetylcholine.

ADD: Attention Deficit Disorder. A generic term that includes a variety of attentional problems.

ADHD: Attention Deficit Hyperactive Disorder in which there is restlessness and impulsive behavior in addition to distraction.

ALS: Lou Gehrig's Disease. A degenerative disease characterized by loss of muscle control, and fatigue that affects the nervous system.

AVS: Audio-Visual Stimulation.

C-2 I-330: Biofeedback instrument made by J&J Engineering.

CAM: Complementary and Alternative Medical Approaches.

CES: Cranioelectrical Stimulation (a form of Bioelectromagnetic Medicine). Cranial-electrical stimulation or "microcurrent stimulation" as in the "alpha-stim" machine is used when there is physical pain or a blockage. Can also help with anxiety and addictive problems when used cranially.

CHADD: Children with ADD (a Parent's Organization).

CNS: Central Nervous System.

CNSQ: Central Nervous System Questionnaire designed by Dr. Len Ochs.

CP: Cerebral Palsy. A severe developmental disability usually occurring perinatally and characterized by one or more sensory-motor and cognitive handicaps.

CT or CAT: Computer Assisted Tomography. A brain and body scanning technique.

DHEA: Di-hydro-epi-andosterone. A benign well-being enhancing corticoid made in the body by the adrenals, or taken supplementarily. Measurable improvements in DHEA are observed with HeartMath training.

DSM IV-r: Diagnostic and Statistical Manual of Mental Disorders-revised.

EDF: EEG Disentrainment Feedback (an early name for the LENS).

EDS: EEG-Driven Stimulation (an early name for the LENS).

EEF: EEG Feedback (an early name for the LENS).

EEG: Electroencephalograph. The brainwave-reading machine discovered and named by Hans Berger in 1924.

EMDR: The Eye Movement Desensitization and Reprocessing discovered by Francine Shapiro used for therapeutic amelioration of traumas and painful memories.

EMF: Electomagnetic Field.

EMG: Electromyograph. A machine that measures and displays muscle tension.

FNS: Flexyx Neuropathy System (an early name for the LENS).

GSR: Skin Galvanometer. A machine that shows a read-out of changes in the skin's conduction of electrical stimuli, a way of measuring stress.

HRV: Heart Rate Variability. A measure of cardiac health and well-being used in HeartMath and other biofeedback protocols.

I-400: Biofeedback instrument made by J&J Engineering.

ILT: Interactive Light Therapy (an early name for the LENS).

IRB: Institutional Review Board. A body that oversees clinical and research activities at many centers or facilities.

ISNR: International Society for Neurofeedback and Research. A professional body for neurofeedback.

LD: Learning Disabled; can be verbal or nonverbal in nature.

LED: Light Emitting Diode.

LENS: Low Energy Neurofeedback System.

MRI: Magnetic Resonance Imaging. A brain and body analyzing technique.

MS: Multiple Sclerosis. A degenerative disease in which the myelin sheath of the nervous system degenerates causing severe impairments in motor control and many aspects of functioning.

NLP: Neuro-Linguistic Programming. A hypnotic and therapeutic system developed by Grinder and Bandler from the work of hypnotist Dr. Milton Erickson.

OCD: Obsessive-Compulsive Disorder. A disorder characterized by an obsession with primarily repetitive thoughts and/or a compulsive urge to enact rituals or other behaviors.

PDD: Pervasive Developmental Disorder. A disorder characterized by a failure to achieve normal sequences of developmental milestones.

PTSD: Post-Traumatic Stress Disorder. The psycho-neurological aftereffects of severe, tragic, or violent experiences.

QEEG: Quantitative EEG.

QRIBb: A test for Lyme Disease.

RAD: Reactive Attachment Disorder. Reactive Attachment Disorder is characterized by the breakdown of social ability of a child. It is associated with the failure of the child to bond with a caretaker in infancy or early childhood.

RFI: Radio-Frequency Interference Filters. Used on earlier models of EEG processors.

rTMS: Repetitive Transcranial Magnetic Stimulation. A form of Bioelectromagnetic Medicine in which a powerful magnetic field is applied to the brain.

RVS: Reactivity-Vitality-Suppression Questionnaire developed by Dr. Len Ochs to assess neurological sensitivity.

SD: Standard Deviation. A statistical measure of variability in neurofeedback that is indicated by a sudden rise or fall of amplitude of brain waves, in the LENS maps indicated by a blue bar on top of a black one in a histogram. A measure of the "life" in a site.

SMR: Sensory-Motor Rhythm type of brain wave 12–15 Hz, used by Barry Sterman to inhibit seizures.

SPECT: Single Positron Emission Tomography. A diagnostic technique.

SQUID: Superconducting Quantum Interferometric Device magnetometers, which monitor the electrical activity of the brain.

SSRI: Selective Serotonin Re-uptake Inhibitor, which seeks to help depressed patients by flooding the system with serotonin, the "feel-good" neurotransmitter. An example of an SSRI would be Prozac or Zoloft.

TBI: Traumatic Brain Injury. Can be structural (long axonal shearing) or functional (involving loss of function or access to certain brain areas because of the brain's own protective mechanism).

TCM: Traditional Chinese Medicine.

TENS: Transcutaneous Electrical Nerve Stimulation. A form of Bioelectromagnetic Medicine used by some physical therapists or chiropractors to relax muscles.

TMJ: Temporomandibular Joint Disorder. A disorder characterized by a tense jaw and/or teeth-grinding.

VNS: Vagal Nerve Stimulation. A form of Bioelectromagnetic Medicine in which an implant is attached to the Vagus nerve (one of the ten cranial nerves) to control some of the side effects of Parkinson's Disease and other problems.

GLOSSARY OF DISEASES/CONDITIONS

ALS: Lou Gehrig's Disease. A degenerative disease characterized by loss of muscle control, and fatigue that affects the nervous system.

Alzheimer's Disease: A problem involving global loss of CNS functioning in people of middle, but not advanced age.

Aneurysm: A brain bleed, usually due to a ruptured blood vessel.

Anorexia Nervosa: A self-starvation pattern characterized by anxieties related to food and eating.

Anxiety: Fearfulness (generalized or acute) that has no obvious cause.

Asperger's Syndrome: A high functioning species of autism.

Attention Deficit Disorder (ADD): A generic term for a disorder that includes a variety of attentional problems.

Attention Deficit Hyperactive Disorder (ADHD): A disorder in which there is restlessness and impulsive behavior in addition to distraction.

Autism: A developmental disorder characterized by an inability to form normal social relationships and/or communicate with others.

Bereavement: Grief over having lost a loved one or significant other.

Bipolar Depression Disorder: A mood disorder formerly known as Manic-Depression, characterized by extremes of depression and mania.

Bulimia: A condition related to anorexia characterized by binge eating and rituals of vomiting.

Cerebral Palsy (CP): A severe developmental disability usually occurring perinatally, and characterized by one or more sensory-motor and cognitive handicaps.

Chronic Fatigue Syndrome: An identifiable syndrome characterized by a loss of stamina and/or functionality.

Dementia: A loss of mental functioning that may be accompanied by poor thinking, delusions, or hallucinations.

Depression: A mood disorder characterized by sadness and hopelessness.

Disassociative Disorder: A "splitting" of the self into one or more parts; walling off or hiding something from oneself.

Dysthymia: A low-grade persistent depression characterized by a loss of zest for life.

Dystonia: Loss of muscle tone or, on the other hand, involuntary spasms or movement.

Epilepsy: Seizure disorder that may involve neurological loss of control due to mild (*absence*) seizures to severe (*grand mal*) seizures.

Epstein-Barr Syndrome: An infectious problem that often degenerates into chronic fatigue or fibromyalgia.

Explosive Personality Disorder: A problem in which people become extremely angry or even violent over relatively insignificant problems.

Fetal Alcohol Syndrome: Neurological deficits that can be quite severe, in the children of mothers who drink while pregnant.

Fibromyalgia: A problem involving fatigue, "fibro-fog," or cognitive cloud, and bodily pain, including "tender points" throughout the body.

Headache: May present as "Cluster," acute and painful but shorter lived; Migraine, which can be both acute and of longer duration with "aura" nausea and photophobia; or Tension, a common, lower-grade, more persistent kind of headache that is often caused by tense neck and scalp muscles.

High Blood Pressure: Can be due to a known physiological cause, as in atherosclerosis, or an unknown cause "essential hypertension."

Irritable Bowel Syndrome: A milder form of "ulcerative colitis" characterized by frequent diarrhea.

Learning Disability: A developmental disability that can be verbal or nonverbal in nature.

Lyme Disease: A disease caused by the spirochete *Borrelia burgdorferi*, which attacks the nervous system and may leave a person weak and in considerable pain.

Manic-Depression: Now called "Bipolar Disorder," characterized by mood instability.

Migraine: see Headache.

Monopolar Depression Disorder: Affective disorder characterized by "depression" but without mood-swings or mania.

Multiple Sclerosis (MS): A degenerative disease in which the myelin sheath of the nervous system degenerates, causing severe impairments in motor control and many aspects of functioning.

Muscle Spasms: Painful involuntary contractions of muscles. One of the few "scheduled" problems for which biofeedback (having demonstrated success) may be billed to third party payers.

Obsessive-Compulsive Disorder (OCD): A disorder characterized by an obsession with primarily repetitive thoughts and/or a compulsive urge to enact rituals or other behaviors.

Oppositional-Defiant Disorder: A refractory behavior pattern in children and adolescents characterized by the attempts of adults to oppose and control the children's behavior.

Osgood-Schlatter's Syndrome: A disorder characterized by growing pains, usually affecting the knees and lower legs in painful ways.

Panic Attack: An acute anxiety disorder involving feelings of imminent disaster or death.

Parkinson's Disease: A degenerative disorder caused by abnormalities in the neurotransmitter dopamine, and the *substantia nigra* of the midbrain.

Paranoia: A fear that others, or secret forces, are plotting against you.

Pervasive Developmental Disorder (PDD): Failure to achieve normal sequences of developmental milestones.

Phobia: Anxiety provoked in a particular situation or environment, i.e., bridges, elevators, closed spaces.

Post-Traumatic Fibromyalgia: Fibromyalgia with accompanying weakness and exhaustion and pain points; often can be traced to an injury of some kind.

Post-Traumatic Stress Disorder (PTSD): The psycho-neurological aftereffects of severe, tragic, or violent experiences.

Reactive Attachment Disorder (RAD): A disorder in which the child is neglected, abused, or both; characterized by emotional abnormalities and lags in development.

Restless Leg Syndrome: An extremely distressing condition in which the legs twitch or jerk involuntarily and may be pain-filled as well. Often sleep-related.

Savant Syndrome: An autistic-like behavior in which the child or adult lacks ordinary social or emotional intelligence but may show close-to-genius abilities in other areas—such as mathematics, memory, calendar calculations.

Schizo-Affective: A DSM IV-r diagnosis for problems that resemble schizophrenia, but also have an associated mood disturbance.

Schizophrenia: A loosely defined category involving bizarre ideas, poor social skills, inappropriate affect or hallucinations and/or delusions.

Seizure Disorder: A disorder wherein the brain or Central Nervous System (CNS) is periodically overwhelmed by extremely high amplitude brain waves, frequently in the theta (4–8 Hz range). Can be severe (*grand mal*) to mild (*absence*). Temporal lobe epilepsy can resemble schizophrenia.

Shaken Baby Syndrome: A type of child abuse by immature or emotionally ill parents or other caretakers, in which there is significant nervous system damage; may include axonal shearing, paralysis, and death.

Stroke: A loss of Central Nervous System (CNS) function, usually due to a restriction in blood flow (clot).

Temporomandibular Joint Disorder (TMJ): A disorder characterized by a tense jaw and/or teeth-grinding.

Tics: Involuntary physical (motor) movement, can include involuntary jerks, grunts, grimaces.

Tourette's Syndrome: A neurological problem of unknown origin characterized by involuntary tics, or verbal expostulations, including obscenities or involuntary "cursing."

Traumatic Brain Injury (TBI): Can be structural (long axonal shearing) or other physical damage, or functional (involving loss of function or access to certain brain areas because of the brain's own protective mechanism).

Ulcerative Colitis: A severe bowel disorder characterized by involuntary diarrhea, intestinal spasms, and gas.

GLOSSARY OF HEALING MODALITIES

Acupuncture: A form of TCM (traditional Chinese medicine) using small needles placed at points along "meridian lines" to alleviate many kinds of problems.

Bioenergetic Therapy: A "neo-Reichian" therapy involving analysis of "character armor"—problems "stuck in the musculature of the body." Developed by Dr. Alexander Lowen.

Biofeedback: A generic term for a therapeutic modality in which information about the person is "fed-back" to them, usually with electronic instrumentation.

Complementary and Alternative Medical Approaches (CAM): Therapeutic practices not currently considered an integral part of conventional allopathic medical practice. Therapies are termed as Complementary when used in addition to conventional treatments and as Alternative when used instead of conventional treatment.

Cranial-Electrical Stimulation (CES): Also known as "microcurrent stimulation" as in the "alpha-stim" machine, used for physical pain or blockage. Can also help with anxiety and addictive problems when used cranially.

CranioSacral Therapy: A type of gentle manipulation of the bony plates of the skull, believed to affect the synovial fluid, often helpful for relaxation or emotional release.

Deep Vascular Relaxation: A type of visualization and attention exercise developed by Dr. Len Ochs to help with peripheral pain, Raynaud's Syndrome, and migraine headaches.

EMDR: The Eye Movement Desensitization and Reprocessing technique developed by Francine Shapiro.

Feldenkrais: A gentle technique of physical manipulation (believed to cause "cortical reprogramming") developed by the Israeli martial artist and teacher Moshe Feldenkrais.

HeartMath: A technique of biofeedback with Heart Rate Variability developed by Dr. Lew Childre.

Interactive Light Therapy (ILT): An early name for the LENS.

Interactive Metronome: A central nervous system "timing" type of biofeedback developed by musician James Cassily.

Jungian Therapy: The depth psychological approach developed by the Swiss psychiatrist Carl Jung, who for a number of years was a colleague of Freud's.

LENS: The Low Energy Neurofeedback System developed by Dr. Len Ochs, using radio waves that "feed back" the person's own "dominant frequency" at an "offset" (variation of that dominant frequency).

Neurofeedback: A subcategory of biofeedback in which the brain or central nervous System is the primary system trained.

Neuro-Linguistic Programming (NLP): A hypnotic and therapeutic system developed by Grinder and Bandler from the work of hypnotist Dr. Milton Erickson.

Nutritional Support: A valuable way of making sure the body has the proteins (amino acids), fats (phospholipids), sugars (glyconutritionals), and vitamins necessary for efficient and healthy functioning.

Open Focus: A technique of expanded awareness involving special visualization of space in and around the body, developed by Dr. Les Fehmi of Princeton Biofeedback Therapy.

Past Life Regression Therapy: While mainstrian psychiatry sniffs at such an unusual idea, it is congenial to the Sanskrit-based cultures that believe in reincarnation. There are serious clinical past-life therapists such as Dr. Brian Weiss *(Many Lives Many Masters)* and Oxford-trained Jungian, Dr. Roger Woolger *(Other Lives Other Selves.)*

Photonic Stimulation: A device first developed by Maurice Bales of CTI (Computer Thermal Imaging) for help with muscle pain, spasms, and weakness. Dr. Len Ochs has designed his own portable model, frequently used in connection with the LENS, but for different problems.

Qi Gong: The most ancient of the Chinese "energy practices," which also include acupuncture, tai chi (a gentle exercise program), and tai chi chuan (a gentle martial art). Stephen Larsen is trained and certified in qi gong and finds it very effective and helpful in particular situations.

Reiki: a form of energy healing whereby the therapist channels life force energy to the recipient through massage.

Repetitive Transcranial Magnetic Stimulation (rTMS): A form of Bioelectromagnetic Medicine.

Rolfing: Neuro-muscular reeducation, a deep massage of the connective tissue, developed by Dr. Ida Rolf.

Sandplay: A modality of "expressive-arts-therapy" developed by Dr. Margaret Lowenfeld and Dora Kalff, a Swiss colleague of Jung's, wherein toy figures and houses, bridges, and fences are arranged into a "world."

Transcutaneous Electrical Nerve Stimulation (TNS): A form of Bioelectromagnetic Medicine used by some physical therapists or chiropractors to relax muscles.

Yoga: An ancient psychophysical technique of meditation and physical well-being developed first in India. SKY or Sudarshan Kriya Yoga is a form taught in Art of Living Courses.

RESOURCES

LENS Practitioner Listings
www.ochslabs.com
A list of LENS practitioners currently working in the United States and in Australia, Germany, and Singapore is available on the Web site www.Ochslabs.com. The list is maintained by Dr. Len Ochs and includes the practitioner's credentials and contact information. Also see Biofeedback Certification Institute of America (BCIA).

Ameriden International
(808) 405-3336
Ameriden.com
One of the major distributors of Rosavin (Rhodiola Rosea), a Russian-discovered adaptogen, which can help with a variety of fatigue syndromes, Lyme Disease, depression, and other problems. Ameriden carries other excellent products for allergy relief, energy for physical performance, and natural treatments for illnesses.

Art of Living, International
www.artofliving.org
A yoga society following the teachings and practices of HH Sri Sri Ravi Shankar, also called Sudarshan Kriya Yoga (SKY). Seminars are taught in many countries around the world and most major cities in the United States.

Association for Applied Psychophysiology and Biofeedback (AAPB)
Wheat Ridge, Colorado
(303) 422–8436
www.aapb.org
A membership body that represents professional practitioners (as does the AMA for medicine, and the APA of psychology or psychiatry). Coordinates regional membership groups such as the Northeastern Biofeedback Society, puts on annual and other conferences, lists and contacts for providers.

Association of Biofeedback Technologies (AIBT)
drmaryjo@sabosystems.com or
www.therippleeffect.com
A training and certifying body directed by Dr. Mary Jo Sabo at Biofeedback Consultants in Suffern, New York.

Biofeedback Certification Institute of America (BCIA)
10200 W. 44th Ave., Suite 304,
Wheat Ridge, Colorado, 80033
(303) 420–2902
A professional nationwide certifying body for practitioners. Maintains lists of certified practitioners and manages "blueprint" for certification requirements.

The Center for Neurofunctioning
Len Ochs, Ph.D.
8151 Elphik Lane
Sebastapol, CA 95472
(707) 396-3598
lochs@earthlink.net
In utilizing the LENS, Dr. Len Ochs deals with traumatic or acquired brain injuries (including those persons in a coma), autism, chronic fatigue, mood problems from depression to bipolar (manic-depression I and II), post-traumatic stress disorders, and ADD and ADHD.

Glyconutrients
Yvonne Cable, M.A.
(845) 657-7010
Nutritional consultants.

HeartMath Institute
Boulder Creek, California
(800) 450-9111
www.heartmath.com
Offers training programs, education, literature, research, and licensure in HeartMath as a one-on-one provider.

Interactive Metronome
www.interactivemetronome.com
Interactive Metronome has their own program for training professionals in IM methods and also has machines used for therapy or training.

International Society for Neurofeedback and Research (ISNR)
www.isnr.org
A professional body for practitioners of neurofeedback as a subspecialty of biofeedback. Puts on annual and other conferences, coordinates research, raises funds, and gives grants for research.

J&J Engineering
Manufacturer of finely calibrated EEG processors and generic biofeedback machines that can be used for the LENS. (For the LENS, however, must be combined with ochslabs proprietary software.) Best to buy from Dr. Len Ochs at www.ochslabs.com.

Life Extension Foundation
(800) 544-4440
www.lifeextension.com
High quality provider of nutritional supplements.

Neurotherapy Center of Washington
7920 Norfolk Avenue, #200
Bethesda, MD 20814
(301) 652-7175
www.neurotherapycenters.com
The Neurotherapy Center of Washington is a research facility that provides treatment to patients with central nervous system disorders including pain and the complications of fibromyalgia, ADD, Chemobrain, depression, and traumatic brain injury.

OchsLabs
Cathy Wills, R.N., M.S.N., C.N.S
www.ochslabs.com
Cathy Wills works with Dr. Ochs to maintain a website where one can find information about training, workshops, current research, and equipment pertaining to the LENS, as well as a list of providers and how to contact them. See also the Center for Neurofunctioning and http://migraine-helpers.com.

Open Focus Training
(609) 924-0782
lesfehmi@ix.netcom.com
Open Focus training is offered by Dr. Les Fehmi at the Princeton Biofeedback Center. Programs are available for professionals in both Dr. Fehmi's alpha synchrony neurofeedback training and the accompanying attentional technique called "Open Focus."

Stone Mountain Center
475 River Road Extension
New Paltz, NY 12561
(845) 658-8083
stonemountaincenter.com
Stone Mountain Center is where Stephen Larsen conducts his practice of the LENS, HeartMath, Psychotherapy, Interactive Metronome, and Open Focus. Contact the center to arrange for a screening or intake interview. Dr. Larsen also coordinates professional training programs around the country and LENS training workshops for professionals biannually at Stone Mountain Center.

ABOUT THE CONTRIBUTORS

Carla Adinaro, A.R.I.A., has a bachelor of arts degree in biology and a bachelor of science degree in history. She has taught riding for thirty years, is a member of the American Riding Instructors Association, and is certified to teach dressage to level 2. She has trained thoroughbred race horses since 1970, has owned a thoroughbred breeding farm, and raised show horses that have won many prestigious horse shows, including Devon in Pennsylvania, Upperville in Virginia and Warrenton, also in Virginia.

Wendy Behary, L.C.S.W., is the founder and clinical director of The Cognitive Therapy Center of New Jersey, specializing in cognitive therapy and schema therapy for narcissism, trauma, and interpersonal conflicts in individuals and in couples. She has supervised and trained clinicians throughout the country in cognitive and schema therapy and is an affiliate and faculty member of the Cognitive Therapy Center and Schema Therapy Institute of New York, under the direction of Dr. Jeffrey Young.

Lynn Brayton, Psy.D., graduated from Florida Institute of Technology in 1988 with a Psychology Doctorate. She has been in private practice in the New Orleans area since 1990, utilizing neurofeeedback, EMDR, and psychotherapy to treat adults and adolescents.

Curtis Cripe, Ph.D., has his doctoral degree in research psychology with an emphasis in neuropsychology, neurodevelopment, and psychophysiology. He also holds a Master's degree in Clinical Psychology and Aerospace engineering. He is board certified in Neurodevelopment, Neurotherapy, and is a Diplomate in Peak Performance. Prior to this he was a top aerospace engineer for NASA's Jet Propulsion Laboratory. He has established five Crossroads Clinics and Centers around the country.

Mary Lee Esty, L.C.S.W., Ph.D., founded the Neurotherapy Center of Washington in 1995 because of the positive treatment results produced by the forerunners of the LENS, which she began using in 1994, as well as the potential offered by the field of traditional Neurotherapy. She specializes in EEG-stimulation therapy and has treated more than 1,300 people with extremely positive outcomes. She offers individualized treatment programs for those with chronic pain or fibromyalgia.

Thomas E. Fink, Ph.D., is a psychologist who is licensed in the state of Pennsylvania and who has practiced general rehabilitation and behavioral psychology for over twenty-five years. He received his Bachelor's degree in psychology from Gettysburg College, Gettysburg, Pennsylvania, and his Ph.D. in cognitive-experimental psychology from Temple University, Philadelphia, Pennsylvania. His current time is divided between an outpatient practice in Harrisburg, Pennsylvania, specializing in EEG Biofeedback; behavioral consultation with several Pennsylvania state hospitals; and working out the theoretical implications of EEG Biofeedback, particularly LENS, on our understanding of mental illness and its treatment.

Sarah Franek, M.T.P., A.I.B.T., was a biofeedback clinician for three years at the Stone Mountain Counseling Center in New York City. She has a Masters degree in Transpersonal Psychology.

Beth Hanna, R.N., has a private neurofeedback practice in Lansing, Michigan and also works as a Registered Nurse for the College of Human Medicine in the Occupational and Environmental Health division of Michigan State University.

Kristen Harrington, M.A., M.F.T., A.I.B.T., is a licensed marriage and family therapist and certified neurofeedback clinician. She is a staff member of the Stone Mountain Counseling Center and works in Kingston, New York. She specializes in using neurofeedback to help couples to more effectively learn to communicate with each other.

Thom Hartmann is the award-winning, bestselling author of fourteen books currently in print in over a dozen languages on four continents, an internationally known speaker on culture and communications, and an innovator in the fields of psychiatry, ecology, and democracy. In the spring of 2003, Hartmann began hosting a nationally syndicated talk show, *The Thom Hartmann Program,* which has been on the air on radio stations from coast to coast and on Sirius Satellite Radio for over two years, and runs from noon to 3 P.M. Eastern Time, originating in Portland, Oregon. The father of three grown children, Hartmann lives in Portland, Oregon, with his wife, Louise.

Sloan Johnson, M.A. Sloane Johnson's early training in the healing arts field was with Dr. Jonathan Miller at Lapis Light Natural Health, a whole systems practice of education and training in America, Taiwan, China, Malaysia, and Singapore. After focusing on neurofeedback, she went on to study with many different pioneers of it, including Dr. Les Fehmi, Dr. Len Ochs, and Pete Van Deusen. She presently has her own practice and, in addition to her work using neurofeedback, she also practices the disciplines of BioExplorer, HEG, pROSHI, and other systems. In January of 2005, she began to include the treatment of dogs and horses in her practice.

Robin Larsen, Ph.D., is an exhibiting artist, art historian specializing in comparative and ritual iconography, and coauthor, with her husband Stephen, of *A Fire in the Mind* and *The Fashioning of Angels.* Also with Stephen, she is founding director of the Center for Symbolic Studies in New Paltz, New York, and has been lecturing internationally for over forty years.

Joan Piper Mader, M.A., is a Masters-level Registered Nurse. She had a cerebral aneurysm in 1986, at age thirty-nine. She was one of the first individuals to receive long-term treatment in the LENS technique via an early prototype of the LENS.

Len Ochs, Ph.D., the developer of the LENS approach, has a Ph.D. in Social Psychology from the State University of New York at Albany, an M.A. in Psychology from Hofstra University in Hempstead, New York, and a B.A. from Muhlenberg College in Allentown, Pennsylvania. He is a former coeditor of *Biofeedback*, the news magazine of the Association of Applied Psychophysiology and Biofeedback in Colorado. At present he has his own private psychology practice and is the President of Ochs Labs, a research and development company exploring the diagnostic and treatment significance of EEG-Driven Stimulation for chronic central nervous system dysfunction.

Karen Schultheis, Ph.D., was a LENS practitioner for about five years in the Dallas/Fort Worth area. She incorporated biofeedback and laser work into her neuropsychology practice, primarily working with patients with CNS and chronic pain problems related to traumatic brain injury, stroke, cerebral palsy, autism, chronic fatigue, and fibromyalgia. After moving to Maui in 2003, Karen became a licensed massage therapist with an emphasis on Upledger's CranioSacral bodywork techniques.

Evelyn Soehner, M.A., earned a Master of Arts degree in Psychophysiology from Lesley College in Cambridge, Massachusetts. She specializes in the treatment of psychophysiological sequelea to central nervous system deficits, injury, and disease. Ms. Soehner and Dr. Fink established Acorn Health Associates, P.C., a private practice offering rehabilitation psychology and EEG neurofeedback, which blends state-of-the-art technologies with a holistic and humanistic approach to biobehavioral healthcare.

Theresa Yonker, M.D., graduated from the Medical College of Ohio at Toledo in 1986. She attended the Albany Medical Center Hospital in Albany, New York, for her internship, Adult Psychiatry Residency, and her Child and Adolescent Psychiatry fellowship, graduating in 1991. She recently opened her own private practice, an Integrative Behavioral Medicine and Psychotherapy Center, called Reflexions, in 2002. She is a Board Certified Child, Adolescent, and Adult Psychiatrist. She is also AIBT certified for LENS neurofeedback. In her practice she incorporates different healing modalities, including HeartMath and guided imagery techniques.

INDEX